PLANNING
URBAN HEALTH SERVICES

ABOUT THE AUTHORS

RUTH ROEMER, J.D., Researcher in
Health Law, School of Public Health,
University of California, Los Angeles, has
been engaged in law practice, legislative
work, and community health service. She is
the author of numerous publications on legal
aspects of organized health services,
including mental hospital admission law,
abortion law reform, fluoridation of public
water supplies, and regulation of health
manpower.

CHARLES KRAMER, M.S., is an economist
with extensive legislative and research
experience in the field of health economics.

JEANNE E. FRINK, M.P.H., Associate
Director for Program Operations, Los
Angeles Regional Family Planning Council,
is now engaged in tackling the problems of
multiple agencies and fragmented health
services described in this book.

MILTON I. ROEMER, M.D., who
contributed the final chapter of this book, is
Professor of Health Services Administration,
School of Public Health, University of
California, Los Angeles; he has worked in,
taught, studied, and written extensively on
the organization of health services in the
United States and other countries since 1940.

The Foreword is by PHILIP R. LEE, M.D.,
Professor of Social Medicine, University of
California, San Francisco and former
Assistant Secretary for Health and Scientific
Affairs, United States Department of Health,
Education and Welfare, 1965-1969.

PLANNING
URBAN HEALTH SERVICES
from Jungle to System

Ruth Roemer
Charles Kramer
Jeanne E. Frink

with a concluding chapter by
Milton I. Roemer

SPRINGER PUBLISHING COMPANY
New York

Library of Congress Cataloging in Publication Data
Roemer, Ruth, 1916-
    Planning urban health services.

    Includes bibliographical references and index.
    1. Medical care—United States. 2. Health plan-
ning—United States. 3. Medical care—California.
I. Kramer, Charles, joint author. II. Frink, Jeanne,
1946-   joint author. III. Title. [DNLM: 1. Comprehensive health care—U.S. 2. Delivery of health
care—U.S. 3. Health and welfare planning—U.S.
WB50 AA1 R67p]
RA395.A3R63   362.1'0973   73-92203
ISBN 0-8261-1650-7

This research was supported by Public Health Service Grant
Number HS 00459 (Geopolitical Jurisdictions and Comprehensive
Health Services) from the National Center for Health Services
Research and Development, U.S. Department of Health, Education,
and Welfare.

Printed in the United States of America

To the Memory of
L. S. GOERKE, M.D.,
Dean, School of Public Health,
University of California, Los Angeles, 1961-1972,
who sponsored the initiation of this study.

CONTENTS

FOREWORD

This is a critically important book because it documents and describes the present state of organized health services in the United States. It examines the problems of fragmentation in the public and private sectors at the national, state, and local levels. It deals thoroughly and objectively with the consequences of the multiplicity of programs, agencies, and providers, each with its own interests, goals, and means of meeting the health care needs of individuals or groups.

The ultimate goal of comprehensive health services should be to improve the physical and mental health of the people served. These services should be so organized as to be available and accessible, continuity of care should be fostered, and there should be sufficient coordination to achieve an integration of needed services. The services should be acceptable to both providers and the people served. There should be due consideration of the social, psychological, and personal aspects of illness, and the health services should provide the means for dealing with these. The system or systems should be sufficiently flexible to adapt to changing biomedical technology, not blindly applying every new technology without prior consideration of the health and economic costs as well as the benefits. Finally, a means of setting priorities, allocating resources in relation to health needs, and controlling costs should be part of any system for the provision of comprehensive health services.

If any illusions are still harbored about how far we are from achieving this reasonable standard of comprehensive health services, this book will quickly dispel them. It documents the problems at the local, state, and national levels as no other study in recent years has done.

Objective evidence, analysis, and rational discussion can now replace intuition and feelings in policy and program decisions about comprehensive health planning, the organization of health care, and its financing. The book provides the basis for independent analysis and the development of policy options that might coincide with or differ from those proposed by the authors. Whether or not one agrees with their proposals for more rational systems of health care, there can be no disputing the evidence that is now available for all concerned with matters to study. The problems that have been created for patients and providers almost defy description. The categorical approach to diseases, patients, and institutions can no longer be supported as a reasonable or rational approach in health care.

Seven years ago in proposing to Congress the program that later became the Comprehensive Health Planning and Public Health Services Amendments of 1966 (PL 89-749), the attempt was made to deal with some of the consequences of twenty years of federal emphasis on categorical approaches to health needs and services. The present state of affairs, as brilliantly and thoroughly documented and described by the authors, shows what a feeble instrument that legislation proved to be in dealing with the forces of fragmentation. The results are summarized succinctly in chapter 8 of this book:

The effects of fragmentation are pervasive, restricting the quantity and quality of services for consumers and limiting the capability of providers to furnish them. Fragmentation contributes to unequal access to care, gaps and inequities in services, a dearth of preventive care, discontinuous and sometimes inappropriate care, and considerable lag in responding to changing needs.

That says it all. But who is responsible? Physicians? Hospitals? Insurance companies? Voluntary health agencies? Government? Consumers? Sad to say, but all of these play a role in a society that venerates pluralism while it bemoans fragmentation and inefficiency.

In the United States we have ample resources available to provide comprehensive health services for the entire population, but the systems of planning, organizing, providing, financing, and paying for services do not provide the means to achieve the basic objectives of a comprehensive health service. Scientific and technological progress, coupled with the social demand for a more equitable distribution of medicine's enlarged potential, have heightened the need for organizational change.

Resistance to change is pervasive and persistent. Forty years ago the Committee on the Costs of Medical Care recommended "that medical services, both preventive and therapeutic, should be furnished largely by organized groups of physicians, dentists, nurses, pharmacists, and other associated personnel. Such groups should be organized, preferably around a hospital, for rendering complete home, office, and hospital care. The form of organization should encourage the maintenance of high standards and the development or preservation of a personal relation between patient and physician." The Committee also recommended that "the costs of medical care be placed on a group prepayment basis, through the use of insurance, the use of taxation, or through the use of both these methods" and "the study, evaluation, and coordination of medical services be considered important functions for every state and local community, that agencies be formed to exercise these functions, and that the coordination of rural with urban services receive special attention."[1] These proposals were strongly resisted. The same forces that resisted change then resist it today.

There is considerable resistance to change among many physicians who wish to retain the solo practice fee-for-service model which seems less and less adapted for meeting the changing health care needs of our society, particularly the needs of the chronically ill, the mentally ill, and the disabled. Resistance to change has been strong among other providers, such as hospitals, nursing homes, and laboratories. Other professions, new in the field of health care, such as psychology, social work, and physical therapy, often wish to pursue the fee-for-service model rather than fitting into an organized system of care.

In financing, the private and public sectors have aggravated the problem with their adoption of piecemeal, categorical approaches to the financing of health services. Governments, at the local, state, and national levels, remain among the major culprits; yet the fragmentative and categorical approaches that characterize government problems are a reflection of the larger problem in the private sector.

The forces that resisted the recommendations of the Committee on the Costs of Medical Care forty years ago can hardly resist the constructive proposals that form the concluding chapter of this book. The evidence now at hand will make many of the old arguments irrelevant. The status quo can no longer be defended now that the problems have been so clearly described. Whether or not one agrees with the conclusions, this book represents a significant contribution in the nation's effort to provide compassionate, comprehensive health services for all.

Philip R. Lee, M.D.
Professor of Social Medicine and
Director, Health Policy Program,
School of Medicine, University of
California, San Francisco

REFERENCE

1. The Committee on the Costs of Medical Care, *Medical Care for the American People*, Chicago: The University of Chicago Press, 1932, p. XVI.

PREFACE

This study concerns the conflict between the fragmented system of personal health services and the goal of comprehensive health care for the total population. We set out to describe and analyze the multiplicity of programs, agencies, and resources providing health services in a single state. In this process, we found that categorical public programs for specific persons, diseases, or services are highly visible and that a similar but more elusive fragmentation characterizes the private sector of health services. More importantly, we found that fundamental to the character of the health service system as a whole are the confused relationships or lack of coordination among multiple providers and agencies within and between the public and private sectors of health care. In fact, a key issue in achievement of the goal of comprehensive health services is, we believe, the capacity of the health service system to build effective relationships among the various components of the system.

This work began in 1969 with preparation of inventories of agencies involved in provision of personal and environmental health services at all governmental levels in the State of California. Analysis of specialized sectors of health service proceeded by means of interviews with representatives of public and private agencies, attendance at meetings of health organizations, examination of reports and documents, and preparation of working charts showing the functions of public and private agencies, according to their own descriptions, at the federal, state, regional, and local levels of government.

The description of the current system of health services is based on information collected in the period April 1969 to December 1972. Of course, many changes took place in health programs and agencies during this time. Some programs altered their direction. Some were abolished. Functions allocated to one agency were transferred to another. The names of some agencies changed. As a result, neither the inventories nor the working charts are reproduced. One set of charts concerned with agencies in the field of mental health is presented to illustrate the extent of fragmentation of functions, although the functions of several of these agencies have changed since the chart was prepared.

During the course of this study, two major reorganizations of health agencies took place in California, and similar reorganizations have occurred in other states and metropolitan areas. On September 1, 1972, a unified Los Angeles County Department of Health Services was established, composed of the former County Departments of Hospitals, Health, Mental Health, and the Office of the County Veterinarian. At the state level, the California existing Departments of Public Health, Mental Hygiene, Health Care Services, and parts of other agencies were also merged into a unified State Department of Health, operational as of July 1, 1973. Frequent reference is made to the former state and county health departments, as well as to the new unified departments, since separate departments of public health, mental health, and hospitals are still typical of many places in the United States. Federal agencies are described generally as of 1971-1972, although these agencies, too, have undergone a number of reorganizations. It is important to note that reorganizations of agencies do not *per se* bring about integrated health services; but, properly implemented, reorganizations can create a framework conducive to provision of comprehensive care in the communities and neighborhoods where services are delivered.

The study has several limitations. First, it is based on data collected in California for the state level and in Los Angeles County for the local level. But we believe that the California experience not only reflects but emphasizes the conditions in other states and localities, even if there are obvious variations. Second, the data emphasize fragmented services provided by public agencies, with less discussion of fragmentation in the private sector, which is well known. Attention is directed here to ways in which public policy can lessen fragmentation in the system as a whole. Third, this report is concerned with personal health services; the results of our work on the multiplicity of agencies in environmental health have been published in the *Milbank Memorial Fund Quarterly*.* Finally, there remains the danger that the details of fragmentation tend to obscure the need for services which categorical programs were designed to meet. In a period of retrenchment, these details may be exaggerated to support uncritical budget-cutting. But fragmentation of health services is not cured by cutting either the scope or the number of public programs. Our plea for rational planning and organization of services is not designed to decrease the total resources allocated to health services but rather to enhance them.

Appreciation is expressed for support of this research by Public Health Service Grant Number HS 00459 from the National Center for Health

---

* Roemer, Ruth, Jeanne E. Frink, and C. Kramer, "Environmental Health Services: Multiplicity of Jurisdictions and Comprehensive Environmental Management," *Milbank Mem. Fund Q.*, Vol. XLIX, No. 4, Part 1, p. 419, Oct. 1971.

Services Research and Development, U.S. Department of Health, Education, and Welfare to the Institute of Government and Public Affairs, University of California, Los Angeles. Particular gratitude is extended to Dr. Harris S. Cohen, whose helpful advice exceeded his role as principal Project Officer.

We have received indispensable help from many people. We acknowledge with deep gratitude our debts to some of these persons:

To Dr. Werner Z. Hirsch, Director, Institute of Government and Public Affairs, University of California, Los Angeles and Principal Investigator of this project, for freedom throughout and assistance as needed.

To the late Dr. L. S. Goerke, Dean, School of Public Health, University of California, Los Angeles and our Co-Principal Investigator, for his unfailing encouragement and support.

To Professor Donald G. Hagman, School of Law, University of California, Los Angeles, for expert advice and help during the year that he served as Acting Director of the Institute of Government and Public Affairs and Principal Investigator of this project.

To Mrs. Velma Pratt and Mrs. Elizabeth Bennett of the Institute of Government and Public Affairs, University of California, Los Angeles, for their patient and helpful administrative services.

To Dr. Lester Breslow, Dean, School of Public Health, University of California, Los Angeles, for having first proposed this subject as calling for study.

To Dr. Saleem A. Farag, Director, Office of Comprehensive Health Planning, California State Department of Public Health, for encouragement and support of studies on planning of environmental and personal health services related to this work.

To Mr. Douglas R. Steele, Chief, Management Services Division, County Administrative Offices, Los Angeles County, for helpful information and insights on numerous occasions.

To Mrs. Pamela S. Brier for her thorough and able contribution in the field of emergency medical services.

To Ms. Sherri Gold for careful and competent preparation of the working charts on which the sector analyses of health services are based.

To Mrs. Marilyn R. Schroeter, Ms. Clarissa Dong, and Ms. Patricia Nicholas for able and patient typing of the manuscript.

To Ms. Mary J. Ryan, Head of the Public Affairs Service Library, University of California, Los Angeles, her associate, Ms. Dorothy V. Wells, and their staff for help in furnishing the enormous number of public documents used in this study.

To the following persons who contributed to the research as members of the staff: Mrs. Geraldine R. Dallek, Dr. Dale Rogers Marshall, Mrs. Hannah C. Sprowls, Mrs. Rhea Schauben, Ms. Susan Anne Cohen, Ms. Laura Lee Glickman, and Alan Zarky.

To Mrs. Lila Berman, Mrs. Marcia Buck, Alfred J. Cavalier, Dr. Robert Davidson, Robert Kimball, Dr. David Michener, Dr. Donald A. Schwartz, Dr. Helen M. Wallace, and Howard A. Worley, for able review and criticism of various chapters of the manuscript.

And, above all, to Dr. Milton I. Roemer, for his prototype study twenty years ago, *Health Services in a County of the United States,* for his generous and unflagging ideas and guidance throughout this research, and for his writing the final chapter—one that we hope will be heeded by health service planners and policy-makers in the years ahead.

All errors and faults are, of course, the responsibility of the authors.

Ruth Roemer
Charles Kramer
Jeanne E. Frink

Institute of Government and Public Affairs
University of California, Los Angeles
April 1973

PLANNING
URBAN HEALTH SERVICES

CHAPTER 1

Fragmentation of Health Services

> *Thus, what passes for United States health policy today is a conglomerate of specific laws, collateral authority in other laws, traditional, but changing divisions of powers among the several levels of government, historical dependence on voluntary associations and individual effort, and a sometimes child-like faith that since no major catastrophes have come to light recently, everything will work out for the best. One hardly needs to catalogue the disadvantages to this kind of implicit health policy, among which the most obvious are fragmentation, incompleteness, and inability to define a point of accountability.*[1]

> Myron E. Wegman, M.D.
> Dean, School of Public Health
> University of Michigan, 1972

In the summer of 1969, the president and the president-elect of the American Public Health Association undertook a tour to examine health conditions in the United States. Investigating typical environmental and medical care situations in widely scattered parts of the country, these public health physicians, who thought they were familiar with health problems, were shocked at what they found. They wrote:

We recall with pain:

—approximately 50,000 persons of the Kenwood-Oakland area of Chicago, who live in rodent- and insect-infested housing, with broken plumbing, stairs and windows. Today, these people pay from one- to two-thirds of their incomes for rent and are served by a total of five physicians in their community — a physician-to-population ratio less than one-tenth of the country as a whole — with the county hospital and clinics eight miles away.

—a 53-year-old American Indian in Great Falls, Montana, veteran of the South

Pacific in World War II, raising a family of six children (and one grandchild, whose father is now in Vietnam) on a pension and what he can scrounge by salvage in a junkyard. He can neither afford to buy food stamps nor return to the hospital for post-cancer treatment—closure of his bowel, which now opens on his abdomen—because his family would not have food while he is gone.

——the farmworker in Tulare County, California, who said that exposure to pesticides from airplane spraying of fields, contrary to regulations and often leading to illness, was frequently not reported. "What's the use?" he asked. "We lose wages going to the doctor, get better in a week usually, and get no compensation, and they don't stop spraying."

——the woman in Tulare County, eight months pregnant, whose Medi-Cal (Medicaid) eligibility had been cancelled last month because her husband had just found a temporary job, thus forcing her to seek care at the County Hospital which previous experience had taught her to hate.

——the young woman in Houston, whose welfare check for a family of eight had been cut from $123 to $23 a month.

——a therapist in the Child Treatment Center, Atlanta, Georgia, where excellent work with youngsters in trouble was underway, but "the main difficulty is that the kids have to go right back to the same life that got them into trouble in the first place, and we can't do anything about that here."

——an "uncooperative" chronic alcoholic who carried a card from Grady Hospital identifying him as an epileptic, but who, a few days before our visit, had occupied the "hole"—a 4 foot by 8 foot solitary confinement cell—in the Atlanta City Prison.

——dead fish floating in the dirty water of the Potomac, the "Nation's River," which flows through our capital city so polluted by untreated and inadequately treated sewage that fish cannot live there, and the spread of human disease-causing bacteria appears as a serious threat.[2]

These findings document graphically the "massive crisis" in health care—in the words of President Nixon in 1969—that afflicts the United States—a crisis in part related to our national health policy, described as lacking coordination, often lacking rationality, and frequently having glaring shortcomings of performance.[3] These features of our national health policy are carried over into the health service system itself. While not all the defects of the health service system can be ascribed to uncoordinated purposes and multiple programs, fragmentation contributes to these defects and often blocks their correction.

A bewildering array of programs, services, and agencies confronts the individual seeking health care in the United States. Listings of federal assistance programs have revealed hundreds of separate health programs at the federal level of government alone, within the Department of Health, Education, and Welfare and other departments.[4] In California, approximately 275 public programs, provided by separate administrative entities within 83 major agencies operating at five governmental levels—federal, state, regional, local, and special district—are concerned with provision of personal health services.[5] These public programs must interrelate with the even more numerous voluntary and private programs, agencies, facilities, and individual providers that furnish segments of health care.

Each program has its special purpose, its sources of financing, its particular eligibility requirements, its own geographic span, and its individual mode of operation. Links among the programs and agencies are, at best, tenuous and variable. Indeed, coordinating mechanisms themselves, where they exist, constitute another layer of specialized agencies. The result is fragmentation of health services—a term that has become so hackneyed that its significance in real life is often obscured.

DEFINITION

Fragmentation of health services may be defined as the division of responsibility for health care among multiple, separate individuals and agencies, each with a categorical purpose, and the whole lacking a coherent policy, an integrated direction, and coordinated relationships. Fragmentation is of two kinds—functional and geographic. Functional fragmentation is the division of responsibility for performance of functions or for provision of services into delimited and separately accountable programs. Geographic fragmentation is the performance of functions or provision of services within numerous but often noncongruent or overlapping geographic areas and political jurisdictions. The antithesis of fragmentation is continuous and comprehensive care.

Fragmentation is closely related to pluralism, the cliché used to describe health services in the United States, which may be defined as multiplicity both of aims and of means. Pluralism applies to all services, whether under public, voluntary, or private auspices. It characterizes both dimensions of the organization of health services—the dimension of economic support and that of modes of delivery. Various sources and mechanisms for financing health services entail multiple standards for services and varying eligibility requirements. Different methods of organizing health services are associated with different amounts and quality of service. Some services, such as voluntary health insurance plans, are organized only along the dimension of economic support, some, such as hospitals and other facilities, only for mode of delivery, and some, such as the Veterans Administration health care system, crippled children's services, and numerous preventive health service programs, are organized along both dimensions.

Pluralistic services are not necessarily fragmented. Many different programs and providers, with differing aims and means, may be welded into an integrated system. Thus, fragmentation of health services does not imply solely the provision of health care by many individuals and organizations, nor does fragmentation mean numerous sites or settings for provision of services. Many places for the provision of services and many different kinds of facilities are required in all societies and particularly in a society as large and as complex as ours. By the same token, fragmentation does not mean provision of the same or similar services by different providers or programs, if all these furnish needed services.

Thus, numerous providers, differing sites for service, and replication of similar services are not the distinguishing features of a fragmented system. The salient characteristic of fragmentation is, rather, the lack of an integrated policy and purpose to govern and link the many parts of the system that provide or assure services to persons needing them. As a result, in a fragmented system each component operates separately and independently, functioning in its own bailiwick for its own ends — an inherently difficult setting in which to build interrelationships and to effect coordination. The measure of fragmentation is thus not what the pluralistic system does, but what it fails to do in providing comprehensive, continuous, and appropriate care for all who need it.

CONTRIBUTING FACTORS

Over the years, organized programs have been developed for specific purposes; as new needs in health care have emerged and been recognized, organized programs have been created to meet these needs. Each program was well intended. Each provides or funds needed services. But the totality has created an accretion of categorical programs and largely autonomous agencies that defies the best efforts to assure equitable and comprehensive care to all. The roots of fragmented health services are to be found in basic political, historical, and scientific-technological forces in American life. Each of these forces has set in motion developments that encourage multiplicity and diversity of services and an accumulation of separate agencies and programs.

Political Factors

Underlying the organizational forms for all services is the pluralistic character of government in the United States and the interplay between the public and private sectors in all spheres. The separation of powers among the federal, state, and local levels of government has divided functions in health services and created overlapping responsibilities and jurisdictions. The federal role in health, grounded in the taxing power and the authority to provide for the general welfare, is fundamental to the direction and emphasis of health services. The police power of the state to protect and promote the public health and welfare is the basis for action by state government, and by local government as a creature of the state. Historically, considerable responsibility for provision of medical care to the poor has been assigned to local government, a responsibility increasingly shared by higher levels of government. Differing boundaries of local government units, the emergence of special-purpose political districts, particularly for environmental services but also for hospitals, and, above all, the strength of the tradition of home rule have tended to emphasize division, rather than unity, of health services.

Interacting with this tripartite governmental framework is the vast voluntary and private sector of health care: physicians and other individual practitioners, voluntary hospitals in nearly every community, mushrooming for-profit nursing homes and other facilities, and programs of numerous voluntary health agencies. In the division between the public and private sectors of health care, government has tended to assume responsibility for the highest risk groups — the poor, the mentally ill, and the chronically ill; others are cared for largely within the private sector. Although increased public financing of services provided by the private sector blurs this distinction, the legacy of voluntarism and of autonomous private agencies is to be found in fragmented services.

Fundamental to political pluralism is the social and group structure of American society, which consists of numerous segments differentiated by professional, occupational, or ethnic background or by association for special purposes. The fragmentation emanating from the specialization of groups influencing separate policy subsystems will not, in the opinion of political scientists, be modified by consolidation or coordination of agencies alone.[6] Certainly, in the field of health services, the melting pot has not melded its contents.

Historical Factors

Historical forces have contributed significantly to the splintering of services. Incremental development of services as new needs and demands have been recognized has characterized the evolution of both public programs and the voluntary and private sectors of health care.

In the public sector, environmental health protection was the earliest service subjected to organization because of the need for a pure water supply, safe milk, and general community sanitation. Communicable disease programs followed. High priority groups — the military and veterans, mothers and children, and later other groups — commanded special attention. With industrialization came new occupational hazards and, as a result, programs to create a safe working environment and to compensate workers for industrial accidents and diseases. In the years following World War II, special programs were created to construct hospitals, to provide care for special groups, such as the mentally ill, the chronically ill, and the aged, and to add new services, such as family planning. Each effort represented needed and expanded services but services provided in categorical and compartmentalized segments.

As governmental programs were developed in response to public awareness of unmet needs, so voluntary programs with specialized purposes emerged from the dedication of individuals and groups vitally concerned with special problems, such as control of tuberculosis, heart disease, cancer, mental retardation, and many other conditions. Their organizational efforts, fund-raising, education, and community services have created a large and energetic world of voluntary organizations devoted to specialized purposes.

Within the private sector of health care, individualism and autonomy dominate with resultant unplanned proliferation of isolated offices, clinics, hospitals, nursing homes, and specialized resources. Both the geographic distribution of physicians and services and the features of private insurance reinforce fragmented services. They contribute to limited access, restricted benefits, and varying quality of care.

Scientific-Technological Factors

Specialization, which proceeds from division of labor and is reinforced by the biomedical revolution, tends to promote high-quality health services, but it also contributes to fragmented care. Emphasis on technology has encouraged multiplication of technical arrangements to deal with particular conditions.[7] Fragmentation is not inherent in specialization, but highly specialized skills and services tend to accentuate fragmented services in the absence of a systematic deployment of specialist skills to apply in an organized manner the knowledge produced by the biomedical revolution to demonstrated human need.

Countervailing Forces

At the same time that powerful political, historical, and scientific-technological forces have propelled the health care delivery system into fractionated segments, countervailing forces drive toward assuring continuity of care, closing gaps, increasing equity in access to services, and improving quality of care. The first of these is the expanding demand for improved health services, as the consumer voice in health affairs has highlighted long-standing inequities in provision of health care to the poor and to minorities. Demand is made more effective by the extension of health insurance. So strong is public insistence on adequate health services that health care is increasingly recognized as a right of all citizens. Second is the changing structure of payment for health services. The growth of private insurance and, since 1965, the vast federal and state spending for Medicare and Medicaid have revealed the high price of a fragmented system not only in money but in the quality of care. Third, the rising cost of health care prompts a new look at the organization of health services. Fourth are new knowledge and changed professional practices. Specialization itself requires coordination. Shortages of professional personnel increase the need to use allied and auxiliary health manpower, which in turn mandates management and direction. The urgency of translating the benefits of science into better health services is widely recognized. The discrepancy between scientific and technological capability, on the one hand, and the organizational means for applying knowledge about health and disease to human welfare, on the other, impels fundamental changes in the system of providing health services.

SIGNIFICANCE

No description or analysis of the American health service system can reveal the full extent of its diversity and complexity, for the mere description of multiple agencies and programs tends to simplify the actuality. The reality for any consumer or administrator of health services is much more intricate than any description can indicate, and full exploration of the ramifications of categorical, segmented programs and services would lead to enormously magnified complexities. Perhaps it may be helpful at the outset, therefore, to summarize what fragmentation of health services means for the lives, health, and well-being of people who need health care.

1. Fragmentation means separation of preventive and curative services. It means that a low-income mother takes her baby to a well-child clinic at a public health center for immunizations and well-baby care but, when the baby becomes sick, must travel to a distant public hospital, waiting in a crowded outpatient department, sometimes for five to six hours, to see a doctor — a different doctor — who will treat her baby. This separation of preventive from curative services applies to both poor and rich alike.

2. Fragmentation means separation of ambulatory care from inpatient

services. It means that a patient who sees a physician in his private office under a welfare medical care program or a physician in a neighborhood health center or a psychiatrist in a mental health center must be shifted to a different system of care for acute or long-term inpatient care for physical or mental illness.

3. Fragmentation means multiple financial or other eligibility requirements. It means that a sick person meeting certain requirements of income, residence, age, or disease is eligible for one kind of health care, while a person with the same or a similar health condition but meeting different eligibility standards is channeled to other services or locations. Neither may be eligible for comprehensive services but only for the treatment of a specified condition.

4. Fragmentation means difficult access to care and a necessity for repeated reentries into the system of care. It means that a person or family requiring different kinds of care must seek out various sources of care and gain entry repeatedly to separate resources. Ready guides to direct the consumer to appropriate resources are generally inadequate or lacking. Some persons who are in need may never be reached at all by the system.

5. Fragmentation means travel time to seek appropriate or specialized care. It means that a person or family requiring a combination of medical, psychiatric, nutritional, rehabilitative, or other services must travel to different places for different services. At best, the need to travel for specialized services is burdensome; at worst, it stands as a barrier to prompt and accessible care.

6. Fragmentation means reliance on multiple sources of financing. It means that a variety of financing mechanisms may be necessary to pay for care for a person or family or to support a single service. Varying amounts of coinsurance, deductibles, and benefit periods may be involved, requiring multiple billing, complex adminstration, and contributions from people unable to pay.

7. Fragmentation means services of uneven quality because of multiple regulatory standards. It means that various public and voluntary agencies divide the functions in regulation of health personnel and facilities according to variable and often inadequate standards and requirements.

8. Fragmentation may mean extravagant duplication of functions. Different levels of government may repeat the same function in health service, or the function may be repeated at the same level of government among different agencies. A quite similar duplication exists in the private sector, in the maintenance, for example, by several hospitals in the same geographic area of the same expensive, specialized services, frequently not fully utilized. Quality of care is rarely enhanced by dispersed responsibility.

9. Fragmentation means isolation of health services from other essential community services. It means that health services are separated from the large range of community services that are intimately related to health:

welfare and social services, employment and training activities, and housing, recreation, and child development programs.

10. Fragmentation means gaps in health service and provision of care according to criteria based on age, income, residence, or kind of disease. It means that legal authority and prescriptions of financing determine health services rather than the sole valid criterion — health needs.

This is not to deny the virtues of fragmentation. Some of the strengths of the current system of health services may be associated with the division of the system into manageable, identifiable segments and programs that command specialized expertise, high technical quality, and dedication to a defined goal. Pluralistic efforts engender some degree of competition to provide the quantity and quality of services needed. These virtues, however, are not unique to a fragmented system and may even be enhanced in alternate patterns of providing care.

OUTLINE

The full impact of fragmented health services can be appreciated only as the structure and functioning of the total system are examined. First is presented an overview of the American health service system, both with respect to its organization and to its financing (Chapters 2 and 3). Next, four sectors of the health service system are described in their historical development and in order to reveal the operation and interrelationships of multiple programs and services provided from public and private resources within defined fields (Chapters 4 through 7). The problems associated with fragmented services are then noted (Chapter 8).

Thus far, the reader will undoubtedly ask himself — as the writers have done — whether the goal of comprehensive health services for the total population can be achieved through some combination, organization, or restructuring of the many separate segments of the health service system. To answer this question, more rational systems of health care that have been proposed for the United States and some that are in operation in other countries are reviewed briefly (Chapter 9). Recognition of the constraints on the development of an ideal system of health care, however, leads to proposal of what is deemed by the authors a feasible and realistic system for the United States in the 1970s (Chapter 10). Explanation of this alternative is designed to point the way toward a conversion from the present jungle of categorical programs and uncoordinated services into an integrated system of comprehensive health care for all.

NOTES

1. Wegman, Myron E., "Policy, Priorities and the Courage to Act," Centennial Presidential Address, American Public Health Association, 1971-1972.

2. Breslow, Lester, M.D., and Paul B. Cornely, M.D., *Health Crisis in America*, A Report by the American Public Health Association, p. v, New York, N.Y., 1970.

3. Wegman, supra note 1. See also Hilleboe, Herman E., M.D., "Preventing Future Shock: Health Developments in the 1960's and Imperatives for the 1970's," The Eleventh Bronfman Lecture, *Am.J. Public Health*, p. 136 at 142-143, Feb. 1972.

4. *Federal Role in Health*, Report of the Committee on Government Operations, United States Senate, made by its Subcommittee on Executive Reorganization and Government Research, 91st Cong., 2d Sess., Report No. 91-809, Apr. 30, 1970; *1969 Listing of Operating Federal Assistance Programs Compiled during the Roth Study*, prepared by the staff of Representative William V. Roth, Jr., H.R. 91st Cong., 1st Sess., Doc. No. 91-177, 1969.

5. Inventory of Agencies Providing Personal Health Services in California, developed in the course of this research project, "Geopolitical Jurisdictions and Comprehensive Health Services," supported by Public Health Service Grant No. HS 00459 from the National Center for Health Services Research and Development, U.S. Department of Health, Education, and Welfare.

6. Walsh, Annmarie Hauck, *The Urban Challenge to Government*, p. 49, Frederick A. Praeger, New York, N.Y., 1969

7. Mechanic, David, "Problems in the Future Organization of Medical Practice," *Law and Contemporary Problems, Health Care*, Part I, Vol. XXXV, No. 2, p. 233 at 237, Spring 1970.

CHAPTER 2

The Tangled Net of Programs

> The tremendous proliferation of Federal assistance programs over the years has resulted in a tangled net of programs which now threatens to negate entirely the basic reason for most of the programs: the delivery of services. The overwhelming need today is to improve the delivery systems: to find means of sorting out the overlapping programs and cutting through the array of technical and administrative requirements to insure that the intended services reach the intended recipients effectively and economically.[1]
>
> Robert H. Finch
Secretary, U.S. Department of
Health, Education, and Welfare, 1969

Each year the "tangled net of programs" becomes more tangled as new programs are added, old ones are redirected, and the functions of public agencies and the private sector become increasingly interrelated. The complexity of the health service system in the United States is the result of the accretion of programs and agencies over the years as new needs in health services have been recognized, of the specialized and categorical character of these services, of the sheer numbers of individuals and organizations that provide health care, and of the lack of a rational pattern for fitting the many parts into an effective whole.

This complicated system, composed of multiple public programs and agencies, a large private sector increasingly dependent on public financing and many diverse voluntary agencies, all functioning at the national, state, regional, and local levels of government, can be described in various ways: by the kinds of persons served, by the nature of services provided, by the varying sponsorships of programs and services, or by the levels of government

11

involved.[2] The primary focus is placed here on the kinds of services provided, with attention secondarily to other features of the system.

This chapter presents an overview designed to show the structure of the pluralistic system of personal health services. It is divided into three main parts: (1) production of resources, (2) provision of services, and (3) social controls.

This overview is supplemented in four succeeding chapters by analyses of sectors of the health services, designed to reveal the functioning of the system and its consequences for health care. Examination of these — each a constellation of programs and services that provide care for specific persons or for specific diseases, or that perform other specific functions — will, it is hoped, illuminate the operation of the system and the interrelationships or lack of interrelationships among its many parts.

Health services may be described by the purposes for which they are organized. This functional classification facilitates description of the multiplicity of segmented programs and services that make up the mosaic of personal health services. A defect of this classification, however, is that it may blur the links or lack of links among different functions, different kinds of services, and different levels of care. To the fragmentation within each of the segments of health services discussed should be added the fragmentation that exists between segments, that is, the separation of preventive services from curative services and of curative from rehabilitative services.

PRODUCTION OF RESOURCES

The basic resources for provision of health services consist of manpower, facilities, drugs and equipment, and knowledge. Each of these resources is produced by multiple entities and in numerous, specialized undertakings. Health personnel are trained in various kinds of schools and facilities, with variable mechanisms for setting standards and providing financing. The many kinds of health facilities are provided by another constellation of private efforts and public programs concerned with the planning, financing, and construction of different kinds of facilities. Drugs and equipment are manufactured and distributed largely through the efforts of private enterprise, with government involvement in standard-setting, inspection, and enforcement of quality controls. New knowledge is produced as a result of research, organized in various settings, financed chiefly by government and by numerous private agencies, and with its results distributed through many publications and organizations.

Programs for Production of Health Manpower[3]

In 1967, 3.5 million persons were employed in more than 125 health occupations and some 250 secondary or specialty designations.[4] These numerous and varied health workers were prepared in different kinds of schools and programs, located in many different places. Fragmentation in production of personnel is not created by differing sites for training; an integrated system of education must have many locations for the provision of training. Fragmentation stems from lack of a consistent, coherent policy for the preparation of health manpower; from differing standards and curricula for training the same kind or level of personnel; from uncoordinated training programs for different levels of the same or similar kinds of personnel; and from unrelated training for related occupations.

Federal Programs.   In recent years, federal support for the preparation of health personnel has expanded enormously. An inventory of health manpower training programs supported by federal funds in 1970 identified 144 separate programs or authorizations, 94 of which were exclusively for health manpower training.[5] In 1972, 12 different federal agencies were involved in manpower training programs, with a total expenditure of $1.1 billion.[6] The principal agencies involved in health programs are the Department of Health, Education, and Welfare, the Department of Labor, and the Veterans Administration, but all 12 federal agencies support the preparation of the same or similar kinds of personnel in separate programs and through various sources of funding with differing prescriptions. Within the Department of Health, Education, and Welfare alone, many separate training programs are administered by more than six separate components of the Department.[7] Table 1 in Appendix I shows the numbers and kinds of personnel aided by training programs of various federal agencies, together with expenditures by each agency.

The objectives of the numerous agencies charged with financial and administrative responsibility for the preparation of health personnel differ so widely that coordination for common goals is difficult. The Manpower Development and Training Act, administered by the Department of Labor, contributes significantly to the supply of manpower below the baccalaureate level. This program proceeds from the objective of providing job opportunities for the disadvantaged. The Allied Health Professions Personnel Training Act, administered by the Department of Health, Education, and Welfare, aids training programs, particularly in community colleges and hospitals, for specified categories of personnel. This program is directed to expanding a pool of manpower that can itself provide important technical services and at the same time boost the productivity of highly trained professionals. For the

Defense Department and the Veterans Administration, training is largely a by-product of the principal health activities of these agencies in providing services. This fractionalization of federal programs in the production of health manpower has accentuated the shortage and maldistribution of health personnel.[8] It contributed to the enactment in 1971 of the Comprehensive Health Manpower Training Act providing for Area Health Education Centers, intended to provide coordinated training of needed health manpower on a regional basis and to relate manpower education to patterns of delivery of care.

State Programs. On the state level, educational programs for health manpower are affected significantly by federal programs and funding. Given this predominant federal influence and the need in all states for more and better health services, it is not surprising that surveys in two states of educational programs for health manpower identified common problems related to fragmentation. Both stressed the need for planning, articulating, and coordinating the training of health personnel provided by public and private institutions.

In California, an investigation in 1967-1968 of educational programs for 35 selected categories of health manpower found a diversity of educational settings for the same or similar categories of personnel; differing educational prerequisites and duration of curricula for the same level of different categories of personnel and, in some cases, even for the same category; multiplicity of standards for accreditation of educational institutions and programs and for certification of personnel; and a lack of a rational and coherent system of education, relevant to the functions these personnel perform or should perform and to the goals of modern health services.[9]

In Michigan, analysis of health manpower needs and educational programs for 26 categories of health workers within the context of the total health care system revealed a need for cooperative planning on a regional basis by educational institutions, health facilities, and professional associations; for joint planning by university medical centers with respect to manpower development; for the creation of health occupation centers for vocational and technical personnel through a consortium of educational resources; for long-range plans based on the concept of developing clusters or "families" of related programs; and for a coordination of roles of educational and health agencies.[10] A response to these problems is the development of Area Health Education Centers, mentioned above.

Local Programs. At the local level of government, educational institutions and county hospitals contribute to the production of health personnel. A wide variety of technically trained allied and auxiliary personnel is prepared in adult education programs of secondary schools and in community colleges. In California, various kinds of health personnel are prepared in one and two-year programs in governmental community colleges. Hospitals, both governmental and voluntary, provide clinical training for several professions requiring a baccalaureate degree, such as professional nursing, clinical laboratory technology, and physical and occupational therapy. Hospitals also train a large variety of aides and technicians for service in their own facilities.

Voluntary Programs. Much of the production of health personnel takes place in private institutions of higher education or vocational training. Voluntary hospitals prepare nurses and provide the clinical training required for a number of professions. Voluntary professional associations also play a large role in determining the quantity and quality of education. A reflection of the substantial support of the private sector for the production of personnel is the contribution of more than $21 million for health manpower training by 153 private foundations in the single year of 1966.[11]

Construction of Health Facilities

In recent years construction of medical facilities has been financed two-thirds by private funds and one-third by public funds. But from 1929 through the late 1950s, public funds had been the chief source of financing for both public and private construction, and they still provide a substantial source for private construction. In fiscal 1972, private construction came to a little more than $3 billion, public construction to more than $1 billion. But public funds directly supplied almost $350 million for private facilities.[12] In addition, public funding programs, such as Medicare, Medicaid, CHAMPUS (Civilian Health and Medical Program for the Uniformed Services), and others, furnished private facilities with some $600 million in depreciation funds available for construction.

Federal Programs. The dominant federal program aiding construction of health facilities has been the Hill–Burton program, administered by the Health Facilities Planning and Construction Service of the Department of Health, Education, and Welfare. From 1947 to 1971, this program provided some $3.7 billion for the construction and modernization of nonprofit health facilities, both public and private, 29 percent of the $12.8 billion total spent on more than 10,000 medical facility construction projects.[13] In addition to grants, the Hill–Burton program also provides guaranteed loans and direct loans to assist the construction, modernization, and replacement of various kinds of health facilities; and project grants are available for the construction of emergency room facilities.

Other federal health programs support the construction of facilities as well. The federal government finances construction of its own facilities for direct provision of services to the military, veterans, Indians, and others. The National Institute of Mental Health aids construction of community mental health facilities and facilities for the treatment of alcoholism and drug dependence. The Rehabilitation Services Administration aids construction and remodeling of rehabilitation centers. Other programs provide construction grants for medical schools and other training facilities for the health professions. \

Non-health agencies also support health facility construction: the Federal Housing Administration of the Department of Housing and Urban Development, the Office of Economic Opportunity, the Department of Commerce, and others.

State Programs.   Several departments of state government are concerned from different points of view with the administration of the Hill-Burton program, the support of construction of specialized facilities, the financing of construction of facilities for specific populations for whom the state has a responsibility, or the reimbursement of hospitals and nursing homes for care, thereby funding depreciation. Multiple, uncoordinated efforts at the state level contribute to the support of construction of facilities.

Local Programs.   At the local level, construction of facilities is supported primarily by private financing from banks, insurance companies, and other investors. A significant source of funds is provided by philanthropic contributions. Departments of county government are involved in construction of county-operated facilities and in matching federal funding. In addition, hospital districts have been formed to finance and build community hospitals in areas where public hospitals are not available.

Production of Drugs, Appliances, Equipment, and Supplies

The important resources of drugs, appliances, equipment, and supplies are, with few exceptions, produced entirely by the private sector. The role of government in development, testing, surveillance, and monitoring the safety and quality of drugs, and to a lesser extent of equipment, is a form of social control discussed below. Government also exercises some influence through its purchases of drugs and equipment for use in public hospitals and through federal and state health care programs.

Drugs.   Drugs and drug sundries take the third largest share of health spending — close to $8 billion in fiscal 1972, or almost ten percent of the national health bill.[14] Spending on drugs outside the hospital setting comes largely from consumers out of pocket; private insurance covers only half the population for drugs, Medicaid pays a small portion, while until recently Medicare barred payment for drugs. Thus the consumer bears the chief burden; among the aged the burden of spending is three or more times that of those under 65; women spend more; the poor under 65 less; the nonwhite far less.[15]

Three factors in drug production, distribution, and use contribute to fragmentation. The usual drug transaction is divisive. Drug production emphasizes a bewildering variety of drugs. Drug distribution contributes to important variations in prescribing practices.

First, the drug transaction is an economic anomaly, for the person who orders the drug does not pay for it, at least not for most prescription drugs. Consumer demand is thus a removed demand of the 300,000 physicians who prescribe drugs, not of the 200 million people who buy and take them. For prescription drugs, the consumer has little if any choice and less knowledge about the products he pays for. For over-the-counter drugs, to which much of his money goes, the consumer has even less to depend on, except inflated advertising claims.

Second is the emphasis of the drug industry on new products. "Drugs" include three different but related industries: bulk medicinals and botanical preparations with some 125 producers; biological products, serums, and vaccines, with an equal number; and pharmaceutical drugs, with about 1100 producers.[16] Pharmaceutical drugs, the largest category, consist of prescribed and over-the-counter drugs. Prescribed drugs are both brand-name drugs and generic drugs. Over-the-counter drugs may be called patent medicines or proprietary drugs.

Since the pharmaceutical revolution, a rash of chemotherapeutic agents, antidepressants, sedatives, hypnotic drugs, antihistamines, hormones, vitamins, enzymes, and other drugs have been developed. Before the 1950s proprietary drugs constituted more than half of all sales; after that time, prescription drugs outstripped them and now constitute more than two-thirds of all sales.[17] Research tends to concentrate on prescription drugs. While investment in research has subsidized many scientists and yielded invaluable contributions to therapy, a considerable amount of research has been characterized as "molecular roulette" — minute modifications of existing drugs. These new products are then protected by patents and trademarks and promoted through intensive marketing to yield the high profits of the drug industry.[18]

Third, the proliferation of new products, many differing only minutely one from the other, contributes to confusion in prescribing practices. Current distributing and marketing methods compound differences in prescribing practices. The market is a narrow one, concentrating on the prescribing physician, who is subjected to costly advertising campaigns in national and state medical journals, mailings of free samples, and regular visits from detail men to promote new drugs. Marketing efforts of drug companies are four times the size of their research efforts,[19] which are frequently cited by producers as a leading factor in the high prices of drugs.[20] Since there are few means of evaluating competing claims of quite similar drugs, the prescribing physician is often unable to distinguish between them.[21] The result is a wide variation in prescribing practices and use of higher priced brand name drugs in place of lower priced generic drugs of equal potency.

Appliances, Equipment, and Supplies.   Production and distribution of appliances, equipment, and supplies are exclusively in the private sector. Expenditures are of two kinds. Consumer expenditures, usually at the direction of physicians, optometrists, or opticians, are frequently not covered by either insurance or public payment programs. In fiscal 1972, expenditures on eyeglasses and appliances came to more than two billion dollars.[22] The other and larger kind of expenditure is by institutions and the professions. Nearly $3 billion a year is spent on medical and surgical equipment by hospitals, physicians, and dentists; more than half is for surgical appliances and supplies, about $300 million for dental equipment, and almost $900 million for surgical and medical instruments.[23]

Although the eight largest producers of such equipment account for more than half of yearly shipments,[24] the large number of small firms in the industry and the great variety of their products have led to increased centralization: cooperative purchasing by hospitals; formation of large wholesalers of medical equipment and supplies, such as the American Hospital Supply Company, to facilitate central purchasing by hospitals; and, with increased technical and electronic equipment, entrance of more of the giants of American industry into the hospital and medical supply field.

The division of functions among numerous manufacturers, wholesalers, retailers, advertisers, and private agencies in the field of production and distribution of drugs and equipment follows the general pattern of American industry, with two notable differences. The first is the economic anomaly noted above for prescription drugs—the separation of prescriber from consumer. The same holds true for any appliance ordered by a physician but paid for by the user. Second, "reasonable cost" formulas in public programs and in private insurance make institutions less cost-conscious in their purchases of equipment. Both these factors weaken the bargaining at the heart of a competitive system, result in duplications, and introduce waste into the system.

Production of Knowledge—Research

Biomedical research is conducted by hundreds of research entities, located in universities—both medical schools and basic science departments—research institutes, hospitals, and pharmaceutical companies. Great independence and autonomy characterize both the objectives and the methodology of this research. The freedom of investigators is limited only by their ability to obtain financial support. To some extent, therefore, federal financing acts as a mechanism for indirectly influencing the choice of objectives by research scientists in public and private institutions.

Proliferating medical discoveries that have advanced the knowledge of life processes, laid bare some of the causes of disease, and led to new modes of treatment are, to a considerable extent, the result of federal support of biomedical research. In 1972, 65 percent of national spending on medical research was federally funded; 27 percent was provided by industry; foundations, hospitals, voluntary agencies, and state and local governments provided the remaining 8 percent.[25] If industrial research, incorporated in the prices of its products, is omitted, the federal effort comes to almost nine-tenths of the total. In 1972, 14 federal agencies spent $1.8 billion on medical research.[26] If all life sciences are included, 19 agencies are involved.[27]

The chief federal agency involved in biomedical research is the Department of Health, Edcuation, and Walfare, particularly its National Institutes of Health (NIH) with 11 categorical Institutes, the Health Services and Mental Health Administration (HSMHA), and the Food and Drug Administration (FDA). NIH also contains the Bureau of Health Manpower Education, the National Library of Medicine, the Fogarty International Center for Advanced Study in the Health Sciences, and a Clinical Center, all of which are involved in performance or support of research. The Division of Research Resources supports institutional and regional research centers. HSMHA is concerned with research in the field of mental health and mental health services and in many aspects of the organization and delivery of health services generally. FDA regulates research in drugs and pharmaceuticals and, as of 1972, contains the Division of Biological Standards, which conducts research on biological serums and vaccines.

While the federal effort in health research is concentrated principally in the Department of Health, Education, and Welfare, other agencies also participate. Although spending considerably below the level of the Department of Health, Education, and Welfare, the National Aeronautic and Space Administration (NASA), the Atomic Energy Commission, the Department of Defense, the Veterans Administration, the National Science Foundation, and the Department of Agriculture all contribute to biomedical research. Much smaller amounts are spent by some ten other agencies.[28] The research goals, missions, and orientation of these agencies differ widely, conceived in 18 or more legislative committees, modified in appropriations subcommittees, overhauled in the budgetary process, and bent to executive priorities and agency requirements.

Fragmentation of programs for biomedical research among 19 different agencies is magnified by the grants mechanisms. In 1971, less than a fifth of expenditures by the National Institutes of Health for biomedical research was for intramural work; more than half of its funds went to universities and colleges; 14 percent went to industrial establishments; and 2.5 percent supported research by foreign scientists.[29] Support is given to 244 regional or national research centers within 125 institutions for clinical investigation, development of biotechnology, and raising of animals for laboratory experimentation, as well as to 400 institutions for biomedical research and training. Of the General Clinical Research Centers funded by the National Institutes of Health, 88 are in hospitals, 79 of them in university medical centers as discrete units.[30] In addition to continued research funding, from 1957 to 1968 some $360 million went to universities to construct research facilities, and hospitals and research institutes received another $63 million for the same purpose. As to the effect of multiple funding programs on the recipient, the Worcester Institute for Experimental Biology, where basic research on fertility by Pincus and Chang produced the first modern contraceptives, reported in one year that it received 65 percent of its budget from 104 different federal grants totalling almost $4 million.[31] Research is also supported by private foundations, such as the Rockefeller Institute, and by many voluntary health organizations.

Few other federal activities, except for training with which it is closely allied, involve such a multiplicity of agencies as does the research enterprise. The dispersal of research, the differing missions of agencies, their competition for funds, and the problems of communication emphasize what has been called an "unmanageable" enterprise by some, "chaos" by others.[32] The 1969-1970 decline in funding sharpens this emphasis. Over the past 20 years, at least six special review commissions,[33] as well as lengthy Congressional inquiries,[34] have called for greater coordination of the research enterprise.

Coordinating Mechanisms. The coordinating apparatus for research as of 1972 consists of several levels. Within each Institute or agency, working committees of scientists, both staff personnel and outside consultants, review grant applications. Each Institute has an Advisory Council, which reviews the work of the Institute periodically. NIH has also appointed an overall Advisory Council. Scientific affairs are under an Assistant Secretary for Science of the Department of Health, Education, and Welfare. Other departments and agencies are similarly staffed with advisory boards and assistant secretaries.

Coordination of the various agencies begins with the President's Science Adviser, aided by a Science Advisory Committee, both staffed by the Office of Science and Technology, created to increase cooperation among federal agencies. Eleven departments and agencies are involved in this Council at the policy level, with representatives of seven other departments attending meetings. Standing committees have been established for specialized fields, and from time to time interagency committees on special problems are formed. Additionally, the National Science Board of the National Science Foundation reviews different fields of research periodically and maintains a registry of scientific personnel. The Science and Technology Division of the Office of Management and Budget oversees and reviews the research and development budgets of the operating agencies; its management division seeks better administration within the research agencies; and its statistical division helps with reporting and statistical activities of each agency. Thus, the very effort to coordinate adds to the multiplicity of agencies involved in the production of knowledge. Moreover, the coordination achieved has had only limited effect on the conduct of research by multiple agencies.

Dissemination of Scientific Information. The results of scientific research are disseminated through many outlets. More than 50,000 scientific and professional journals publish papers in specialized fields. Growing numbers of knowledgeable science writers report discoveries and developments, even in advance of their publication in scientific journals. The curricula of basic education programs for health professionals disseminate new scientific findings. Continuing education programs in numerous fields and the Regional Medical Programs transmit scientific developments to health practitioners. Conferences dealing with specific problems are organized to encourage application of research findings to the world of practice. Hospital staffs, local and state medical societies, and other professional associations sponsor special meetings to keep their members abreast of new knowledge. Governmental agencies—the Smithsonian Institution, the Library of Congress, the Department of Commerce, various divisions of the Department of Health, Education, and Welfare, and the quasi-governmental National Academy of Sciences, to mention but a few—disseminate the results of biomedical research to the health and scientific community, to industry, and to the public at large. No single repository of the findings of biomedical research has been established.

PROVISION OF SERVICES

The focus of this study is on personal health services; the vast field of environmental health protection is beyond its scope. But the importance of the environment to health and well-being requires at least brief mention of the basic environmental services that have a direct and intimate effect on the health of people. These services may do as much or more to assure health as do all medical care services.

Environmental Health Protection

Environmental health activities consist of direct provision of services, such as a pure water supply or a sewage disposal system, and of programs of social control, such as food and drug surveillance, milk and meat inspection, housing, restaurant, and recreational sanitation. Direct services may be provided either by private companies or by governmental entities. For example, waterworks systems may be established and operated by private corporations, public utilities, or by municipal or county governments. Garbage disposal systems, likewise, may be operated by any of these agencies or by a combination of local government and private collection companies. In-plant health services concerned with the air, noise, and safety conditions in industry are operated to varying degrees by each company, subject to federal and state regulation. Thus, the elements of a healthful environment may be provided by government, by the private sector, or by a combination of the two.

Measures of social control affecting environmental health services are almost exclusively governmental. The task of monitoring the quality of working and living conditions is enormous, and understandably it requires multiple and varied resources.[35] An inventory of agencies concerned with environmental health services in California revealed nearly 500 separate programs at the federal, state, regional, county, and city levels of government.[36] In each field of environmental health, be it food and drug control, health aspects of housing, or occupational safety, multiple programs under the auspices of both health and non-health agencies at all governmental levels perform categorical functions concerned with environmental health.

Personal Preventive Services

A wide range of environmental, educational, nutritional, and social measures contributes to prevention of illness. Although these measures outside the system of personal health services are basic, this review emphasizes preventive services in organized programs of personal health service.

Federal Programs.   Personal preventive services are woven into an array of categorical programs for special population groups—low-income mothers and infants, Indians, migrants, military dependents, federal employees, preschool children, and workers—and for particular diseases—communicable, addictive, and chronic. Federal agencies also perform certain general functions directed at the prevention and control of disease, such as international and national epidemiological surveillance and evaluation, national nutrition surveys, consumer protection activities, development of clinical laboratories, and preparation of educational materials dealing with health, safety, and nutrition.

State Programs. The categorical organization of preventive activities for particular persons and particular diseases originating at the federal level is reflected at the state level by dispersal of such functions and services among eight state agencies in California. The State Department of Public Health administers services for migrants and Indians and provides support of prenatal and well-child care for low-income mothers and infants. Responsibility for preventive services for children is shared by three state departments — Public Health, Social Welfare, and Education — and by local school districts, which enforce mandatory vision and hearing screening and immunization requirements for school-age children.[37] Casefinding, immunizations, screening clinics, testing programs, consultation, health information, education, and community outreach for particular diseases and target populations are lodged haphazardly in other programs of the Departments of Education, Industrial Relations, Health Care Services, Social Welfare, Mental Hygiene, Motor Vehicles, and Public Health. Interagency councils on smoking and health, tuberculosis, family planning, alcoholism, and drug abuse have been formed to improve communication among public programs and those of voluntary and private organizations at the state and local levels.

County Programs. The county health officer is the public official with mandated responsibility for the organization of the array of preventive health activities. Nevertheless, such preventive functions as casefinding, immunizations, quarantine, education, outreach, laboratory analysis, and epidemiological surveillance are performed also by other county agencies, city agencies, school districts, courts, physicians, hospitals, voluntary organizations, and private groups. While the multiplicity of agencies performing any one of these functions results in varied preventive activities in many settings that reach large numbers of people, this very diversity impedes systematic referral and follow-up. No agency has the capacity to identify the gaps, let alone fill them.

Geographically, in Los Angeles County 23 public health districts, 11 mental health regions, 24 municipal court districts, 96 school districts, 20 family aid districts, the local chapters and divisions of hundreds of voluntary agencies, and 76 cities — only one of which is the City of Los Angeles with its many communities — define the multiple boundaries for preventive services. Distribution throughout the county of 490 clinical laboratories, approximately 12,000 physicians, and numerous other providers magnifies the task of coordinating casefinding and preventive services.

Voluntary and Private Programs. Preventive services are, of course, provided by private physicians in the regular course of medical practice. Individual voluntary hospitals, too, provide immunizations, screening tests, and X-ray examinations. Professional associations lend their authoritative voices to educational campaigns for the prevention of disease. Voluntary health organizations devoted to the control of specific diseases place great stress on preventive measures, such as proper diet and exercise to prevent heart disease, early detection of cancer, and education on smoking and health. Each of these organizations has national, state, and local components, so that preventive activities of a single disease-specific voluntary agency are carried on at multiple levels. In addition, important preventive services are provided by many prepaid group health plans and by union health and welfare programs.

Some notion of the magnitude of the voluntary health movement is provided by the estimate that there were 100,000 voluntary health and welfare agencies in the United States in 1960.[38] In 1963, these agencies, excluding the Red Cross, were estimated to have at least 500,000 members of committees and boards, with annual expenditures of more than $800 million.[39] In 1969, 16 large voluntary health agencies that were members of the National Health Council, the coordinating council of voluntary health agencies, had nearly 9 million volunteers involved in the activities of their 11,000 state and local affiliates.[40] These agencies had 188 committees with a total of 2,034 members. On their national boards were 1,406 persons. Multiplicity is thus a feature of voluntarism as well as of government.

Ambulatory Care

This component of the medical care system covers both general ambulatory care, diagnostic and therapeutic, and specialized ambulatory services for particular conditions. The varied settings for the provision of ambulatory care include individual physicians' offices, hospital emergency rooms and out-patient departments, health department clinics, school and college health services, private group practices, health maintenance organizations or prepaid group practices, neighborhood health centers, Indian and migrant health centers, and free-standing clinics, such as cancer detection centers, free clinics, and other specialized clinics.

Federal Programs. The functions performed by the federal government affecting organization of ambulatory care include support for the operation of facilities, direct provision of service, purchase of service, financial assistance for state and local programs, and promotion of new organizational patterns through grants and contracts. Each of these functions is subdivided among programs for designated segments of the population, specified conditions, or specialized services. Although much federal funding is channelled through state agencies, several federal programs bypass state government to provide support directly to county, city, or nonprofit agencies.

The federal government is thus a participant in, as well as a sponsor of, community health services.

State Programs. Ambulatory services in California are provided by categorical public programs—some authorized by federal legislation but structured and administered by state departments and others initiated by state agencies—and by the vast private sector including individual, group, and institutional providers of care. As public funds are increasingly used to purchase or reimburse services from the private sector and to provide essential health care for all segments of society, the distinction between public and private services is no longer so clear as in the past.

The functions of the various state departments related to the provision of ambulatory care include technical and financial support for the provision of care to special groups or for special diseases, licensing of personnel and facilities, quality control of services provided in public programs, and demonstration of improved methods of organizing services. These functions are dispersed among a variety of agencies. The State Departments of Public Health, Mental Hygiene, and Rehabilitation develop state plans for facilities and services of various specialized kinds—rehabilitation, mental health, mental retardation, and emergency services. Health agencies are joined in these efforts by agencies with other missions, such as the Departments of Social Welfare and Corrections and the state system of higher public education.

Other agencies, including the Department of Industrial Relations, the Workmen's Compensation Board, the crippled children's program, and the Department of Rehabilitation, utilize local panels of providers for medical diagnosis, evaluation, and treatment. By far the largest program for ambulatory services is the Medicaid program, called Medi-Cal in California, which reimburses private practitioners and institutional providers for approved services rendered to a portion of the state's medically indigent. A few contracts with prepaid group practices and medical foundations have been approved to demonstrate and develop more efficient and effective methods of organizing ambulatory and hospital care. Under the county option portion of the Medi-Cal program, counties are assisted by the state without federal aid in providing outpatient care to the medically indigent who do not qualify for care from private providers.

County Programs. Within Los Angeles County, ambulatory services are operated by federal, state, and county agencies. The Veterans Administration and the Department of Defense operate outpatient clinics for their patients. Federal, state, county, and city employees may have insurance coverage for services provided by individual physicians or by prepaid group practices. The federal government supports directly one neighborhood health center, two demonstration projects for mothers, infants, and children residing in defined areas, and 12 Community Mental Health Centers. County and state departments sponsor, in addition to preventive services, clinic and out-patient hospital care for adolescents, crippled children, the mentally re-tarded, mentally ill, and parolees; for control of venereal disease, tubercu-losis, drug dependence, alcoholism, and for smoking withdrawal; and for dental, psychiatric, rehabilitation, emergency care, and family planning services. Numerous separate systems, with multiple sources of funding, varying eligibility criteria, and different standards of care provide these services.

Voluntary and Private Programs. Despite this multiplicity of govern-mental programs providing, financing, or shaping ambulatory care, this segment of health services is furnished mainly by the private sector. In contrast to institutional care, which is highly organized, the major portion of ambulatory care is not provided in organized programs but rather by individual physicians and other practitioners in their private offices. An increasing proportion of ambulatory care is provided by voluntary hospitals, industrial clinics, multi-specialty groups, and clinics sponsored by voluntary agencies. Until recently, ambulatory care was a limited benefit of health insurance policies and even now is less well covered by insurance than is in-patient care. Thus, the financing mechanism tends to reinforce and per-petuate the basic fragmentation of ambulatory and hospital services.

Hospital Care

In California, 541 general hospitals, with 74,000 beds, served a population of 20 million in 1970. These hospitals range in size and services from facilities of fewer than 20 beds, providing limited medical and surgical services, to large medical centers with 500 or more beds and at least 25 specialized services.[41] Most numerous at 244 voluntary, nonprofit hospitals with 42,000 beds, followed by 124 state and local governmental hospitals with 20,000 beds, and 173 for-profit hospitals with 12,000 beds. In addition, 10 state mental hospitals and 10 facilities for the mentally retarded, some of them serving both groups, and 55 specialized hospitals for maternity care, tuberculosis, alcoholism, and other conditions made up the full complement of hospitals. Numerous federal, state, and local programs directly affect the services provided by this most expensive component of the health care system.

Federal Programs. The role of the federal government in hospital care includes direct provision of services, purchase of hospital care, promotion of hospital planning and hospital standards, and support of innovative patterns of organizing hospital and health care. These functions are performed by at least ten divisions of the Department of Health, Education, and Welfare and four other federal departments or agencies.

Federal hospitals provide direct services to selected segments of the population; veterans, the military, Indians, and others. Hospital care is purchased or partially financed for larger segments of the population through a variety of federal programs, each with its own eligibility criteria, reimbursement formula, service limitations, and standards of care. Thus, hospital care is purchased for military dependents under the CHAMPUS program of the Department of Defense, for veterans with service-connected conditions in hospitals close to their homes by the Veterans Administration, and for crippled children whose conditions qualify for treatment under the federal-state crippled children's program. The largest programs for financing hospital care are Medicare, administered by the Social Security Administration, and Medicaid, administered by the Social and Rehabilitation Service of the Department of Health, Education, and Welfare and by participating state governments.

Various federal programs are concerned with planning, developing, and improving the quality of hospital services. These programs are discussed in connection with the production of resources and social controls. Probably one of the most significant federal efforts related to the provision of hospital care is encouragement of innovation in management and organization of hospital services. Manpower training programs, promotion of health maintenance organizations, and demonstrations of functional relationships between hospitals and other community health resources all have an impact on the provision of hospital care.

State Programs. State functions in provision of hospital services include operation of state mental hospitals and other state facilities, purchase of hospital services, and technical assistance in the provision of general and specialized hospital services. Planning and licensing of health facilities, functions essential to the provision of services in which the state has a paramount role, are discussed below in connection with social controls.

Operation of hospitals for the mentally ill and the mentally retarded has traditionally been a state function. Although the ambitious program of community care for the mentally ill undertaken in California has reduced the census in these hospitals, inpatient care remains largely a state responsibility. The state also operates specialized facilities for tuberculosis, alcoholism, and drug dependence and facilities for special groups in the population, such as prisoners.

The state purchases hospital services indirectly through its contribution to the state employees' health benefits program and directly through various programs, such as the crippled children's program, Workmen's Compensation, the state rehabilitation program, and the state Medicaid program (Medi-Cal) for categorical welfare recipients and the medically indigent. These programs are administered by several departments, and each program establishes its own criteria for the quality of care to be purchased.

The state health agency provides limited technical assistance for hospital care. Development of specialized services in hospitals has occurred largely on an ad hoc basis, with a resultant duplication and maldistribution of scarce resources. For example, although the principle of locating expensive and complex services on a regional basis has been recognized in California legislation with a provision for up to four kidney dialysis centers,[42] 38 other hospitals provide this service and are not part of the regional plan. A state report in 1970 revealed that while 18 of these facilities operated at less than full capacity, 144 patients in California were waiting for this vital service.[43]

Cancer therapy units, similarly, reveal unplanned development of highly specialized and costly resources. A study conducted in Southern California in 1970-1971 found that 78 hospitals with radiation therapy equipment were operating the equipment at approximately 75 percent capacity. When current plans have been put into effect, the installed megavoltage equipment will be sufficient to service twice the population of this area.[44] One medium-sized city in California had the foresight to set up a committee a few years ago to determine the need for supervoltage units. The committee recommended one supervoltage unit as adequate for the population. That city, however, now has three such units.

Neither the State Plan for Hospitals nor the facility licensing regulations take account of the need for specialized services. Functional relationships and cooperative arrangements between individual hospitals or between hospitals and other health care services for efficient utilization of specialized resources are not yet within the purview of the state plan, although priority is assigned under the 1970 amendments to the Hill-Burton program to projects providing comprehensive health care.

County Programs.   Local governments provide hospital care for the poor, generally in large county hospitals, that are often overcrowded and geographically inaccessible to the poor whom they serve. In most counties, hospital services are functionally and organizationally independent of preventive health care and of the social and supportive services provided to the same indigent population by other agencies. In some counties, the lack of public or private facilities has led to formation of special hospital districts, with taxing powers to build and maintain district hospitals that serve the entire population.

Functional linkages between public and private hospitals exist in Los Angeles County primarily for emergency services. The Los Angeles County Department of Hospitals contracts with approximately 75 voluntary hospitals throughout the county to provide emergency care easily accessible to the patient. Such emergency care is paid for by the patient or by the county if the patient is unable to pay.

For both public and private hospital services the linkages between the hospital component and ambulatory, extended, or other specialized care are lacking or ill-defined. With the establishment of a single county health agency in 1972, implementation of a projected system of ambulatory service centers in the neighborhoods where people live, linked to public and voluntary hospitals, has begun. Although such a system of referrals and linkages will apply only to public medical care, it should serve to demonstrate the benefits of coordinated services.

Voluntary Hospitals. The bulk of general hospital care is provided by voluntary, nonprofit hospitals, as indicated by the numbers of facilities and beds above. Voluntary hospitals are the principal resources for meeting the general hospital needs of the population, for diagnosing and treating serious illness, and for providing continuing education for physicians and other health personnel. In this important role, they have been virtually autonomous, except for minimal standards set by the licensing laws, conditions required for obtaining federal funds for construction, and recently requirements in about 20 states for prior approval of construction or modification of facilities. Since 1965, the most important governmental influence on voluntary and private hospitals has been the required Conditions of Participation of the Medicare program and, to a lesser extent, the requirements of the Medicaid program for reimbursement of hospital care.

Long-Term Care

Long-term care is provided in various kinds of public, voluntary, and private institutions. In California, these include 1,000 nursing and convalescent homes with 88,000 beds, nine state-operated hospitals, 78 long-term facilities for the mentally ill and retarded, three county tuberculosis hospitals,[45] and licensed, residential, out-of-home care facilities for all age groups.[46] Each of these providers, catering to differing needs and groups in the population, is affected by the programs and activities of many public agencies. Formal linkages to ambulatory care facilities and general hospitals are highly variable and frequently lacking.

Federal Programs. The functions of the federal government related to long-term care, similar to its functions in general hospital services, concern direct provision of care and purchase of care. Planning of facilities and setting of standards are matters of social control, discussed below. The Veterans Administration both provides and purchases nursing and domiciliary care for veterans. CHAMPUS purchases care for dependents of the military. Both Medicare and Medicaid purchase nursing home and extended care services for designated segments of the population. The requirements of these programs for quality and cost controls and for certification of facilities affect standards of long-term care facilities generally.

State Programs.   The state is also a major purchaser of long-term care through various programs—Medi-Cal, Aid to the Totally Disabled, Old Age Assistance, Aid to Families of Dependent Children, community mental health services, crippled children's services, regional centers for the mentally retarded, and the Youth Authority. Payment rates and standards established for these placement programs by separate agencies lack both consistency with each other and coordination with the activities of the licensing agencies. Placement of persons in specialized facilities is made on a regional basis by some state agencies providing direct services, for example, the Alternate Care Services Unit of the Department of Mental Hygiene for persons leaving state mental hospitals and the Department of Rehabilitation and the regional centers for the mentally retarded for persons requiring services in these respective fields.

County Programs.   At the county level, the various federal, state, and county programs, the services organized by the private sector, and the variety of public and private systems for financing long-term care all converge. In Los Angeles County, the Department of Hospitals operates a large chronic disease hospital, a geriatric hospital, and long-term rehabilitation centers; the state operates four mental hospitals serving the area; and the Veterans Administration operates five large centers to provide long-term care for chronic and psychiatric conditions. Private and voluntary providers operate the rest of the extended care services for the county's population. Their services are purchased or reimbursed by (1) federal programs—directly by Medicare, CHAMPUS, and the Veterans Administration and indirectly through Social Security Disability Insurance; (2) state programs—by Medi-Cal, Workmen's Compensation, the Community Services Division of the Department of Social Welfare, the Department of Rehabilitation, and the regional centers for the mentally retarded under the Department of Public Health; (3) county programs—by the Department of Public Social Services for the disabled, blind, aged, and dependent children, the Probation Department, and the crippled children's services; and (4) private sources—by hospital and disability insurance and out-of-pocket payments by individuals or families.

The variety of programs requiring some extended care services is striking. More striking is the variation in reimbursement formulas, record and patient identification systems, restrictions on length of stay or quantity of service, and certification requirements and standards of care. The whole creates difficulties in assuring placement of an individual at the most appropriate level of care and in assuring transfer of each patient and his records from general hospitals or other services at the time when it is beneficial to the patient and efficient for the system. The inadequate number of residential care facilities for the mentally ill, retarded, and handicapped persons, and for children and the aged, means that many unlicensed facilities are certified by placement agencies (the County Departments of Public Social Services and Probation and the Community Services Division of the State Department of Social Welfare) in order to meet their own needs for resources.[47]

The Private Sector. The operation of nursing homes and long-term care facilities is largely conducted by the private sector. While some religious and other nonprofit organizations operate facilities for the aged and the chronically ill, the bulk of these facilities are commercial undertakings. These for-profit facilities show great variability in their standards and services. They are subject to minimal requirements concerning staffing and medical and nursing care. Licensing requirements pertain mainly to physical facilities, safety, and sanitation. It was not until 1972 that licensure was required in California for board and care facilities for persons aged 16 to 64. Enactment of the Medicare and Medicaid laws served to raise standards by requiring nursing homes and extended care facilities to meet specific conditions to be eligible to receive patients covered by these programs. In the absence of effective controls on allocation of resources, however, these programs also encouraged overbuilding of private, long-term care facilities in anticipation of governmental reimbursement for care.

SOCIAL CONTROLS

Many mechanisms, programs, and agencies exert control over the quality and costs of health services.[48] These controls are both governmental and voluntary. Understandably, the governmental role in social controls is prominent, but both legally required and voluntary measures regulating services are to be found coexisting in nearly every field of health service. Social controls consist of three kinds of measures: (1) those constituting prior approval as a condition of functioning in a particular capacity, such as licensing; (2) those constituting a form of on-going surveillance over performance in the provision of health services; and (3) those relating to allocation of resources, usually described as planning. In order to show the interrelationships of social controls provided by different levels of government and the private sector, social controls are reviewed according to the above three basic types, with mention of the federal, state, local, and voluntary roles operative for each type.

Prior Approval

Various governmental and voluntary programs impose some form of prior approval as a condition of providing health services. Licensure is, of course, the principal governmental mechanism constituting prior approval; it is the process by which a governmental agency grants permission to persons or facilities to function in a certain capacity by certifying that the applicant meets certain minimum qualifications or standards. Other official mechanisms for prior approval are essentially variations of the licensing mechanism.

Since licensure of both personnel and facilities is a state function, the federal government applies the mechanism of prior approval only in the operation of various federal programs of health service. Thus, the Medicare program specifies Conditions of Participation for various kinds of facilities; only with such approval may facilities be reimbursed under the program. Similarly, other federal programs purchasing health services specify other conditions that must be met; the Veterans Administration requires certain standards in nongovernmental facilities from which it purchases long-term care; CHAMPUS specifies other requirements for providers whom it reimburses. Even when a program, such as crippled children's services or vocational rehabilitation services, is jointly funded by federal and state funds, the federal government specifies standards for facilities and personnel for participation or reimbursement.

At the state level, the many different categories of health personnel and the various kinds of health facilities are subject to numerous separate personnel and facility licensing laws administered by different agencies. In California, licensure of health personnel is administered by ten occupational licensing boards within the State Department of Consumer Affairs and the State Department of Public Health. Licensing of facilities is conducted by three state departments — Public Health, Mental Hygiene, and Social Welfare — with a fourth, Health Care Services, involved in setting standards for certification of facilities and group prepayment contracts under Medi–Cal. Drug formularies under some Medicaid programs constitute a form of prior approval.

At the regional level, new construction or alteration of health facilities may require approval by areawide Comprehensive Health Planning agencies. By 1972, about 20 states had enacted legislation requiring certificates of need as a condition for the construction of new facilities. Under California's legislation, if the areawide planning agency disapproves construction of the facility but the construction is nevertheless undertaken, the facility cannot be licensed for one year.

At the local level of government, health agencies exercise prior approval through the mechanisms of contracts and licensure. In Los Angeles County, contracts between the county and voluntary hospitals for emergency services and contracts with voluntary agencies for community mental health services impose social controls on the quality of those services. Also, in this very large county, licensure of health facilities and of radiation equipment is a function of the county by contract with the state.

Voluntary mechanisms for social control that take the form of prior approval include certification or registration of personnel and accreditation of educational institutions and programs and of health facilities. Certification or registration by voluntary organizations that an individual meets predetermined standards is conducted by all the specialty boards in medicine, now integrated in the American Board of Medical Specialties, formed in 1970 to replace the loose federation of separate boards that had existed formerly,[49] and by numerous professional associations for their respective categories. For some occupations, several agencies share or compete for the role of certification. The American Registry of Radiologic Technologists and the American Registry of Clinical Radiography Technologists both register radiologic technologists.[50] Four organizations perform this function for clinical laboratory personnel, each according to its own standards.[51] For those occupations for which licensure is also required, such as physical therapy, clinical laboratory technology, and radiologic technology in some states, surveillance of qualifications is fragmented among both governmental and nongovernmental agencies.

Accreditation of educational institutions and programs is predominantly private and is conducted by numerous specialized agencies. The most noted agency is the Council on Medical Education of the American Medical Association, which accredits educational programs for 15 health occupations in collaboration with various professional groups.[52] In addition, 20 other agencies accredit educational programs in health fields.[53] And two agencies accredit the accreditors—the National Commission on Accrediting and the U.S. Commissioner of Education. This multiplicity of accrediting mechanisms and agencies means that different agencies establish different standards for education of the same or similar occupations. A single educational institution or program may have to meet various standards of several accrediting agencies and prepare for several accreditation reviews. Although accreditation is performed by private groups, it has the force of law because of the frequent requirement in licensing laws that the applicant must have graduated from an accredited school or program; yet the accreditation process operates with limited public accountability.[54] In 1972, a major national study of accreditation of selected health educational programs recommended rationalizing the jungle of accrediting programs and agencies and establishing a single, recognized quasi-governmental accrediting commission with strong public accountability to oversee the accrediting process.

Accreditation of health facilities by the Joint Commission on Accreditation of Hospitals is a powerful form of prior approval. So widespread has been its acceptance that it has come to be recognized in federal law as a standard for participation in Medicare and several other federal and state programs.

This brief review of various mechanisms of social control that exercise prior approval of personnel, educational programs, and health facilities, while by no means comprehensive, perhaps suffices to show the categorical nature of this form of technical control. Each form of approval is specific to the jurisdiction of the program or function to which it is related. The result is an uneven mosaic of diverse controls.

Surveillance of Performance

This form of social control applies both to the quality and to the cost of health services. Exercised by multiple agencies in various governmental and voluntary programs, surveillance of performance may be directed to a specific end or may operate generally to promote the quality of care.

The federal government incorporates surveillance of different kinds in the operation of its health programs. In direct programs of the federal government, such as the Veterans Administration, on-going controls are exercised in the form of administrative supervision. In programs in which the federal government purchases care from private providers, such as Medicare, surveillance is provided over costs by requiring that charges be based on reasonable costs and customary fees, as defined in various regulations; responsibility for exercising this surveillance is delegated to fiscal intermediaries, but ultimate authority rests with the U.S. Social Security Administration. In the same program, quality promotion as a social control is illustrated by the requirement that extended care facilities, in order to participate, must have transfer agreements with general hospitals.

One of the most elaborate forms of surveillance by the federal government over performance is found in the field of food and drug control. At least eight federal agencies are involved in the surveillance of various aspects of the production and distribution of drugs. The Food and Drug Administration within the Department of Health, Education, and Welfare has the broadest concern in the development of new drugs, control of experimental drugs, setting of standards for the production of drugs, and monitoring their quality. The Food and Drug Administration has powers to control virtually every stage of drug production. It approves protocols of investigation, reviews animal test procedures and results, examines new drug applications, inspects processes and plants, reviews advertising claims, tests results of clinical investigations, and requires substantial evidence of efficacy.

Other agencies within the Department of Health, Education, and Welfare perform other functions. The Division of Biological Standards supervises the production of biologicals, serums, and vaccines. The new National Institute of Safety and Occupational Health monitors hazardous substances in production processes, including those of the drug industry. The Consumer Protection Agency oversees product safety. Several programs of federal health care provide some surveillance through their purchase of drugs.

Non-health agencies are also involved in the surveillance of performance in the field of drugs. The National Bureau of Standards has developed standards of purity for fine chemicals used in drug manufacturing. The Federal Trade Commission has powers over advertising of nonprescription drugs and administers the Fair Trade Practices Act, regulating the prices of fair-traded, brand-named drugs. The Bureau of Customs within the Treasury Department is concerned with the importation of drugs and consults with the Food and Drug Administration on proper identification of drugs for imposition of customs duties as well as on their safety and purity. Still another agency is the quasi-governmental National Academy of Sciences-National Research Council, which has been engaged for some years in study of the efficacy of about 3,000 drugs, both old and new; from time to time it issues reports on drugs tested.

Still another federal program for the improvement of the quality of health services is the Regional Medical Programs. Originally designed to promote regionalization of services for heart disease, cancer, stroke, and related diseases, as implemented this program, with 100 percent federal financing, has been directed toward improving the quality of health services through continuing education of physicians, training of other health personnel, and demonstrations of new mechanisms for the delivery of health services.

A very recent example of federal surveillance is the requirement, enacted in 1972, for Professional Standards Review Organizations (PSROs) to be established nation-wide for monitoring the Medicare and Medicaid programs. While limited initially to review of inpatient hospital services, it obviously lays the groundwork for general surveillance of physician's care in all settings.

At the state level, various agencies are engaged in the surveillance of performance in specialized fields. The State Department of Public Health monitors and provides technical assistance to local health departments on public health services generally. The State Department of Industrial Relations (in most states the Department of Labor) conducts factory inspections to assure industrial safety and prevent accidents. The State Department of Rehabilitation provides surveillance of alcoholism control programs. The State Department of Education oversees educational programs for various health occupations. Another illustration is seen in the monitoring of health insurance plans by state departments of insurance—a field in which the potential, however, is far greater than the practice.

At the local level, surveillance of performance is illustrated by the county health department's inspection of a host of environmental matters—housing, restaurants, markets, dairies, milk pasteurization plants, and many other features of the living and working environment of the population. The Department of Mental Health provides surveillance of the quality of community mental health services in child guidance clinics and other agencies that have contracted to provide services.

Examples of voluntary surveillance of the quality of services are the numerous mechanisms within hospitals for surgical tissue committees, pathological review of deaths, mandatory consultations, medical audits, and continuing education, all designed to promote the quality of care. The inspections involved in the accreditation of health facilities by the Joint Commission on Accreditation of Hospitals is another measure of surveillance. Medical and other professional societies monitor the quality of care by setting standards for professional ethics. Although this device has been abused on occasion, it has served to control advertising and other activities deemed deleterious to patient care. A voluntary mechanism for cost controls is the process of claims review conducted by voluntary insurance plans.

Thus, the multiplicity of mechanisms for the surveillance of performance operates at all levels, governmental and voluntary. Moreover, in many fields, such as food and drug control, all three levels of government as well as the private sector may exercise surveillance over performance.

Planning

Many categorical programs for the development of resources or provision of services, whether for specific populations or specific diseases or providing more comprehensive services, build in a component for planning. Ordinarily, each program can be planned only within the confines of its scope. Beyond such planning efforts, there are specific programs focused on planning, mainly in the sense of deliberate allocation of resources in some rational manner.

At the federal level, the best example of planning as a form of social control is the Hill-Burton program for the support of the construction of facilities, which mandates state plans for hospitals aided by such grants. Over the years since 1935, most of the federal grant-in-aid programs for categorical purposes (maternal and child health services, venereal disease control, chronic disease services, and so forth) have required "state plans" as a condition. Most recently, the federal Comprehensive Health Planning Act of 1966 provides, among other things, for grants to the states for planning of all kinds of personal and environmental health services. As implemented, the Comprehensive Health Planning program has given emphasis to the planning of all health facilities, a broadening of the planning authority previously provided only for federally aided health facilities.

At the state level, most organized planning efforts have been developed pursuant to federal grant programs. Thus, to give an example beyond those noted above, a state plan for emergency medical services is mandated by the National Highway Safety Act. State mental hospitals, however, have long required extensive state planning independent of federal legislative action. The new unified State Department of Health in California will have the capability to coordinate planning and other separate functions related to health services.

At the regional level are various categorical planning efforts. In California, planning of services for the mentally retarded on a regional basis is particularly advanced. As areawide Comprehensive Health Planning agencies have gained experience in planning, efforts are being made to develop comprehensive regional plans for health facilities and services.

At the local level, planning is undertaken by each department of county and city government. With the merger of the principal county health agencies, the new County Department of Health Services in Los Angeles will have an overall responsibility for planning integrated health services. In addition, a major role in planning health services in Los Angeles County is played by the office of the Chief Administrative Officer of the county through its power to review budgets of county departments and its responsibility to carry out the policy of the elected officials of the county. Strong county government acts as an integrating force in local planning, enlisting cooperation not only of official agencies but of the many segments of the private sector as well.

This overview of the organization of the provision of health services tells only half the story. The other half concerns the dimension of financing. In the next chapter attention is turned to the pluralistic system of financing health services through a mixture of various forms of public and private spending.

NOTES

1. Letter of Robert H. Finch, Secretary, U.S. Department of Health, Education, and Welfare to the Senate Committee on Government Operations, Hearings before the Subcommittee on Intergovernmental Relations of the Senate Committee on Government Operations on Intergovernmental Cooperation Act of 1969, p. 28, 91st Cong., 1st Sess., Sept. 1969.

2. See Roemer, Milton I. and Ethel A. Wilson, *Organized Health Services in a County of the United States,* Federal Security Agency, PHS Pub. No. 197, Washington, D.C., 1952.

3. See Kramer, C. and Ruth Roemer, *Health Manpower and the Organization of Health Services,* Institute of Industrial Relations, University of California, Los Angeles, 1972 (processed).

4. Pennell, Maryland Y. and David B. Hoover, *Health Manpower Source Book 21,* p. 1, PHS Pub. No. 263, Washington, D.C., 1970.

5. *Inventory of Federal Programs that Support Health Manpower Training* (Lucy M. Kramer, Ed.), p. iii, DHEW Pub. No. (NIH) 72-146, U.S. Department of Health, Education, and Welfare, Nov. 1971.

6. *Special Analyses, Budget of the U.S. Government, Fiscal Year 1972,* p. 153, U.S. Government Printing Office, Washington, D.C., 1971. The number varies from year to year. *Special Analyses* for the previous year notes 10 federal agencies (p. 151), whereas 14 federal agencies were reported in *Federal Role in Health,* Report of the Committee on Government Operations, U.S. Senate, made by its Subcommittee on Executive Reorganization and Government Research, Report No. 91-809, p. 11, 91st Cong., 2d Sess., 1970.

7. *Special Analyses, Budget of the U.S. Government, Fiscal Year 1972,* supra note 6 at 171, Table K-15.

8. Statement of Dr. James Shannon, formerly director of the National Institutes of Health, in *Federal Role in Health,* supra note 6 at 521-525:

> The Federal contributions to health manpower production suffer from a peculiar type of fractionalization . . . there seems to be a lack of general awareness that the simple and

modest extension of the present programs, even when coupled with new programs aimed at the evolution of new careers, will not resolve the combination of shortage and maldistribution in any reasonable period of time . . . decisive executive action is called for. . . . Such a review would require an examination of the commitment of the Federal Establishment for manpower production, including Federal contributions to higher education in general. Such a review could lead to a restructuring of the educational underpinning of many health occupations and professions . . . make full use of the Nation's educational base as well as its health institutions, and provide systems of training and education which not only satisfy the urgent current needs, but provide the upward mobility within some of the health occupations.

9. Reeder, Leo G., Ruth Roemer, and Hannah C. Sprowls, *Education of Health Manpower in California, A Survey of Programs for Preparing Selected Categories of Personnel,* Report for the California Committee on Regional Medical Programs, Survey Research Center, University of California, Los Angeles, 1968 (processed).

10. *Education for Health Care in Michigan, Report of the Citizens Committee on Education for Health Care,* Education for Health Care Publications, Series 1, No. 5, Michigan Department of Education, Lansing, Michigan, 1970.

11. *A Special Report to the National Advisory Council,* Regional Medical Programs Service, p. 23, Continuing Education and Training Branch, Regional Medical Programs Service, Health Services and Mental Health Administration, Department of Health, Education, and Welfare, May 11-12, 1971.

12. Cooper, Barbara S. and Nancy L. Worthington, "National Health Expenditures, 1929-1972," *Social Security Bull.,* Vol. 36, No. 1, p. 7, Table 3, Jan. 1973.

13. *Special Analyses, Budget of the United States Government, Fiscal Year 1974,* p. 146; *Major Federal Aid Programs for Hospitals,* American Hospital Association, Chicago, Illinois, 1970.

14. Cooper and Worthington, supra note 12 at 7, Table 2.

15. Task Force on Prescription Drugs, *Final Report,* p. 2, Table 1, Feb. 1969; *The Drug Users,* U.S. Department of Health, Education, and Welfare, p. 21, Table 21, Dec. 1968.

16. Task Force on Prescription Drugs, *The Drug Makers and the Drug Distributors,* Background Papers, pp. 4-5, U.S. Department of Health, Education, and Welfare, Dec. 1968.

17. Task Force on Prescription Drugs, *Final Report,* supra note 15 at 7.

18. See *The Drug Makers and the Drug Distributors,* supra note 16 at 116-119 and Harris, Richard, *A Sacred Trust,* Penguin Books, Inc., Baltimore, Md., 1969.

19. *The Drug Makers and the Drug Distributors,* supra note 16 at 14, Figure 14.

20. Id. at 45-49.

21. Id. at Chapter 8; *Administered Prices/Drugs,* Part IV, Report of the Committee on the Judiciary, U.S. Senate by its Subcommittee on Antitrust and Monopoly, Chapters 10-12, pp. 165ff., 87th Cong., 1st Sess., June 27, 1961.

22. Cooper and Worthington, supra note 12 at 7, Table 2.

23. U.S. Department of Commerce, Bureau of Foreign & Domestic Commerce, *U.S. Industrial Outlook,* p. 164, 1971; *Statistical Abstract of the U.S. 1972.*

24. Ibid.

25. *Special Analyses, Budget of the U.S. Government, Fiscal Year 1973,* p. 157, Office of Management and Budget, Washington, D.C., 1972.

26. Ibid.

27. Derived from National Science Foundation, *Federal Funds for Research, Development and Other Scientific Activities, Fiscal Years 1970, 1971, 1972,* Surveys of Science Resources Series, Vol. XX, NSF 71-35, 1972.

28. Ibid.

29. Id. at 94.

30. *Departments of Labor and Health, Education, and Welfare and Related Agencies Appropriations,* Hearings before the Committee on Appropriations, U.S. Senate, 92nd Cong., 2d Sess., Part 3, p. 2507, 1972.

31. *Research in the Service of Man,* Hearings before the Subcommittee on Government Research of the Committee on Government Operations, U.S. Senate, 90th Cong., 1st Sess., p. 159, 1967.

32. Statement of Dr. Daniel Hornig, Presidential Science Advisor in *Centralization of Federal Science Activities,* Report to the Subcommittee on Science, Research and Development of the Committee on Science and Astronautics, H.R., 91st Cong., 1st Sess., p. 80, 1969.

33. The outstanding special reports are: *Medical Research Activities of the Department of Health, Education, and Welfare,* Report of the Special Committee on Medical Research appointed by the National Science Foundation at the Request of the Secretary of Health, Education, and Welfare, Washington, D.C., 1955 (Long Report); *The Advancement of Medical Research and Education,* Final Report of the Secretary's Consultants on Medical Research and Education, Department of Health, Education, and Welfare, Washington, D.C., 1958 (Bayne-Jones Report); *Federal Support of Medical Research,* Report of the Consultants on Medical Research to the Subcommittee on the Departments of Labor and Health, Education, and Welfare, Senate Committee on Appropriations, Washington, D.C., 1960 (Jones Report); *Federal Support of Basic Research in Institutions of Higher Learning,* Report of the Committee on Science and Public Policy, National Academy of Science, Washington, D.C., 1964 (Kistiakowsky Report); *Biomedical Science and its Administration—A Study of the National Institutes of Health,* Report to the President of the NIH Study Committee, Washington, D.C., 1965 (Woolridge Report); *Report of the Secretary's Advisory Group on the Management of NIH Research Contracts and Grants,* Department of Health, Education, and Welfare, Washington, D.C., 1966 (Ruina Report); *Scientific and Educational Basis for Improving Health,* Report of the Panel on Biological and Medical Science of the President's Advisory Committee, Washington, D.C., 1972.

34. These date back many years, starting with the Kilgore Subcommittee of the Senate Committee on Military Affairs in 1945. More recently, for example, see *Coordination of Federal Agencies' Programs in Biomedical Research and in Other Scientific Areas,* Report of the Committee on Government by its Subcommittee on Government Operations and International Organization, U.S. Senate, 87th Cong., 1st Sess., 1961; *Science, Technology, and Public Policy during the 90th Congress,* Report of the Subcommittee on Science of the House Committee on Science and Astronautics, July 1969; *Centralization of Federal Science Activities,* supra note 32; *National Commission on Health Science and Society,* Hearings of the Subcommittee on Government Research of the Committee on Government Operations, U.S. Senate, 90th Cong., 2d Sess., 1968; *Research in the Service of Man,* Subcommittee on Government Research of the Committee on Government Operations, U.S. Senate, 90th Cong., 1st Sess., 1967.

35. See *Future Directions for Health Services, County of Los Angeles/1970,* Review of the Program of the Los Angeles County Health Department, undertaken at the request of the Los Angeles County Board of Supervisors, p. 58, American Public Health Association, Community Health Action Planning Services (Malcolm H. Merrill, M.D., Director of study), Los Angeles, 1970.

36. Roemer, Ruth, Jeanne E. Frink, and C. Kramer, "Environmental Health Services, Multiplicity of Jurisdictions and Comprehensive Environmental Management," *Milbank Mem. Fund Q.,* Vol. XLIX, No. 4, Part I, p. 424, Oct. 1971.

37. State of California, Department of Public Health, *A Report to the 1970 Legislature on Reimbursement of Public School Health Services in California,* Jan. 1970. School-age children received health care from school districts in 1968-69 in the amount of $38.4 million and another $3 million from local health departments, but the amount and types of services were highly variable among the districts, with variable contributions from local health departments.

38. *Voluntary Health and Welfare Agencies in the United States, An Exploratory Study by*

an *Ad Hoc Citizens Committee* (Robert H. Hamlin, M.D., Study Director), p. i, The School-masters' Press, New York, N.Y., 1961.

39. Hanlon, John J., *Principles of Public Health Administration*, p. 669, C.V. Mosby Company, St. Louis, Mo., 1964.

40. Personal communication from Peter G. Meek, Executive Director, National Health Council, New York, N.Y., June 1972.

41. Guide Issue—Part 2, *Hospitals*, Vol. 45, No. 15, Table 3, p. 478, Aug. 1, 1971.

42. Cal. Health and Safety Code, secs. 417-417.6 (Supp. 1971).

43. State of California, Department of Public Health, *Chronic Renal Disease and its Treatment, California Statistical Data, 1970,* Table 9, Information from Chronic Hemodialysis Facilities, California, Dec. 1970.

44. Hanson, Gerald Peter, *Organization of Radiation Therapy Services Related to Outcome,* Abstract of Doctoral Dissertation, School of Public Health, University of California, Los Angeles, 1971.

45. State of California, Department of Public Health, *Hospitals, Nursing Homes and Related Health Facilities Licensed by the Bureau of Health Facilities Licensing and Certification,* Annual Listing as of March 13, 1970.

46. State of California, Human Relations Agency, Standards and Rates Unit, *Survey of Out-of-Home Care Beneficiary Needs,* 1969.

47. In 1968-1969, there were 112 licensed child care institutions in California with capacity to care for 3,746 children, but an estimated 9,876 children required placement in the single program of Aid to Families with Dependent Children—nearly three times more children than spaces available. This number does not include children requiring placement by other agencies in other programs. See McClellan, Ruth, "Where Are the Resources to Meet the Need?" paper presented to the California Association for Mental Health, Sept. 1970.

48. See Roemer, Milton I., "Controlling and Promoting Quality in Medical Care," *Law and Contemporary Problems, Health Care,* Part I, p. 284, Spring 1970.

49. Faulconer, Albert, M.D., "Can Specialty Boards Respond to Change?" *J.A.M.A.,* Vol. 218, No. 9, p. 141, Nov. 29, 1971.

50. *Report on Licensure and Related Health Personnel Credentialing,* p. 131, U.S. Department of Health, Education, and Welfare, Office of Assistant Secretary for Health and Scientific Affairs, DHEW Pub. No. (HSM) 72-11, June 1971.

51. Forgotson, E. H., R. Roemer, and R. W. Newman, "Legal Regulation of Health Personnel in the United States," *Report of the National Advisory Commission on Health Manpower,* Vol. II, Appendix 18, U.S. Government Printing Office, Washington, D.C., 1967.

52. *Report on Licensure and Related Health Personnel Credentialing,* supra note 50 at 12.

53. *Accreditation of Health Educational Programs, Part One: Working Papers,* Table 1, Study of Accreditation of Selected Health Educational Programs, Washington, D.C., Oct. 1971.

54. See Table 5, "Provisions of State Licensing Statutes governing the Approval of Educational Programs for Selected Categories of Health Personnel, 1970," *Accreditation of Health Educational Programs, Part II, Staff Working Papers,* Study of Accreditation of Selected Health Educational Programs, Washington, D.C., 1972.

CHAPTER 3

Pluralistic Financing

The worst way to finance health care is by categorical grants. Categorical grants tend to attract programs to where the money is rather than where the need is . . . rather than developing services on a broad basis so that people get the services they need, categorical grants tend to stimulate programs that match the money that is available.[1]

—James G. Haughton, M.D.
First Deputy Administrator
Health Services Administration, City of New York, 1968

Five money streams pay for health care: three major streams proceed from consumers directly, from their insurance, and from public programs and two minor streams from philanthropy and from industrial health services. The source of all these streams is the citizen-taxpayer-consumer, through direct payments to providers, insurance premiums, payroll deductions, regressive property and sales taxes, more progressive income taxes, and donations. In the space of 40 years, the main streams of funding have undergone radical changes without producing comparable changes in the way in which services are delivered.

The most significant change has been the deepening commitment of public — chiefly federal — programs to assume more of the financial burden of health care. Public funding, once limited to public health protection and caring for special groups, now underwrites a substantial share of medical services for more than a fourth of the population. It also supports the major portion of biomedical research and training of health workers, and it shares in the construction of health facilities. From little more than 13 percent of health spending in 1929, the public portion has tripled to 39.4 percent in 1972.[2]

Also significant is the declining role of direct spending by consumers — a result of the growth of collective financing through private insurance and public programs. The consumer paid nine-tenths of his medical care bill in

1929; today he pays little more than a third directly out of pocket. Philanthropy and industrial health services now account for only 1.4 percent of the bill, a decrease from 2.6 percent in 1929.[3]

THE RISE IN TOTAL SPENDING

National health spending has risen from $3.6 billion in 1929 to $83.4 billion in 1972, per capita spending from $29 to $394. Spending on health has doubled its share of the national product, from 3.6 percent to 7.6 percent, in these years.[4] (See Table 2, Appendix I, National Health Expenditures.) Each of the main streams of funding has contributed to this increase but at unequal rates. Within the private sector, insurance has risen at a rate of seven or eight times that of consumer, out-of-pocket spending. Within the public sector, federal spending increased ten times compared with the rate of state and local spending. The most decisive increase came after enactment of the Medicare and Medicaid programs in 1965 and their implementation in 1967; together, these two programs accounted for half of public spending on health in 1972.[5] The specific forces behind increased spending for personal health care are mainly more people using more of a better product at higher prices.

What stands out is the increased spending, both overall and per capita, on hospital care. Since 1929, while per capita spending for all health services increased 13 times, spending on hospital care increased about 30-fold, whereas spending on physicians' services increased only nine and one-half times and on dental services six times. Forty years ago, per capita spending on physicians' services exceeded spending on hospital care; by 1972 it was less than half. This long-time trend continues in the period of Medicare and Medicaid. Since 1969, per capita spending on hospital care has more than doubled, while spending on all other medical services rose at less than three-fourths that rate.[6] Medicare has resulted in more hospital days for the elderly, but with little appreciable increase in physician visits outside the hospital.[7] Medicaid has similarly increased hospitalization for the poor and their use of physicians and dentists but, even more, their use of outpatient hospital services and of nursing homes.[8]

THE PRICE RISE AND COST ESCALATION

Of greatest concern has been the rise in medical care prices. A prevalent view is that the sudden infusion of Medicare and Medicaid funds created such sharp increases in demand that, in the absence of proportionate increases in supply or changes in the way that services are delivered, prices escalated. This is only partially true. The disproportionate rise in medical care prices long antedates these major public funding programs. In the postwar inflation of 1946 to 1960, when the consumer price index for all items was rising at the rate of 3 percent per year on the average, the medical care price index rose 4.2 percent per year. Between 1960 and 1967, when there was a pronounced decrease in the rate of inflation, the disparity increased: the consumer price index for all items rose at a diminished rate of 1.6 percent per year, but the medical care index, although its rate was also declining, was still 3.2 percent per year. And in the period between 1967 and 1971, when Medicare and Medicaid funding became most potent, while the consumer price index rose at a rate of 4.8 percent per year, the medical care index rose 6.6 percent per year.[9]

The long secular rise in medical care prices is the largest single factor in the rise in total spending on health, exerting more influence than does the increase in population or increased use of a technically improved medical product. Between 1950 and 1972, spending on personal health care rose by $55 billion; 47.2 percent of this rise was attributable to the rise in prices.[10] Between 1965 and 1972, 52 percent of the $38.4 billion increase in medical care spending was due to the rise in prices.[11] This rise is most dramatically manifest in the rise in hospital daily charges, to a lesser extent in physicians' fees, and still less in dental fees.

From 1946 to 1960, hospital charges rose at an average annual rate of 8.3 percent, at almost twice the rate of all medical services; from 1960 to 1967, hospital daily charges rose at a rate of 7.8 percent and from 1967 to 1971 at a rate of 13.5 percent per year, which is almost double the rate of physicians' fees. The index of physicians' fees has also shown a secular rise, although not so great as hospital daily service charges. From 1946 to 1966, physicians' fees rose an average of 3.4 percent and 3.3 percent per year but doubled that rate between 1966 and 1971. Dentists' fees rose 3.2 percent per year from 1946 to 1960, slackening to 2.5 percent between 1960 and 1966, and then accelerating to 5.8 percent between 1966 and 1969 and 6.1 percent per year between 1969 and 1971.[12]

Three features of the funding mechanisms and the direction of both private insurance and public programs tend to acceleratte price increases. First is the concentration of both programs on high-cost hospitalization, whereas those health services that are not so funded, such as drugs, show the least price escalation. Second, both insurance and Medicare and Medicaid pay "reasonable costs" and "usual and customary" fees. These are essentially cost-plus payments, acting as disincentives to cost reduction or increased efficiency and positively to stimulate price increases. A third factor relates to the organization of the delivery system. Neither private insurance nor Medicare or Medicaid has exercised effective controls over organization and utilization. Medicare, the largest federal program, explicitly accepted the given organization of services and disavowed any interference with it;[13] only recently have limited steps been taken to influence the delivery system. The private insurance system is geared to existing organizations. Both are indeed "third parties" in the sense of acting as conduits for money flows, rather than exercising the prerogatives of consumer-buyers to influence the character of services.

PRIVATE SPENDING

Private funds, directly and through insurance, furnish two-thirds of all health spending. Private spending differs, however, from the direction of public spending. Hospital care accounted for 30 percent of all private funds in 1972 and 50 percent of public funds; 37 percent of private funds but only 13 percent of public funds went for professional services. Nursing home care took 3 percent of private spending, 6 percent of public funds. The contrast is sharpest in spending on drugs, claiming 15 percent of the private dollar but only 2 percent of the public. Less than one-half of one percent of private funds went for research, against 6 percent of public funds. Private funds bore, however, a larger share of health construction.[14]

The Consumer

National income has reached spectacular heights. In dollars of constant purchasing power, disposable personal income (after taxes) has doubled since 1950; on a per capita basis it has risen by three-fifths.[15] As personal income rises, a larger share goes for services. Medical care, viewed as a necessity, consumes a larger portion. Since 1950, private spending on medical care has risen by 50 percent, exceeding the proportionate increase in all other forms of consumer personal spending.[16] Unequal distribution of personal income is reflected in unequal receipt of medical care; the poor, the aged, and particularly the blacks in both groups, who are poorer, have fewer visits to doctor and dentist despite more days of restricted activity, fewer physical and prenatal examinations, and a larger pool of unattended ills.[17] The supply of services to these groups is also lower and less accessible than is that of more advantaged segments of the population. Out-of-pocket spending by consumers is currently directed to filling the gaps in private insurance and public programs, as described below.

Private Insurance

In 1972, $18 billion in private insurance benefit payments provided one-fourth of total health care expenditures and about 43 percent of the consumer's health bill. Insurance paid for 37 percent of the total bill for hospital care and physicians' services but for only 5 percent of the cost of all other services.[18] Although private insurance coverage has risen steadily, this coverage is still uneven. In 1971, it provided protection for about three-fourths of the civilian population for hospital and surgical care, part of the cost of physicians' in-hospital visits for 72 percent of the population, and X-ray and laboratory services for 71 percent of the population. Smaller numbers are covered for out-of-hospital services: 47 percent for physicians' office and home visits, 52 percent for nursing home care.[19] Coverage for mental illness is growing, but it still provides fewer benefits than coverage for physical illness and with more restrictions.[20]

The extent of coverage varies. By 1971, private insurance was paying close to four-fifths of the consumers' cost of hospitalization. But in the same year insurance met less than half the cost of physicians' services. And for all other services, including drugs, dental services, nursing home care, visiting nurses, and home care—despite the growth of coverage in recent years—private insurance met only 6 percent of the consumer's costs.[21]

The structure of private insurance, the multiplicity of its plans, and the direction of its spending have been fragmenting forces in health care. Sponsorship may be through providers, such as the 75 Blue Cross plans and the 72 Blue Shield plans (hospital and physician organized); through the 700 commercial insurance companies writing group health policies and the 1,000 companies writing individual policies; or through the many consumer, employer, and joint employer–employee plans or trust funds. Each sponsor may be specialized as to the form of medical practice it generally funds—whether solo practice, reimbursed by the Blues and commercial insurance companies, or group practice, favored by consumer and employer–employee funds, such as Kaiser, Group Health Association, or Health Insurance Plan of New York; and some group practices are provider-sponsored, such as Ross-Loos in California.

This cross-classification of insurance plans by type of sponsorship and mode of service may be further defined by the manner of consumer benefit and form of payment to the physician. Two principal forms of benefits are indemnity, which provides a fixed allowance for each service, permitting the physician to charge the difference between his normal fee and the allowance paid by insurance, and service benefits, which pay only agreed-upon amounts as full payment. Some 43 Blue Cross and Blue Shield plans offer a mixture, paying full coverage fees for those with incomes below a certain level and indemnity payments for those above these levels. Physicians may be paid either on the more usual fee-for-service basis, by capitation, or on salary. The indemnity and service payment division is closely related to the division between solo and group practice.[22]

Private insurance has performed a significant service in taking on a share of the burden of medical care costs, particularly for catastrophic illness in the working population. It pays for about one-fourth of personal health care costs, amounting to two-fifths of total private spending. Although, as noted, it has taken up much of the economic burden of hospital care, almost half of physicians' care, and much smaller proportions of all other services, private insurance is far from comprehensive and is characterized by well-known deficiencies: it is incomplete in coverage and benefits; it has failed to contain costs and may even have pushed them higher; and it has contributed little to improving the organization of services.

With respect to coverage and benefits, private insurance avoids the high-risk groups: the aged, the poor, and those with chronic conditions. In 1971, while 80 percent of the civilian population under 65 were covered for hospital care, only 51 percent of those over 65 were so covered. The poor and the low-income worker are also not covered—only 36 percent of those under 65 with incomes under $3,000 per year had some insurance coverage for hospitalization, as compared with 93 percent of those with incomes above $15,000.[23] A fifth of the population has no coverage at all. Benefits are incomplete. Co-insurance and deductibles are common features of most insurance plans, thrusting the burden back on the consumer. The temporarily unemployed loses his insurance. Private insurance fails to cover preventive care, periodic examinations, or rehabilitation; instead, it concentrates on payment for hospital care. In 1971, almost two-thirds of all insurance benefits went for hospital care, somewhat less than a third for physicians' services, and only 5 percent for all other services.[24] The lack of coverage for preventive care is singular, since insurance companies have traditionally been concerned with the avoidance of unnecessary risks to health, and many of the large companies have excellent accident and illness prevention campaigns.

Private insurance has shown little capacity to control costs of providers. Usual, customary, and provider-fixed fees, with their built-in incentives for cost escalation, are generally accepted. Some notable experiments have sought to curb costs, usually through improved management and accounting practices, but little control is exercised over quality of care.[25]

Perhaps most serious has been the failure of private insurance to affect the organization of services. Prepayment is designed to relieve consumers of paying lump sums during illness and to make services available when needed. But limited coverage, lack of preventive care, deductibles, coinsurance, and indemnity payments tend to nullify both objectives of prepayment. The insurance industry has only begun to address itself to the problem of improved organization of services.

By contrast to the bulk of commercial private insurance, prepaid group practice plans combine prepayment for illness with improved organization of services. Group practice plans, about evenly divided between community based and employer–employee–union based, covered some 5 million persons in 1971, double the number covered in 1953.[26] These plans tend to furnish comprehensive care, to show less hospitalization and surgery than indemnity plans and the Blues, and to demonstrate economies of scale.[27] Their contributions to lower costs and more comprehensive care are the cornerstones of the health maintenance organization (HMO) concept.

PUBLIC SPENDING

In 1972, some 20 or more federal agencies spent $21.6 billion on medical and health-related activities, in contrast with a total of less than $100 million spent in 1928-1929.[28] The growth of federal health spending has increased the public share and altered federal-state-local contributions. This growth reflects the commitment to a broadened federal role in assuring health care of the general population and in repairing deficiencies in the supply of health services in the private sector.

Federal Spending

Federal spending may be divided into several sectors: (1) spending on production of resources—construction of facilities, education and training, and research; (2) spending on medical services provided directly by the federal government to selected beneficiaries; (3) financing of indirect services; (4) financing of preventive services and traditional public health functions; and (5) relatively new spending to improve the pattern of organization of services. The largest amounts are federal financing of vendor payments, followed by funding of direct services, research, training, preventive measures, construction, and organization.[29] (See Table 3, Appendix I, Federal Health Expenditures by Function.)

1. Production of Resources. Federal spending for medical facilities in 1971-1972 came to $600 million, of which $200 million went for facilities of the Defense Department and the Veterans Administration and $400 million for public and private facilities. In 1972, of the $4.1 billion spent on construction of health facilities, a fourth went for publicly owned facilities and three-fourths for privately owned facilities to which public funds, through seven federal agencies, contributed about ten percent of construction costs.[30] Private construction is also aided through the estimated $600 million depreciation allowed in Medicare and Medicaid reimbursement formulas.[31] The recent shift in Hill-Burton funding from direct construction aid to loans and loan guarantees, although tending to lower interest costs for hospital construction supported in this way, will require increased cash flow from patient fees (see Chapter 7).

Federal spending to assist in the training of medical, nursing, dental, and allied health manpower, an item not usually included in statistics on health spending, has risen from $800 million in 1969 to $1.3 billion in 1972 through four principal agencies: the Departments of Health, Education, and Welfare, Defense, and Labor and the Veterans Administrations.[32] Federal spending on health and medical research by 19 federal agencies came to $1.8 billion in 1972, comprising nine-tenths of the total spent for research by all public and private agencies, including private foundations, hospitals, and medical schools but excluding research by industry.[33]

2. Direct Services. Several major federal programs provide direct medical care. The distinguishing character of these programs is the relative comprehensiveness of care they provide for their special beneficiaries. Public Health Service hospitals and clinics, two narcotics establishments, a leprosarium, and hospitals on Indian reservations had a total budget of some $440 million in 1971, up from only $8.5 million in 1929. They provided ambulatory and hospital care to 132,000 Coast Guard personnel and dependents, 200,000 seamen, 400,000 American Indians, and thousands of other beneficiaries.[34] Despite the many virtues of this relatively integrated system, both the executive and legislative branches of government are moving to dismantle it by removing care to institutions in the private sector.[35]

Approximately 200 Defense Department hospitals and clinics provide care for some 2.9 million members of the armed forces, retirees, and dependents and spent $1.8 billion in 1972, in contrast to $29 million in 1929.[36] About $2.25 billion was spent by 166 Veterans Hospitals, 100 long-term care units, and 200 outpatient clinics for a wide range of veterans' services. In 1929, the Veterans Administration spent less than $50 million. Some care is also purchased from private physicians and nursing homes, but seven of every ten dollars goes for the hospitalization of veterans. Expanded services will be provided in the future with new authorization for care for non-service-connected disabilities — an important contribution to general medical care for a particular segment of the population. Spending by both Defense and Veterans hospitals contributes significantly, also, to the training of medical and allied health personnel.

3. Federal Financing Programs. Some ten federal agencies furnished more than $15 billion in 1971 to purchase medical and hospital services, in addition to the nearly $300 million contributed to health benefits for federal employees. The four major federal funding programs are as follows.

The Civilian Health and Medical Program for the Uniformed Services (CHAMPUS) spent some $400 million to provide medical and hospital care for dependents of servicemen, annuitants, and their dependents. Most care is purchased from private physicians and hospitals, but some 20 percent of the beds in Defense hospitals and 40 percent of outpatient visits in military establishments are for military dependents, retirees, and annuitants.[37] Although

CHAMPUS, like private insurance, requires some coinsurance and has deductibles, it provides more comprehensive services than other major funding programs. It provides dental services, care for mental as well as for physical illness, and a special program for the mentally retarded and physically disabled for its eligible population, estimated to be about 6 million persons.[38]

The two largest spending programs, Medicare and Medicaid, are directed to the neediest groups in the population substantially neglected by the private sector, for generally neither the aged nor the poor can finance needed health care. Both programs operate through vendor payments, largely to private providers, paid through fiscal intermediaries in much the same manner as private insurance. Both stress hospitalization — 65 percent of the Medicaid dollar goes for in-hospital care as does 67 percent of the Medicare dollar. Although both programs have been costly and have had little impact on improving the organization of services, they have made available more and better health care to the aged and the poor.

Medicare is a national program, administered by the Bureau of Health Insurance of the Social Security Administration as part of the Social Security system. State agencies are delegated the task of certifying facilities; paymaster functions are performed by insurance carriers. Financially, Medicare is divided into two systems. Part A of Title XVIII of the Social Security Act, Hospital Insurance, is prepaid insurance derived from payroll taxes levied as part of the Social Security tax on employees and employers equally. All persons eligible for Old Age Security payments are automatically eligible for Hospital Insurance, with the usual exemptions of government employees under separate systems. Part B, Supplementary Medical Insurance, requires application by those over 65 and a monthly payment, matched by federal payments from the general treasury. Supplementary Medical Insurance is therefore largely paid by the beneficiary, usually through deductions from his Social Security payment, after his retirement when his income is vastly reduced. In 1972, premium payments by beneficiaries of Supplementary Medical Insurance came to 44.5 percent of expenditures for this part of the program and to 14.2 percent of the entire Medicare program.

The differing principles of these twin programs under Medicare have fragmenting effects on services. Hospital Insurance requires a deductible that has risen from $40 to $60, copayment after 60 days that has risen from $10 to $15 a day, and after 90 days from $20 to $30 a day. Supplementary Medical Insurance requires a deductible of $60 before payments are made under Medicare and 20 percent copayment by the beneficiary, in addition to the monthly premiums that have risen from $3 to $5.80. Other exclusions or limitations affect payments for out-of-hospital drugs, dental services, stays in extended care facilities, and care in mental institutions. In addition, of course, payroll deductions have also been increased and the maximum wage that is taxed has been raised.[39]

Legislation enacted (P.L. 92-603) has made significant changes in Medicare to expand coverage, to permit new forms of delivering services, to monitor quality of care, and to coordinate standards for Medicare with those of other programs. Medicare has been extended to cover the disabled who have been on the Social Security rolls for at least two years and also individuals under 65 who are currently or fully insured under Social Security—and their spouses and dependent children—who require hemodialysis or renal transplantation for chronic kidney disease. Persons eligible for Medicare may choose to have their care provided through a health maintenance organization. The legislation also mandates establishment of Professional Standards Review Organizations (PSROs), discussed below, to be responsible for comprehensive and on-going review of services. Various provisions coordinate standards and services of Medicare with those of Medicaid and federal employees' health plans. P.L. 92-603 thus addresses some of the most glaring fragmenting features of Medicare.

Unlike Medicare, *Medicaid* is an adjunct of the welfare system and shares that system's almost incorrigible fragmentation—fragmentation by political jurisdiction, by eligibility requirements, by income and welfare levels, and by types of services and benefits. Medicaid consists of 53 different programs, administered by 53 states and territorial jurisdictions. The variable means test, determined, qualified, and administered by each participating state, is the gate or barrier to entry. Medicaid varies in numbers covered, in benefits, services, and limits. The federal government matches from 50 percent to 83 percent of state costs geared to state income levels and expenditures. By 1972, combined federal and state–local outlays amounted to $7.6 billion, rising from $2.5 billion in 1967, and serving almost 20 million beneficiaries. The federal share in 1972 was $4.1 billion, with the states and local governments furnishing $3.5 billion.

The Medicaid program of Title XIX of the Social Security Act separates two groups of eligibles: those who receive cash assistance under state welfare programs and those deemed medically needy, with incomes less than a third above the state welfare level. Both groups must be categorically bound, that is blind, disabled, aged, or having dependent children. These welfare-bound categories thus exclude two classes of the poor: those not categorically bound, such as persons between 21 and 64 who live in families with dependent children and AFDC—Aid to Families with Dependent Children—families, and the poor or low-wage workers with incomes immediately above the 133 and ⅓ percent welfare level. As of 1970, 25 states had not included the medically needy in their Medicaid programs.[40] Thus of the 17 million beneficiaries in that year, 12.2 million were in Group I—the cash assistance group —and only 4.2 million in the medically needy Group II class. By 1972, 77 percent of payments under Medicaid went to the cash assistance groups.

Some indications of the variability and fragmentation of the program may be noted. Eight states, with only one-third of the nation's poor, accounted for 75 percent of the total spent in 1971. Thus, in the understatement of a budgetary document, "a substantial unmet need for medical assistance for the poor continues to exist in many areas."[41] For example, 29 states provide no payments for patients in tubercular hospitals; 33 states provide no payments for clinic services; 6 states make no provision for laboratory services, even though these are among the five federally mandated services, as are prescribed drugs, which are not included by five states.[42] The greatest fragmentation has been in mental care, with states authorized to provide benefits to patients in mental institutions only for those over 65. This age fragmentation in the Medicaid program has now been corrected by the enactment of P.L. 92-603, but new forms of fragmentation have been introduced with imposition of premiums, coinsurance, deductibles, and cost-sharing.

An adjunct of an outmoded welfare system, Medicaid is caught up in multiple means test requirements, resulting in high administrative costs and repeated eligibility determinations. Persons move back and forth across the eligibility line. The recent increases in Social Security payments to the aged, the blind, and the disabled have rendered many persons ineligible under varying state determinations for either medically needy or cash assistance programs and hence for Medicaid benefits, despite the federal injunction that beneficiaries should not lose their eligibility for Medicaid.[43] For several hundred thousand aged, who have the highest medical costs, the loss of Medicaid is far greater than the gain in Social Security cash payments.

Nevertheless, Medicaid has brought substantial benefits to those it has served and, on the whole, has provided a wider range of services than has Medicare, including nursing home services, dental services, and prescribed drugs. Indeed, Medicaid has plugged the gaps for those services to the aged poor under Medicare. In 1972, Medicare paid $216 million for nursing home care, while Medicaid paid over $1.8 billion, its second highest vendor payment, largely for the aged. In 1970, Medicaid paid almost $200 million for prescribed drugs for the aged, $18 million for dental services, and $27 million for other care which was not furnished under Medicare. Although the aged constituted less than one-fifth of Medicaid recipients, payments on their behalf came to about 40 percent of all Medicaid payments.[44]

Federal Employees' Health Benefits are provided to some eight million federal employees and their dependents and annuitants in five types of health insurance plans, including some group practice plans. The contribution of the federal government increased from $121 million to $249 million between 1961 and 1971, but its share declined from 37 percent to 23 percent, so that employee contributions have risen from $200 million to $817 million.[45] New legislation has increased the federal share to 40 percent since 1971. Benefits vary with the type of plan chosen and are limited by coinsurance and deductibles as in private insurance.

4. Preventive and Public Health Services. Numerous categorical programs are designed to prevent and control disease. While some $800 million was spent on these programs in 1971, total health spending on disease prevention and control, environmental health, and consumer safety by all agencies came to no more than 3.3 percent of all federal health spending.[46] Maternal and child health programs accounted for $235 million of federal spending in 1972, other public health activities for $823 million.[47] These include a wide variety of programs concerned with communicable and chronic diseases and with special services, such as health education, social work, and public health nursing. Despite the movement towards separate environmental protection agencies, spending of the Environmental Protection Agency on health has been only one-fifth of its limited budget.

5. *Innovative Patterns of Organizing Health Services.* Spending for neighborhood health centers, for Community Mental Health Centers serving defined catchment areas, for comprehensive maternal and child health demonstrations, and for several other innovative forms of providing ambulatory care is a minor portion of total federal spending. In 1971, a total of 527 health centers of various kinds spent $338 million of federal funds, estimated to rise to 639 centers with federal spending of $439 million in 1972.[48] Despite increasing assistance to Comprehensive Health Planning agencies, Regional Medical Programs, and emergency medical care, these and other programs designed to improve the delivery of health services represent no more than one and a half percent of total federal spending for health.[49]

Recent federal legislation mentioned above (P.L. 92-603) gives some inkling of the power of the federal purse to effect improvements in the system of delivering health care. The legislation provides for the designation of Professional Standards Review Organizations (PSROs), consisting of large numbers of practicing physicians, usually 300 or more, in a local area to review standards of care in institutionalized cases under Medicare and Medicaid. Additionally, the legislation indirectly encourages support for health maintenance organizations through authorizing prepayment for care under Medicare and Medicaid. Both these measures represent a departure from the provisions of earlier legislation, which barred change in the manner of providing care.

State and Local Spending

Traditionally, state and local financing of health services has been addressed to two purposes. The first is provision, for all persons in the community, of public health services including environmental protection, inspection of food and drugs, control of communicable diseases, and licensing of health personnel and facilities. These functions of health departments have both widened to include new categorical programs of personal health services, such as family planning, alcoholism, and drug abuse programs, and narrowed, as environmental agencies have taken over functions in air and water pollution control formerly handled by public health agencies. The second purpose is provision of care too costly for most individuals or avoided by the private sector. The state cares for the mentally ill and retarded, the tubercular, and many requiring long-term care unavailable in the private sector. The counties and municipalities operate public hospitals and outpatient clinics, largely for the poor. The overcrowded and often underfinanced municipal hospital still remains the last—sometimes the first and only—resort of the poor.

In 1971-1972, state and local government spent $11.3 billion from their own sources, about 13 percent of the national total, up from $378 million in 1929 and more than three times their 1960 spending. Federal grants and projects, together with medical contributions, supplemented this sum with another $5 billion—a figure which should be compared with virtually no federal aid in 1929 and about $400 million in 1960.[50] State and local spending on health, although rising steadily, is lower than spending for education, highways, and welfare. Federal aid to state mental hospitals—traditionally a state responsibility—and to local public hospitals has always been minimal. Following these major costs are state and local contributions to Medicaid, which in this period came to $3.6 billion nationally, augmented by $4.1 billion in federal funds. The basic public health protection of the total population constituted less than ten percent of state–local spending, subsidized by varying amounts of federal aid. Maternal and child health services and vocational rehabilitation, aided materially by federal grants, and the self-supporting programs of workmen's compensation and unemployment compensation disability insurance[51] are other major activities. Apart from state mental institutions, the bulk of state–local spending for services takes place in the local communities. The variability of federal aid is noted in the following account of health spending in California.

In California in 1970-1971, the latest year for which comparable data are available, more than $2.5 billion flowed through state and local government health agencies, of a total spent by all private and public agencies of more than $7.5 billion.[52] This "spending" by government agencies represents a gross flow that combines federal, state, local, and private user funds in a complex of intergovernmental and interagency transfers and transactions. While excluding federal direct spending on services or grants for research and training to private institutions, it does include that portion of federal financing, such as Medicare and Medicaid, that goes to state and local agencies as vendor payments but often appears as general revenues. More than half this sum was spent by 12 state agencies; a considerable portion of this goes to the counties. About a third was spent by the 58 counties (the dominant form of local government in California); some 100 special hospital and ambulance districts spent about 7 percent; and the few cities with health agencies spent about 2 percent.[53]

The sources of these funds were different. Only a third of the total came from state funds, about one-fourth from county funds, lesser portions from cities, about one-seventh from user charges; federal aid came to about one-fourth. The special hospital districts, like voluntary hospitals, were supported mainly by patient fees from both private and public sources, apart from federal aid for construction and small amounts from district taxes.

*State Spending on Health in California.** The largest single state-local spending was the more than a billion dollars spent through the Department of Health Care Services for vendor payments under Medi-Cal, the California version of Medicaid, to which the federal government contributes about half. Combined with this program is one known as "county option," paid for largely by the counties with state support, which finances care for indigent persons who do not qualify for Medicaid. In 1970-1971, the federal share of Medi-Cal came to $553 million, the state payments were $489 million, and payments by the counties were $215 million.

Four groups received care paid for by these Medi-Cal funds — more than 2 million public assistance or cash grant recipients, about 75,000 who qualify for cash grants but do not receive them, almost 150,000 medically needy, and some 200,000 county option indigent persons who do not qualify for Medi-Cal. The first three groups are linked to the four welfare categories. As in the national program, the largest sum goes for hospitalization, and the highest per capita costs are incurred for the medically needy and the aged, although both groups constitute a smaller proportion of the total.[54]

Administration of Medi-Cal is handled principally by the State Department of Health Care Services; its regional offices throughout the state have recently (formerly a county function) been assigned responsibility for processing requests for prior authorization of those procedures for which this is required. Additionally, three other state departments — Public Health, Mental Hygiene, and Social Welfare — each have some role in the program. Eligibility determination is conducted by 58 county welfare departments, and three main fiscal agents are involved in reimbursement of providers.

In the effort to cut the costs of this expensive program, three principal methods have been adopted. One consists of restricting eligibility; a second involves reducing benefits, for example limiting outpatient visits and elective surgery. A third method consists of enrolling Medi-Cal beneficiaries in prepaid group health plans at a lower than average per capita cost. Unfortunately, there is some evidence that the latter has been undertaken with

*The major state departments concerned with health were combined into a single State Department of Health, effective July 1, 1973. This description applies as of 1971-1973, prior to reorganization.

inadequate safeguards to guard against the quality hazard of under-servicing.[55]

If the Medi-Cal program is excluded, the largest expenditure by a state department was made by the State Department of Mental Hygiene. In 1971, this department spent a gross of $322 million, or a net of $293 million after deducting reimbursements from other departments and special federal projects.[56] The entire amount came from the state general fund initially, with little federal aid, except for construction funds and special research projects. The counties contributed to the cost of county patients in mental hospitals; about $1.5 million came from Medicare payments; and some $47 million from Medi-Cal payments, in addition to patient fees. With the shift of mental patients out of state institutions, a larger proportion of this department's outlay now goes to the counties for community care, paid for 90 percent by the state and 10 percent by the counties, for net costs above patient and other fees. Only a small portion of this state contribution flows from the counties to the federally supported Community Mental Health Centers, although a larger amount is anticipated as federal staffing aid declines.

In 1971, the State Department of Public Health spent $75 million gross, or $64 million net. Of this sum, the state supplied $37 million, while federal funds came to almost $25 million for the many public health programs. Federal subsidies or grants vary with programs—from the entire amount to assist construction of facilities, five-sixths of the alcoholism rehabilitation services, half the funds for assisting administration of local health departments, to less than one-sixth of funds for crippled children's services. Of this combined state fund, $47 million went to county and local health departments, including approximately $9 million of Hill-Burton funds that went to voluntary hospitals and other institutions.[57]

In 1971, the Department of Rehabilitation spent some $20 million on health-related activities, mostly in rehabilitation of alcoholics, narcotics users, the mentally retarded, and the mentally ill. The Department of Rehabilitation receives the largest proportion of federal funds of any state department and is fully reimbursed (approximately $7 million annually) by the Social Security Administration for determining eligibility for the federal disability program.

Seven other departments of the state, spending some $60 million mostly from state funds, are involved in health spending. The Department of Education conducts schools and special classes for the developmentally disabled, including the blind and the deaf, and supports school health services in the school districts. The licensing boards for health professionals, to be transferred to the new consolidated Department of Health, receive support from fees and licenses. The State Department of Veterans Affairs operates a veterans' home for medical and domiciliary care of veterans, in part paid by federal funds. The Department of Industrial Relations conducts a safety and accident prevention program throughout California industry, supported almost entirely from state funds. The Department of Agriculture, in cooperation with federal and county agencies, inspects food, dairy, and meat processing. The Department of Corrections and the Youth Authority provide medical and surgical care in correctional institutions and camps and provide psychiatric care of parolees, almost entirely from state funds.

Two health benefit programs — Workmen's Compensation and Unemployment Compensation Disability Insurance — are established by state legislation as forms of social insurance under state regulation, although state expenditures are minimal. Workmen's Compensation, financed solely by employers, provides medical benefits for work-connected disability and disease, in addition to partial replacement of lost wages. It is supervised by the Department of Industrial Relations; insurance is usually through private carriers, self-insurance, or a state fund, with rates regulated by the State Department of Insurance. In 1969, Workmen's Compensation paid out more than $160 million in medical costs, about evenly divided between hospital charges and fees paid to physicians and other providers. More than four of five workers in the state were covered.[58]

The State Disability Insurance program, one of only seven in the nation, including the nationwide program for railroad employees, is managed by the State Department of Human Resources Development, paid for by a tax of 1.1 percent on employee wages up to $7,400, and includes persons covered by unemployment compensation insurance. In 1969, some $312 million was contributed by more than five and one-half million employees, including farm workers, out of a total state employment of 8 million, covering non-work-connected disability. About $35 million was paid out for medical benefits, mostly for hospital stays paid at a flat daily rate of $12 for up to 20 days in a disability period. Insurance is provided predominantly through a state fund or (for about 5 percent of covered persons) through private plans.[59]

Although the state and local governments contribute toward their employees' health benefits, the contribution is contained within departmental wage budgets and is considered private insurance. The state, through its Public Employees Retirement System, contributes $16 a month per employee towards health benefit plans chosen by its 200,000 employees. Other public agencies may join this system, which permits employees to choose from 21 plans, including four major medical plans. Total premium costs in 1971-1972 came to $53 million. In addition, 22,000 annuitants were covered at a cost of $4.3 million. Similar plans are financed by county governments, cities, school districts, and other special districts for their employees.[60]

Health Spending in Los Angeles County. The effect of these many streams of funding and the multitude of programs at national, state, and local levels on total health spending in a large metropolitan county is revealed by a special analysis of expenditures in Los Angeles County.[61] In 1968-1969, nearly $2.25 billion was spent for health services in this county of seven million people living in an area of 4,000 square miles. Of this total (which includes some construction of facilities for public programs but omits expenditures for research and training), after eliminating duplications and transfers of funds, the public sector provided some 20 percent of the services delivered, while the private sector provided 80 percent. The sources of funds were different—approximately 40 percent of the funds came from public sources, 60 percent from private sources.

Within the public sector, the principal service agencies were three county departments that have since been merged—the Departments of Hospitals, Health, and Mental Health. Several other county departments are also involved in health activities—the Department of Public Social Services, which conducts eligibility determinations for the Medi-Cal program and supervises board and care facilities; the Sheriff's Department, which maintains a medical staff for jail inmates; the Department of Adoptions; the County Superintendent of Schools; the office of the Medical Examiner; the Department of Senior Citizens' Affairs; the County Veterinarian (also included in the new merged County Department of Health Services); the Air Pollution Control District; and the Probation Department.[62] Of all these, the largest is the County Department of Hospitals, with three large medical centers and five specialized hospitals, almost entirely supported by county-raised funds. The Health and Mental Health Departments receive substantial support from federal and state funds.

The next largest provider of public services was the federal government, through its extensive Veterans Hospitals and clinics located in the county, a Public Health Service clinic, and two military establishments. The state government provided direct services in two mental institutions within the county and through mental retardation and rehabilitation centers, as well as through district offices of the State Department of Health Care Services. Federally funded, autonomous Community Mental Health Centers and a neighborhood health center, funded by the U.S. Office of Economic Opportunity, also provided health services in their areas. In addition, a few cities in the county provided emergency ambulance services, three had their own health departments in part supported by the county, and two autonomous hospital districts served small populations in the county.

The largest provider of services in the private sector consisted of approximately 150 voluntary and proprietary hospitals. In addition, there were 400 nursing homes, 12,000 physicians, 3,500 dentists, thousands of other practitioners, and a wide range of allied and auxiliary personnel in the county.

When funds for health services are traced back to their original sources, the largest public source—more than one-fourth of the total—was the federal government through Medicare, its share of Medicaid, CHAMPUS, federal Community Mental Health Services, and funding of state and local activities. State and county governments provided less than half the amounts spent by the federal government. Within the private sector, individuals contributed the largest share, insurance probably a somewhat smaller share, and philanthropy and industrial spending on in-plant medical services contributed the remainder.

This analysis of expenditures for health services in Los Angeles County in 1968-1969 indicates that about 55 percent of all spending by public and private health agencies in the county was for curative services by hospitals, nursing homes, physicians, and other providers; for rehabilitation activities; and for drugs and appliances. An estimated 16 percent was spent on the detection of illness, including diagnosis, testing, laboratory services, investigation of communicable diseases, and similar activities. Almost 24 percent of all spending was for ancillary services, a large proportion of which was for administration, clerical activities, and related services. Hence, only 5 percent of all spending in the county went for preventive services, including environmental and consumer protection, occupational health services, immunization, health education, and family planning.[63]

FINANCING AND FRAGMENTED SERVICES

The multiplicity of sources of financing that has grown up over the years is inextricably interwoven with categorical and fragmented health services. In a sense, this multiplicity should not matter if the delivery of services were integrated. In fact, however, the many sources of money create multiple prescriptions and specialized preconditions that inhibit the development of an integrated system for the provision of comprehensive care.

It can be argued that the multiplicity of sources of financing yields a greater overall allocation of resources for health. The United States, with its pluralistic system, spends about seven percent of its Gross National Product on health, whereas the United Kingdom, with its unitary source of funding, spends only four to five percent. But the high expenditure associated with multiple sources of financing may well be a wasteful use of resources. Much of this high expenditure is probably extravagant precisely because of the lack of coordination and planning in use of financing.

It is generally agreed that the goal is comprehensive health care for the total population. But multiple sources of funds and the large sums spent have not resulted in effective and efficient organization of services, nor in an adjustment of supply and demand, nor in the equitable distribution of services. In short, the basic dichotomy between the financing and the organization of services is central to the crisis in health care. The failure to provide an adequate national financing system with leverage to rationalize organization of services perpetuates fragmented care with its inadequacies and inequities.

NOTES

1. Testimony of James G. Haughton, M.D. in *Health Care in America*, Hearings before the Subcommittee on Executive Reorganization of the Committee on Government Operations, U.S. Senate, 90th Cong., 2d Sess., Part 2, p. 773, July 1968.

2. Cooper, Barbara S. and Nancy L. Worthington, "National Health Expenditures, 1929-1972," *Social Security Bull.*, Vol. 36, No. 1, p. 5, Table 1 and p. 16, Table 5, Jan. 1973.

3. Id. at 16, Table 5.

4. Id. at 5, Table 1.

5. Id. at 5, Table 1, and 9, Table 3. Medicare's $8.8 billion and Medicaid's $7.6 billion, of total public spending of $32.9 billion.

6. Id. at 12, Table 4. From 1965-1966 to 1971-1972, per capita spending on hospital care went from $71.59 to $155.38, whereas per capita spending on all other personal health services rose from $122.72 to $211.83, or 73 percent.

7. See Green, Jerome and Jacl Scharff, "Use of Medical Services Under Medicare," *Social Security Bull.*, Vol. 34, No. 3, p. 3, March 1971; West, Howard, "Five Years of Medicare — A Statistical Review," *Social Security Bull.*, Vol. 34, No. 12, p. 17, Dec. 1971; and Perringill, Julian M., "Trends in Hospital Use by the Aged," *Social Security Bull.*, Vol. 35, No. 7, p..3, July 1972.

8. Calculated from Merriam, Ida C. and Alfred M. Skolnik, *Social Welfare Expenditures under Public Programs in the United States, 1929-1966*, Table 3-13, p. 230, Social Security Administration, Office of Research and Statistics, Research Report No. 25, Department of Health, Education, and Welfare, 1968. See also, Cooper and Worthington, supra note 2 at 9, Table 3; *Special Analyses of the Budget of the United States Government, Fiscal Year 1973*, p. 165, Executive Office of the President, Office of Management and Budget, 1972; *Numbers of Recipients and Amounts of Payment under Medicaid and Other Medical Programs Financed from Public Assistance Funds*, Tables 1-5, Social and Rehabilitation Service, Office of Program Statistics and Data Systems, National Center for Social Statistics, Department of Health, Education, and Welfare, 1972; and *Health Characteristics of Low Income Persons*, Publication (HSM) 73-1500, Series 10, No. 74, Department of Health, Education, and Welfare, 1972.

9. *Medical Care Costs and Prices: Background Book*, p. 3, Social Security Administration, Office of Research and Statistics, Publication DHEW (SSA) 72-11908, Department of Health, Education, and Welfare, Jan. 1972.

10. Rice, Dorothy P. and Barbara S. Cooper, "National Health Expenditures, 1929-71," *Social Security Bull.*, Vol. 35, No. 1, pp. 8-9, Jan. 1972.

11. Cooper and Worthington, supra note 2 at 13.

12. *Medical Care Costs and Prices*, supra note 9 at 10, Table 1.

13. The Social Security Act, Title XVIII, Sec. 1801 provides: "Nothing in this title shall be construed to authorize any Federal officer or employee to exercise any supervision or control over the practice of medicine or the manner in which medical services are provided. . . ." Similar provisions appear in the Hill-Burton Act and the Regional Medical Programs legislation.

14. Cooper and Worthington, supra note 2 at 7-8 and Table 2.

15. *Economic Report of the President*, p. 213, Table B-16, Jan. 1972.

16. *Statistical Abstract of the United States*, p. 315, Table 513, Bureau of the Census, U.S. Department of Commerce, 1972.

17. See Roemer, Milton I. and Arnold I. Kisch, "Health, Poverty, and Medical Mainstream," *Power, Poverty and Urban Policy* (Bloomberg, Warner, Jr. and Henry J. Schmandt, Eds.), p. 181, Vol. 2, Urban Affairs Annual Reviews, Sage Publications, Inc., Beverly Hills, Ca., 1968. Kosa, John, Aaron Antonovsky, and Irving Kenneth Zola, *Poverty and Health:*

A Sociological Analysis, Harvard University Press, Cambridge, Mass., 1969.

18. Roemer and Kisch, supra note 17 at 14.

19. Mueller, Marjorie Smith, "Private Health Insurance in 1971: Health Care Services, Enrollment, and Finances," *Social Security Bull.,* Vol. 35, No. 2, p. 3, Feb. 1973. See also Reed, Louis and Willine Carr, *The Benefit Structure of Private Health Insurance, 1968,* Social Security Administration, Office of Research and Statistics, Research Report No. 32, Department of Health, Education, and Welfare, 1970; the annual *Source Book of Health Insurance,* published by the Health Insurance Institute, New York, showing higher estimates of coverage.

20. *The Cost of Mental Illness, 1968,* Statistical Note 30, Table 3, National Clearing House for Mental Health Information, Survey and Reports Section, National Institute of Mental Health, Oct. 1970, for estimate of insurance payments for mental health care; and Mueller, supra note 19 at 18, Table 17 for total benefit expenditures. See also, Scheidemandel, Patricia L., Charles K. Danno, and Raymond M. Glasscote, *Health Insurance and Mental Illness,* Joint Information Service of the American Psychiatric Association and the National Association for Mental Health, Washington, D.C., 1968.

21. Mueller, supra note 19 at 21.

22. See Roemer, Milton I., Donald Du Bois, and Shirley W. Rich, *Health Insurance Plans: Studies in Organizational Diversity,* School of Public Health, University of California, Los Angeles, 1970, for analysis of types of plans; Reed and Carr, supra note 19.

23. See *Age Patterns in Medical Care, Illness and Disability, U.S. 1968-1969,* p. 17, Publication (HSM) 72-1026, Vital and Health Statistics, Series 10, No. 70, Department of Health, Education, and Welfare, Apr., 1972.

24. Mueller, supra note 19 at 16-17 and Table 15. In 1971, out of the total of private insurance payments of $17.9 billion, $11.4 billion went for hospital care, $5.5 billion for physicians' services, and $1 billion for all other health services.

25. See discussion of controls by McNerney, Walter J., "Improving the Effectiveness of Health Insurance and Prepayment," *Private Insurance and Medical Care,* Conference Papers, Social Security Administration, Office of Research and Statistics, Department of Health, Education, and Welfare, March, 1968.

26. Mueller, supra note 19 at 14, Table 12.

27. Id. at 12, footnote 4. See also *Towards a Comprehensive Health Policy for the 1970's: A White Paper,* pp. 31-35, Department of Health, Education, and Welfare, May, 1971.

28. *Special Analyses of the Budget of the United States Government, Fiscal Year 1973,* supra note 8 at 176, Table K-17 and Cooper and Worthington, supra note 2 at 9, 16.

29. *Special Analyses of the Budget of the United States Government, Fiscal Year 1973,* supra note 8 at 176, Table K-17.

30. Cooper and Worthington, supra note 2 at 7, Table 2; *Special Analyses of the Budget of the United States Government, Fiscal Year 1974,* pp. 158-159, Table J-26, Office of Management and Budget, Executive Office of the President, Washington, D.C., 1973.

31. Muller, Charlotte, "Program Elements of Federal Laws on Financing of Health Facilities," *Am. J. Public Health,* Vol. 60, No. 2, p. 305, Feb. 1970, for an excellent discussion of reimbursement formulas and depreciation. The $600 million estimate is later, made by Dr. Vernon E. Wilson, Administrator, Health Services and Mental Health Administration, in Senate Hearings before the Committee on Appropriations, Departments of Labor and Health, Education, and Related Agencies Appropriations, *Fiscal Year 1973,* 92nd Cong., 2d Sess., Part 2, p. 2043, 1972.

32. Cooper and Worthington, supra note 2 at 15.

33. Id. at 7 and *Special Analyses of the Budget 1974,* supra note 30 at 158-159, Table J-26.

34. *Special Analyses, Budget of the United States, Fiscal Year 1971,* p. 159, Office of Management and Budget, Executive Office of the President, Washington, D.C., 1970.

35. *Special Analyses, Budget of the United States Government, Fiscal Year 1972,* p. 161, Office of Management and Budget, Executive Office of the President, Washington, D.C., 1971;

testimony of Secretary Richardson, *Departments of Labor and Health, Education, and Welfare Appropriations for 1973.* Hearings before a Subcommittee of the Committee on Appropriations. House of Representatives, 92nd Cong., 2d Sess., Part 1, pp. 110, 155, 157, Feb. 1972.

36. Skolnik, Alfred M. and Sophie R. Dales, "Social Welfare Expenditures, 1971-1972," *Social Security Bull.*, Vol. 35, No. 12, p. 14, Table 7, Dec. 1972; *Special Analyses, Budget of the United States, Fiscal Year 1971*, supra note 34 at 159.

37. *CHAMPUS 14th Annual Report, Calendar Year 1970*, Office for the Civilian Health and Medical Program of the Uniformed Services, U.S. Department of the Army, Denver, Colorado, 1971.

38. Id. at 21, Table 14.

39. P.L. 92-603, Title II for various changes in Medicare and summary in *Social Security Bull.*, Vol. 36, No. 1, p. 1, Jan. 1973.

40. See *Medicaid's 52 Programs, Characteristics of State Medical Assistance Programs under Title XIX of the Social Security Act*, Department of Health, Education, and Welfare, Social and Rehabilitation Service, Assistance Payments Administration and Medical Services Administration, Publication (MSA-PA), 49-71, 1970.

41. *Special Analyses of the Budget of the United States Government, Fiscal Year 1971*, supra note 34 at 158.

42. From *Medicaid's 52 Programs*, supra note 40.

43. P.L. 92-603, Sec. 249E provides for continued eligibility for medical assistance of those who received increased Social Security payments. The California State Department of Health Care Services, however, cut off full medical benefits for about 10,000 aged, blind, and disabled persons receiving the Social Security increase, declaring them ineligible for cash assistance, reducing them to the medically needy group, and thus requiring personal co-payments for care. The California Rural Legal Assistance Office of the National Senior Citizens Law Center, aided by the National Health Law Program, brought a class action to invalidate the Department's action. The Regional Office of HEW upheld the view that the transfer from needy to "medically needy" status was invalid. In Dils v. Geduldig, Los Angeles Superior Ct., No. C-44371, Dec. 27, 1972, the 10,000 Medi-Cal recipients, denied health care financing, were restored to full Medi-Cal benefits.

44. For 1972, see Cooper and Worthington, supra note 2 at 9, Table 3. For 1970, see *Numbers of Recipients and Amounts of Payment under Medicaid and Other Medical Programs Financed from Public Assistance Funds*, supra note 8 at 3.

45. *Special Analyses of the Budget of the United States Government, Fiscal Year 1971*, supra note 34 at 158; *U.S. Civil Service Commission Annual Report 1971*, Appendix E, Health Benefits Program, p. 67, Washington, D.C., 1972; and *Federal Employees Health Benefits Program, Highlights of First Decade of Operation, July 1960-June 1970*, Committee Print No. 5, 92nd Cong., 1st Sess., printed for the use of the Committee on Post Office and Civil Service, House of Representatives, March, 1971.

46. *Special Analyses of the Budget of the United States Government, Fiscal Year 1974*, supra note 30 at 158-159, Table J-26.

47. Cooper and Worthington, supra note 2 at 9, Table 13.

48. *Special Analyses of the Budget of the United States Government, Fiscal Year 1973*, supra note 8 at 168.

49. Id. at 176, Table K-17.

50. Derived from Skolnik and Dales, supra note 36 at 14, Table 7; see also Dales, Sophie R., "Federal Grants to State and Local Governments, 1970-1971," *Social Security Bull.*, Vol. 35, No. 6, p. 30, Table 1, June, 1972; and *Special Analyses of the Budget of the United States Government, Fiscal Year 1974*, supra note 30 at 223-224, which estimates federal grants to state and local governments, including research grants to institutions as well as health manpower training at $6 billion in 1972 actual outlays.

51. Ibid.

52. Compiled from *California Governor's Budget* and *Supplements, 1972-1973* and *1973-1974;* State Controller, *Annual Reports of Financial Transactions Concerning Counties in California, Fiscal Year 1970-1971; Concerning Cities, Fiscal Year 1970-1971; Concerning Special Districts, Fiscal Year 1970-1971; Concerning School Districts, Fiscal Year 1970-1971;* Sacramento, Calif., 1972; and *California Statistical Abstract, 1972,* Department of Finance, Sacramento, Calif., 1973. Discrepancies are explained by differences in reporting procedures of the separate sources. Estimates of total spending on health are from national health expenditures. An earlier distribution of state and local spending, for 1966-1967, is found in *Alternative Fiscal Models for Tax and Revenue Sharing in California,* A Report of the Council on Intergovernmental Relations, Sacramento, Calif., Jan. 1969.

53. Ibid.

54. *1972-1973 Governor's Budget, Program Budget Supplement,* supra note 52 at 809-816.

55. Nelson, Harry, "Investigations of Prepaid Health Programs Asked: Possible Fraud in Some Cases Hinted by Los Angeles County Unit," *Los Angeles Times,* Feb. 24, 1973, p. 1; Ross, Leonard, "The Urgent Need to Control the Quality of Prepaid Plans for Medical Care," *Los Angeles Times,* Jan. 25, 1973; California Council on Health Plan Alternatives, "California Medical Group (CMG) Evaluation Report," Burlingame, Calif., Dec. 7, 1972 (processed).

56. *1973-1974 Governor's Budget, Budget Supplement,* supra note 52, Vol. II., pp. 51-53.

57. *1972-1973 Program Budget Supplement,* supra note 54 at 902-938.

58. *California Statistical Abstract. 1972* supra note 52 at 31-32. For detailed studies of state laws and their shortcomings, see *The Report of the National Commission on State Workmen's Compensation Laws,* Washington, D.C., July, 1972.

59. *California Statistical Abstract, 1972,* supra note 52 at 66; State Department of Human Resources Development, *The California Unemployment Compensation Disability Fund, 1969,* Statistical Handbook on Disability Insurance, Actuarial Report, Aug. 6, 1970; Greenfield, Margaret, *Meeting the Costs of Health Care, The Bay Area Experience and the National Issues,* p. 9, Institute of Governmental Studies, University of California, Berkeley, 1972; *Historical Statistics for Five Temporary Disability Insurance Programs, 1942-1969,* U.S. Dept. of Health, Education, and Welfare, Social Security Administration, Office of Research and Statistics, Research and Statistics Note No. 17-1971, DHEW Pub. No. (SSA) 72-11701, Dec. 20, 1971.

60. *1973-1974 Governor's Budget, Budget Supplement, Vol. I,* supra note 52 at 231 and 511; Greenfield, supra note 59 at 66ff.

61. See Kramer, C., "Fragmented Financing of Health Care," *Medical Care Review,* Vol. 28, No. 8, p. 922, Table 8, Aug. 1972. For details and sources, see chapters on health spending in Los Angeles County in Sonenblum, Sidney and Charles Kramer with Meredith Slobod Crist and Robert Augur, *Local Government Program Budgeting for Urban Health Care Services,* Institute of Government and Public Affairs, University of California, Los Angeles, 1973.

62. See *Future Directions for Health Services, County of Los Angeles/1970,* Review of the Program of the Los Angeles County Health Department, undertaken at the request of the Board of Supervisors, American Public Health Association (Malcolm H. Merrill, M.D., Director of study), Ch. III, Los Angeles, 1970.

63. *Local Government Program Budgeting for Urban Health Care Services,* supra note 61.

CHAPTER 4

Maternal and Child Health Services: Programs for Provision of Services to Specific Persons

> *What is amazing is that any low-income family can produce the necessary combinations of age, economic status, geographic residency and appropriate state of health or disease, at the proper place and time to obtain care for its children.*[1]

Leslie Corsa, Jr., M.D.
Bruce Jessup, M.D.
California State Department
of Public Health, 1962

From the earliest days in the United States, promotion of the health of mothers and children has had a high priority in public health activities. Maternal health is a goal in itself. Recognition of the importance of the mother's health for perinatal and infant mortality, prematurity, birth defects, mental retardation, and a host of more subtle disabilities in the child has intensified attention to maternal health services.[2] Similarly, the desire for healthy children and the recognition that the early years of childhood are critical for the mental and physical development of the adult have led to numerous child health and health-related programs for children and youth. These programs are both voluntary and governmental.

HISTORICAL BACKGROUND

In the United States, as in other nations, concern with the health of mothers and children spurred development of general public health services, including sanitation measures, pasteurization of milk, control of communicable diseases, nutrition programs, and visiting and public health nursing services.[3] New York established a State Board of Health in 1797 to investigate communicable diseases and inspect sanitary conditions. The following year New York City established a Board of Health, prompted in large measure by the unsanitary living conditions of the poor that particularly affected the health of women and children. The formation of the State Board of Health in Massachusetts in 1868 is attributed to revelation by Lemuel Shattuck in 1845 of "shocking infant and maternal mortality" and widely prevalent communicable diseases and to emphasis in the famous Shattuck Report of 1850 on the necessity for an effective public health organization to deal with community health problems. The first unit in a local health department specifically devoted to child health, the Division of Child Hygiene, was established in the New York City Department of Health in 1908.

Voluntary Programs

Some of the earliest maternal and child health services were the result of voluntary, rather than of governmental efforts.[4] Not the consumer or the poor but socially conscious individuals, groups, and physicians were aroused to action by the squalor of the industrialized city and by the poverty, privation, and poor health rampant there. The institutions and agencies they set up, some with small beginnings, grew to encompass a wide variety of organizations: hospitals, visiting nurse associations, diet kitchens, milk stations, settlement houses, well-baby clinics, maternal health clinics, and agencies concerned with specific diseases or social problems. A dominating influence in many of the voluntary organizations was concern with the health of mothers and children in the poverty areas of large cities. These voluntary agencies pioneered the way for the development of maternal and child health programs by official agencies.

Governmental Programs

Contemporary with immunizations and sanitation measures to stem epidemics and attack unsanitary living conditions was the movement for social reform and welfare legislation. A response to the evils of rapid industrialization and the vast migrations of people into the slums of big cities, this movement resulted in legislation to improve working conditions for women and to ban child labor. State industrial safety acts and factory inspection acts were designed to protect the millions of women working in tenement sweatshops and children working in factories and underground mines. The first child labor legislation, prohibiting employment of children under ten years of age, was passed in Pennsylvania in 1848 and in New York in 1849. Between 1905 and 1907, several states enacted protective labor legislation for women and children. In 1907, a 19-volume Congressional study of working conditions for women and children in industry aroused horror in the nation. In 1908, the United States Supreme Court upheld the constitutionality of an Oregon law prohibiting the employment of women in industry for more than ten hours a day. In 1909, the first White House Conference on the Care of Dependent Children was held. Proposals at this conference urged establishment of a federal agency "to investigate and report upon all matters related to the welfare of children and child life among all classes of people."[5]

Against this background, the U.S. Children's Bureau was established as an independent agency in 1912. From its inception, the Children's Bureau was a crusader for mothers and children. During its more than half-century of existence—until its functions were distributed among other agencies in 1969 —the Children's Bureau gave leadership to the many governmental and voluntary efforts concerned with child health and welfare. It provided a focus for child health and welfare programs at the federal level of government. In the judgment of an eminent medical and public health historian,

By holding unswervingly to a broad conception of child welfare as concerned with all the social aspects of child life, by insisting on the use of qualified personnel in all programs, and by encouraging communities in the local and state level to develop maternal and child welfare programs, the Children's Bureau has played a leading role in developing these aspects of community life in the United States.[6]

Perhaps the signal accomplishments of the Children's Bureau are related, at least in part, to its broad mission, addressed to the totality of health and living conditions of mothers and children.

From the earliest days, the federal government embarked on the path of dividing authority for services related to children. The Department of Labor was established in 1913, and its Division of Industrial Hygiene and Sanitation, concerned with working conditions in factories, was formed in 1914. When the Child Labor Law was passed in 1917, however, the Children's Bureau was assigned responsibility for its enforcement. The intent of this assignment was to enforce the ban on child labor, but as a result responsibility for working conditions in factories was divided between the Department of Labor and the Children's Bureau. Moreover, responsibility was further fragmented by the roles of state and local agencies in industrial health services.

In a separate sphere, within the educational system, responsibility for the school lunch program was developing at state and local levels. In 1935, federal impetus was provided through assistance from the Surplus Commodities Corporation of the U.S. Department of Agriculture, and in 1946 this assistance was formalized by enactment of the National School Lunch Act. Nutrition education stemmed from the Public Health Service, the Children's Bureau, and the U.S. Department of Agriculture.

The school health movement also developed within the educational system as a natural concern of parents and the schools. Starting in the 1870s with sporadic physicians' examinations of children for infectious diseases, school health services grew to include physical examinations, vision and hearing testing, immunizations, and nursing services. Massachusetts set the precedent for lodging responsibility for school health services with the state Department of Education, partly because many local health departments were poorly staffed.

The first federal legislation for the protection of the health of mothers and children was the Maternity and Infancy Act of 1921, commonly known as the Sheppard-Towner Act. This law provided for federal grants-in-aid to the states for maternal and child health demonstration services and launched a program of federal-state cooperation, which was carried out until 1929, when the program failed to secure further appropriations. Nevertheless, the pattern had been set for federal grants-in-aid and for demonstration programs.

In 1935, the cornerstone of current maternal and child health programs was enacted — Title V of the Social Security Act — providing grants to the states for support of maternal and child health services of state health departments and through the states to local health departments. Special grants for the care of crippled and handicapped children were provided, and the crippled children's program developed from this support. In some states, the crippled children's program was administered by the department of public health and in others by the department of public welfare. In fiscal year 1969, programs of state and local health services, aided by Title V funds, provided maternity medical clinic services to 337,000 mothers in the United States, maternity nursing services to 515,000 others, and family planning services to 329,000 women, while more than a million children were served in well-child conferences.[7] In fiscal year 1970, 490,000 children received crippled children's services.[8]

On the foundation of federally funded maternal and child health programs were added other federal programs over the years — in 1938 regulation of minimum standards for child labor; in 1943 the Emergency Maternity and Infant Care Program (EMIC) providing maternity and infant care for wives and children of servicemen (1943-1949); in 1946 grants to the states for mental health services for children; in 1950, under the amendments to the Social Security Act, expanded benefits for maternal and child health services, crippled children's services, and child welfare; in 1955 mass vaccinations against poliomyelitis; in 1956 a general medical care program for dependents of military personnel (CHAMPUS); and in 1962-1963 a host of measures, including federally supported clinics for domestic migratory workers and their dependents, expanded community immunization programs against communicable diseases, increased support for child welfare services and day care centers, a program specifically for care of the mentally retarded, and a new National Institute of Child Health and Human Development within the National Institutes of Health.

In the last decade, incremental additions were made to the pyramid of maternal and child health services. Title XIX of the Social Security Amendments of 1965 (Medicaid) provided funds to pay for medical care for dependent children under the Aid to Families of Dependent Children program (AFDC). Vastly expanded support for family planning services was provided in various programs. The Child Health Act of 1967, included in the Social Security Amendments of that year, provided support for family planning services, as did the welfare provisions of Title IV of the Social Security Act, the maternal and child health grants under Title V of that Act, and the projects funded by the Office of Economic Opportunity.[9] Finally, several demonstration programs of comprehensive health care were established — Maternity and Infant Care projects (1963), medical and dental services for preschoolers under the Head Start program (1964), neighborhood health centers supported by the Office of Economic Opportunity (1964), and Children and Youth projects (1965).

MATERNAL HEALTH SERVICES

Maternal health services consist of numerous programs for prenatal care, delivery, postpartum care, and family planning services, as well as for general medical care, administered by various public agencies at different levels of government and by voluntary groups. Categorical services are so much the ingrained pattern that even in a program established for the express purpose of providing the full range of maternity and infant services the provision of maternity care may be separated from the provision of birth control services. Dr. Helen Wallace reported this fragmentation in a Maternity and Infant Care project as follows:

> I recently visited an M & I project which was, on the whole, a very good one. In this project, there were certain half-days of the week which were "M & I sessions" — i.e., where pregnant women could receive maternity care. In addition, there were certain other half-days where women could receive family planning information, counseling, and supplies. I asked, "What would a woman do if she came for family planning help on the day of an M & I session?" and was told that she would be referred to a family planning session which met 2 days later. When asked if she might be provided with family planning help at the M & I session, I was told that this could be done "if there was an emergency." I then asked how one defined "an emergency," and there was some consternation about this. The reverse of the above situation is also

true — the pregnant woman who first comes to a family planning program is told to return on the day the M & I session meets. As part of an MCH Center, it seems to me that preconceptional and interconceptional care, including family planning, needs to be made available to all who need such care, regardless of age, marital status, economic status, etc.[10]

Federal Programs

Four major agencies of the federal government and numerous special divisions within these agencies are involved in a series of quite unrelated endeavors to provide maternity care to needy and high-risk groups. These activities subsidize categorical programs, authorize specific services, set diverse standards, support care for special groups of mothers or separate programs for special diseases, buy medical care, provide direct services, require separate state comprehensive plans, strengthen resources for care, or contribute to improved living conditions. As implemented, the various programs of the Department of Defense, the Department of Health, Education, and Welfare, the Department of Housing and Urban Development, and the Office of Economic Opportunity, through its Office of Health Affairs, bear virtually no relationship to each other.

Examination of the many parts of the U.S. Department of Health, Education, and Welfare concerned with one or another aspect of maternity care reveals the multiplicity and complexity of these programs, separately subsumed under the umbrella agency for health services within the Department of Health, Education, and Welfare — the Health Services and Mental Health Administration (HSMHA). One branch of HSMHA administers categorical grants to the states for maternal and child health services authorized by Title V of the Social Security Act. These basic grants support prenatal clinics, hospital services, postpartum care, and family planning services for low-income mothers. Other branches subsidize similar maternity services for migrant families and for American Indians. Federal employees and their dependents receive direct services. Mental health services are the responsibility of the National Institute of Mental Health and rehabilitation services of the Rehabilitation Services Administration. Welfare services, including the tax-supported Medicaid system, which accounts for the largest portion of federal expenditures for mothers and children,[11] are the concern of other branches. Services for mothers and infants may be found tucked into many broad programs of HSMHA, such as the Regional Medical Programs and the Comprehensive Health Planning program, and of other agencies and departments as well.

By contrast with these segmented programs, a number of recent programs are designed to provide integrated, comprehensive care to designated recipients. These include the 52 federally funded Maternity and Infant Care projects; the 65 comprehensive neighborhood health centers sponsored by the Office of Economic Opportunity, some of which have been transferred to the Department of Health, Education, and Welfare; the family health centers sponsored by the Department of Health, Education, and Welfare; the community health networks of the Office of Economic Opportunity; and the Model Cities program providing an integrated approach to the planning and delivery of the range of services, including health services, necessary for the economic and social growth of an underdeveloped neighborhood. But even these comprehensive programs are not integrated with other existing programs. Although the Comprehensive Health Planning program was designed to consolidate categorical health programs and federal financial assistance to the states, maternal and child health programs funded by Title V of the Social Security Act were not originally included within its purview.

Even more at variance with these tentative experiments in comprehensive health services is the Medicaid program, which promotes fragmentation in at least two ways. First, it limits reimbursement for care to rigidly defined categories of recipient. Second, at the expense of preventive measures, it favors reimbursement for treatment of episodic illness on a fee-for-service basis, including costly hospitalization, without requirements for appropriate and continuous care. In response to this second feature of the program, an expert advisory group recommended that state medical assistance plans assign priority to care of patients during the first, second, and third trimesters of pregnancy, to post-delivery services for mothers, and to care for infants up to the age of one year.[12] Little has been done to relate the maternity services provided under Medicaid to other maternal health services, particularly those provided by health departments and funded by Title V of the Social Security Act. Rather than mobilizing the total array of resources necessary to prevent diseases of social, economic, and physical deprivation, Medicaid treats the health effects of poverty in an already overloaded private medical care system.[13]

State Programs

The purpose of federal grants to the states for maternal health services is not only to channel financing to the local level but also to enable the states to develop comprehensive plans and to ensure provision of adequate services in all areas of the state. The state plan for maternal and child health, in allocating Title V funds to the communities and in requiring certain basic services, is designed to effectuate this purpose.

Other comprehensive state plans in California, within and outside the State Department of Public Health, also provide health services for mothers. Within the Department of Public Health are statewide plans for public health services, for the prevention of mental retardation and services for the retarded, and for the construction of hospitals and other medical facilities. The Department of Health Care Services administers the state medical assistance program and the Department of Mental Hygiene the state plan for community mental health services. The Departments of Rehabilitation and Social Welfare develop plans for rehabilitation, family social services, family income maintenance, and food stamp assistance. Although designed to achieve comprehensiveness in their respective fields, these plans actually fragment services at the delivery level because of categorical requirements in each field.

One reflection of the extent to which current activities fall short of the goal of comprehensive, or even adequate, maternal health services is the fact that 22 percent of the women in California whose deliveries were paid for by the Medicaid program in 1967 received poor prenatal care; 4 percent received no prenatal care, and 15.2 percent received care only in the third trimester, with no statement as to the care received for 2.7 percent.[14] Even though no cash barrier blocked access to medical care for this group, the system of health services, particularly the lack of preventive services in the Medicaid program, failed to assure adequate care for at least one-fifth of these Medicaid recipients. The percentage of women receiving inadequate prenatal care is much larger if the universe of poor women, rather than that of Medicaid recipients, is taken as the base. For example, of the 1,024 women delivered at the largest county hospital in California in the month of July 1968, 26 percent had received no prenatal care whatever before coming to the hospital for delivery.[15]

County and City Programs

Health services for mothers are the result of a chain of programs at all governmental levels, but it is at the local level of government that the full impact of fragmented programs is felt. In Los Angeles County, health care for mothers may involve contact with at least four major county departments: Health, Hospitals, Mental Health, and Public Social Services. If the woman is in need of home health services to avoid hospitalization, or nutritional supplements to assure normal development of the fetus, other agencies — governmental and voluntary — must be involved. Contacts with each agency may include repeated intake screening, eligibility determinations, medical or social history-taking, physical examinations, preventive services, ambulatory care, or hospitalization.

The County Health Department, as recipient of Title V funds through the State Health Department, has operated prenatal clinics and separate well-child conferences at 23 district health centers and 28 sub-centers throughout the county. Of the women served in these clinics in 1967-1969, 80 percent were delivered at one of the three county hospitals.[16] Despite this shared patient load, before September 1972 continuity of care had not been developed.* No common record system existed for the County Departments of Health and Hospitals, and no formalized mechanism had been established for relating the work of the physicians, nurses, and social workers in each department to the patients receiving services from both departments. If a complication of pregnancy arose in a woman receiving prenatal care at a Health Department clinic, the patient was referred to the county hospital or to a private physician, if she was eligible for Medicaid. A separate visit to another provider was necessary. Medical care was not available at the health resource most readily accessible to the patient in the neighborhood where she lived. Following delivery at the county hospital, the patient might return there or go to the Health Department clinic for her postpartum checkup.

Inadequate communication between the Department of Hospitals and the district health centers of the County Health Department prevented public health nurses from identifying high-risk women and infants in need of special supervision. The single liaison nurse stationed at the county hospital obviously could not provide the necessary links with 23 health districts serving thousands of women a year. Despite the risk of pregnancy during the postpartum period and the undesirability of closely spaced pregnancies, family planning services have been offered mainly in special family planning clinics, requiring separate visits. Similarly, well-child conferences were held at clinic hours different from those of prenatal and family planning clinics. Should the infant, another sibling, or the mother require even minimal medical treatment, another visit to a hospital clinic or physician outside the Health Department was required.

Moreover, public health nutrition programs were impeded by the difficulty of obtaining food supplements. County agencies had not integrated the food supplement program with other health services despite widespread under-nutrition in the low-income population.[17] The one exception was a special arrangement to provide food supplements for Maternity and Infant Care (MIC) patients between the MIC project funded by Title V of the Social Security Act and the neighborhood health center funded by the Office of Economic Opportunity.

Fortunately, these segmented functions within and across departments were beginning to change even in advance of the merger of the county departments concerned with health. Contraceptive services are now provided at the time of the postpartum checkup, either at the county hospital or at a com-

---

*A single County Department of Health Services consolidating the county departments of hospitals, health, and mental health and the office of the county veterinarian became operational in Los Angeles County on September 1, 1972. The previous multidepartmental picture is described, however, because it is typical of many counties in the United States and because the benefits of merger may not be achieved for some time.

munity-based clinic to which the patient is referred. The categorical clinics of the Health Department are being combined into multipurpose clinics. Rigid adherence to preventive services in public health clinics is being altered to allow some medical care. Experience of the federally funded Maternity and Infant Care (MIC) project, providing comprehensive services for high-risk, low-income women and their infants up to one year of age in two health districts with a large number of high-risk patients, has shown substantially reduced perinatal death and prematurity rates.[18] It has demonstrated the feasibility of replacing discontinuous efforts of different local departments with continuous, comprehensive care at least within a defined target area.

These straws in the wind herald major changes in the provision of public medical care in Los Angeles County. Implementing the recommendations of two distinguished study groups,[19] the County Board of Supervisors acted to merge the main county departments concerned with health into a single, unified health agency. Not included in this merger is the Department of Public Social Services, thus continuing the separation of social services from health services, except for the activities of public health social workers. The plan is to provide both preventive and curative services to eligible persons in comprehensive ambulatory care centers in neighborhoods close to people's homes. Linked to back-up hospitals, both governmental and voluntary, the health centers are intended to be a means for overcoming the long-standing fragmentation of preventive, ambulatory, and hospital services in the public sector.

Voluntary and Private Programs

The voluntary agencies concerned with the health of mothers are legion. The most numerous are, of course, the private, nonprofit hospitals providing maternity services. Health agencies, such as the visiting nurse associations, provide care for mothers. Welfare agencies, such as the family service associations and homes for unmarried mothers, are involved. Some services are provided by church groups and service clubs. Some agencies are concerned with both the health and welfare aspects of motherhood, such as groups concerned with pregnancy in teen-age girls. Professional associations perform important roles. For example, the regional maternal mortality committees of the California Medical Association study every maternal death in the state and thus provide important information for the development of maternal health programs.

FAMILY PLANNING SERVICES

The rapid expansion of family planning services in the last decade has been associated with the creation of new agencies and the development of multiple programs designed to reach the many women and men who are as yet unserved. With more than four million low-income women in the United States not served through identified organized family planning programs in 1969,[20] a system of specialized clinics with high visibility was promoted. These clinics, however, are not in a position to take advantage of the opportunities for family planning services in the normal course of providing health services to family members. The urgent need to launch the broadest possible effort, and the strong motivation of health workers in this field, have tended to accentuate separation of family planning services from the general health care system.

Federal Programs

Family planning services began as a function of voluntary agencies, principally Planned Parenthood–World Population. As the concept of birth control gained acceptance, governmental agencies have provided increasing support for organized programs. Before the enactment of the Family Planning Services and Population Research Act of 1970, the federal government supported family planning services through five main programs. The U.S. Department of Health, Education, and Welfare provided (1) grants to the states for maternal and child health services requiring family planning as an essential program and additional assistance under the Comprehensive Health Planning program; (2) project grants to private and public nonprofit agencies for family planning services; (3) reimbursement to providers of family planning services under Medicaid; (4) financial assistance for voluntary family planning services required to be offered to appropriate public assistance recipients; and (5) the U.S. Office of Economic Opportunity provided project grants for family planning services as a special priority program. This segmentation of programs is so well known that federal support for family planning programs is customarily described as Title V, Title IVa, Title X, and Title XIX funding.

The Family Planning Services and Population Research Act of 1970 not only authorized a massive infusion of funds for services, research, training, and development of educational materials, but it also provided for the centralized administration of all programs of the U.S. Department of Health, Education, and Welfare by an Office of Population Affairs, with the director having direct line authority over all family planning service and research programs of the Department. This feature of the legislation reflects the search for comprehensiveness and integration within this categorical field.

State Programs

California was one of the first states to enact legislation encouraging provision of family planning services in public health programs.[21] Since 1965, every organized health department has been required to provide family planning services, although the kinds and amounts of service have varied among counties and even among health districts within a single county. Federal requirements specified that at least six percent of maternal and child health funds had to be used for family planning services; thus a basic floor for services was fixed. County welfare departments were required to provide information, education, counseling, and referral for appropriate welfare clients. A provision in the California Welfare Reform Act of 1971 provided for the appropriation of $1 million in state funds, to be matched by $3 million in federal funds, for voluntary family planning services for welfare recipients or potential recipients.

The main state agencies responsible for family planning services are the Departments of Public Health, Social Welfare, and Health Care Services. Other departments, such as the Departments of Mental Hygiene and Corrections, may provide these services in their institutions.

In 1967, in an effort to overcome fragmentation of family planning services provided by numerous public and voluntary agencies, the State Department of Public Health gave support to the formation of the California Interagency Council on Family Planning. Composed of representatives of governmental and voluntary agencies and concerned individuals, the Council undertook to promote coordination of the many efforts in this field and to strengthen family planning programs throughout the state.

County Programs

In Los Angeles County, family planning services have been provided by two main county agencies—the Department of Health and Hospitals, with the Department of Public Social Services determining eligibility and referring patients for care. In addition, voluntary agencies, private hospitals, and physicians provide a large volume of services. In October 1971, 12 agencies operating at 60 different locations provided most of the subsidized services in the county.[22] The Health Department, which formerly had provided family planning services only in selected district health centers, by 1971 had expanded its clinics to offer family planning services in all 23 districts and at 37 locations.[23] These governmental, voluntary, and private agencies served approximately 59,000 medically indigent women in 1971,[24] compared with 28,000 in 1969.[25] Despite the doubling of the number of women served in two years. there remained in October 1971 an estimated 144,630 medically dependent women of child-bearing age desiring and needing birth control who were not served.[26]

Perhaps better than any other field of health service, the field of family planning illustrates both the advantages and disadvantages of organizational diversity. On the one hand, the many governmental and voluntary family planning agencies command a high degree of dedication from highly motivated health professionals and community organizers. Each agency can exercise its special talents in the field. On the other hand, such efforts without central coordination result in segmented medical care, overlapping geographic service areas with some communities not served, difficulty in following patients between agencies, gaps in populations served, duplications in community outreach, inequities in special services, lack of consistent data, and competition for trained manpower and financial assistance rather than efficient distribution and use of these scarce resources.

As a response to the proliferation of organizational efforts in this field, the Los Angeles Regional Family Planning Council was formed in 1968 to coordinate planning, funding, and training of personnel for family planning services. This federation of the major public and private providers of family planning services has been expanded to include not only providers but also consumers and affiliate members. As the officially designated recipient of family planning grants from the federal and state governments, this Regional Council has leverage to guide the extension of services to all geographic areas of the county and to all ethnic and age groups. It holds the financial carrot to promote special functions, such as education, follow-up services, research, and evaluation. The funds can be used to encourage specific agencies with special capabilities and resources to redirect their interests from a narrow focus to the full spectrum of family planning services. The Council has the potential for undertaking the joint training of personnel and joint public education programs, for the development of a unified system of evaluation of services, and for boosting the capacity of smaller agencies to provide increased services. What remains to be seen is whether a voluntary agency, such as the Los Angeles Regional Family Planning Council, can provide the impetus not only for the effective coordination of multiple programs but also for the integration of family planning services into the regular medical care of families.

CHILD HEALTH SERVICES

Child health services are generally organized by the various age groups served: infants, preschoolers, school children, and youth. Each of the many programs provides defined services, specifies conditions of eligibility that must be met, operates in designated geographic areas, or is financed in different ways with varying prescriptions. As the seventh White House Conference on Children noted in 1970,

> Many excellent health care programs are now available, offering *some* services to *some* children. . . . But none of the existing programs delivers all of what is needed for all children who need it. Some of the gaps are immediately apparent. For example, there is no systematic way of keeping track of the health needs of a child from the time he leaves the hospital a few days after birth until he enters the school system. . . . A second group of candidates for sustained neglect are children of the "near poor". . . . And even families whose budgets can accommodate continuing health care for their children are plagued by fragmentation of that care, unpredictable availability of health manpower, and the prospect of insupportable catastrophic illness [Italics in original].[27]

Neonatal and Infant Care

Programs for neonatal and infant care are tied to programs of maternal health services, and the same fragmentation that characterizes public medical care for mothers is true of services for newborns and infants. Originating at the federal level with categorical grants, demonstration projects, and varying payment mechanisms, the fragmentation is carried through the state level of government until it is translated into separate, specialized, and discontinuous services at the local level.

For low-income families, well-child care is provided either in public health clinics, funded under Title V of the Social Security Act, or in voluntary hospitals or private physicians' offices with reimbursement from Medicaid, if the family is eligible, or from some other public program. Care for sick babies has not been available in public health clinics generally but has been provided either in public hospitals, voluntary hospitals (intensive care units and services for low birth-weight infants), or private physicians' offices, with various payment mechanisms. Treatment is rarely available in the neighborhood where the family lives but requires travel to a distant hospital, child care arrangements for other children, and long waits to see a doctor.

Public medical care has thus traditionally separated preventive and therapeutic services for infants, a dichotomy deplored for years and one that, hopefully, will be remedied in Los Angeles County by the merger of the county departments of health and hospitals. (The excellent pattern of comprehensive services demonstrated by the Maternity and Infant Care or MIC projects should become the universal pattern. It should be extended to cover preschool and school-age children.) Further fragmentation exists if the baby has a crippling condition which qualifies for crippled children's services. All health services are separate from nutrition services, except that a public health nurse or nutritionist in the health department may advise mothers on the feeding of infants. Advice without nutritional supplements, however, may be futile.

Services for Preschool Children

The maze of programs in the field of child health services is complex because three streams of programs—in health, education, and welfare—attempt to meet the needs of children. Many special-purpose efforts have been undertaken under various auspices to prevent or correct physically or mentally handicapping conditions, to minimize or reverse the effects of malnutrition and deprivation, and to provide compensatory and enrichment programs for children from poor families.[28] Each program has its own requirements. The result has led to a patchwork of programs for selected children or selected conditions.

Federal Programs.   At the federal level, services for preschool children are supported by programs in five federal departments (Agriculture, Defense, Health, Education, and Welfare, Housing and Urban Development, and Labor) and by the Office of Economic Opportunity. Many of these programs, such as Title V of the Social Security Act and Medicaid, serve both infants and older children. By contrast with maternal and infant care, in the field of health services for preschoolers and older children, the Offices of Education and Child Development of the Department of Health, Education, and Welfare play an important role in providing grants to educational agencies for health, mental health, nutrition, and special education services in low-income areas.

Fragmented services, in a sense, are the result of incremental progress. Every advance represents the addition of a new program and increased fragmentation. For example, federal legislation for day care centers serving preschoolers and older children requires the centers to assist parents in carrying out a plan for medical and dental care for their children. The centers may provide funds for those not eligible for Medicaid or may arrange free or part-pay care, but they have little capacity to redirect delivery of health services into a comprehensive form. In a significant interagency effort to unify standards for all day care centers receiving federal funds from any of seven different sources, federal interagency day care requirements have been promulgated by the Federal Panel on Early Childhood.[29]

Two innovative programs for comprehensive care for children are exceptions to the general pattern of fragmented services, although they, too, are fragmented in serving limited groups of children. Project Head Start serves preschoolers exclusively. The Children and Youth projects serve children up to the age of 18 from selected poverty communities.

Project Head Start, launched by the Office of Economic Opportunity as an effort to break the cycle of poverty, came as an indictment of previous inattention to the crucial preschool period and to the importance of the child's home and social environment in any developmental program. The findings of initial medical and dental examinations of Head Start children, about four years of age, revealed major gaps in prior health care. More than one-third of the mothers reported that the child had not seen a physician for any reason in the two years before care under Head Start. Only one in four of the children had ever seen a dentist; 40 to 90 percent, depending on whether their drinking water was fluoridated, had dental caries. About half had not been immunized for diphtheria, smallpox, or polio, and seven percent failed the vision screening test.[30] The new feature of Project Head Start was provision of complete medical and dental care for the child, not merely screening, diagnosis, and referral to a nonexistent family doctor or dentist. Unfortunately, however, such care is not available once the child enters school.

The demonstration Children and Youth projects, funded directly under Title V of the Social Security Act, were similarly designed to provide comprehensive services for preschool and school age children in low-income areas where health and social services are inadequate.[31] The intent was to substitute for fragmented, categorical services health care focused on the whole child that would assure comprehensive, accessible, high-quality, coordinated, and continuous services, both preventive and curative. At the end of fiscal year 1970, 412,000 preschool and school age children were registered in 58 operating projects.[32] For these children, at least, the projects, which became part of state maternal and child health plans in 1972, have provided care for neglected conditions, substituted combined prevention and treatment for episodic care, decreased hospital admissions, and improved dental health.[33] Average cost per child per year is approximately $125.

State Programs.   At the state level, five main departments are involved in health or health-related services for preschool children: the Departments of Public Health, Mental Hygiene, Health Care Services, Social Welfare, and Education. Among the many activities of the Department of Public Health for this age group are immunization programs, administration of the crippled children's program, and services for the mentally retarded. The Department of Mental Hygiene is concerned with mental health services for children and the Department of Health Care Services with payment for medical care for eligible children. The Department of Social Welfare has broad responsibilities in the administration of the food stamp program, setting of standards for day care services, and conduct of child welfare services, such as adoption and care of children in foster homes. The Department of Education and its Office of Compensatory Education are involved in a preschool education program that requires provision of limited health services.

This diffusion of responsibility at the state level entails split authority and deficiency in services. For instance, new programs of compensatory education, including day care centers, Developmental Centers for Handicapped Minors, the California Preschool Education Program, and migrant day care centers, all have a health component, administered by education or welfare agencies. These specialized programs for children from low-income families provide physical examinations, immunizations, and tuberculin testing, but a plan has not been formulated for comprehensive care and follow-through of defects found by the program. Follow-up care is not provided in compensatory education programs unless the children are eligible for Medi–Cal or unless the agency or school district provides or arranges for medical care. Even the screening program for children authorized by Medicaid fails to ensure appropriate treatment for conditions detected through this screening.

Another example of fragmentation concerns nutrition programs under the jurisdiction of three state departments (Public Health, Social Welfare, and Education), with similar fragmentation at the local level. Food stamp programs, managed by social welfare departments for eligible households, are not integrated with school lunch programs or with health department programs in nutrition and child health. The reduced price or free school lunch programs operate at the discretion of each school district, with no school lunch program in many districts. Preschoolers account for 30 percent of children in need and cannot be reached even through the limited school lunch programs. Eight percent of the three- to five-year-olds screened for the state's largest preschool program were found to be suffering from gross nutritional neglect.[34] For these children, food supplement programs at school may be too late.

County Programs. At the local level, various agencies and programs provide health services for preschool children: departments of county government, public and voluntary hospitals, and specialized governmental and voluntary agencies. Since many of these agencies also provide care for older children, only special problems concerning the health of preschoolers are mentioned here.

Before the merger of the various county departments concerned with health, children over the age of two years could receive only immunizations and some dental care from the Health Department. Well-child conferences of the Health Department in 130 locations throughout the county serve about two-thirds of the children from poor families under age two,[35] but children over age two were excluded for fiscal reasons. Certainly, no sound medical reason justifies cutting off health supervision at this age, and two cities in the county continue well-child services to the age of five. Attendance of preschool children at well-child clinics declines sharply after completion of immunizations, confirming the need for a combination of prevention and treatment for low-income families with urgent health problems.[36] Dental treatment is provided in Health Department clinics to needy children between ages two and six and up to age 13 if they are seen initially before their seventh birthday.

The multiplicity of agencies administering various programs of preschool services has created other problems. Head Start, the California Preschool Education Program, day care centers, Children's Centers, Developmental Centers, and compensatory education programs are each under different and separate sponsorships. Head Start is administered by 19 delegate agencies; one of these is the county Office of Superintendent of Schools, which alone operates Head Start programs in 18 separate school districts. The California Preschool Education Program is administered by each participating independent school district. Day care services are under the county Department of Public Social Services, various school districts, and nonprofit agencies. Children's Centers are under the jurisdiction of the Los Angeles City School District and other school districts. Developmental Centers for Handicapped Minors and the compensatory education programs under the Elementary and Secondary Education Act are separate programs that are also operated by independent school districts or jointly in cooperation with the county Superintendent of Schools.

Neither the Health Department nor the Department of Hospitals has defined the relationship of its public medical services to the services being arranged and purchased by the Head Start program, the day care agencies, the Children's Centers, and the compensatory education program. The two exceptions to this fragmentation are the county-wide immunization programs, conducted by the Health Department through the schools and the preschool programs, and the consultation provided by the Health Department to the largest of the Head Start agencies. Many child development and enrichment programs, lacking links to health agencies, have had to become organizers, as well as purchasers, of medical care. None of these educational agencies has the authority, budget, or expertise to look beyond the specific needs of its own programs, but this responsibility has fallen to them by default or by reason of the limited jurisdiction of the health agencies.

Moreover, most of these programs maintain contact with the child only for a limited period of time, varying from eight weeks to perhaps a year or more. The short-term arrangements made by different agencies, operating under different auspices, with varying regulations, and always with financial limitations, preclude continuity in health services through the formative years. Any gains achieved by a single program are easily lost through this lack of continuity.

Services for School Children and Youth

The main source of fragmentation in child health services is the division of responsibility between health agencies and the educational system. The school as a natural locus for the provision of child health services has led to an assumption of responsibility for some health services by the school system. Health is a primary objective of modern education,[37] and therefore the schools have been willing to provide some health services. Lacking, however, are effective linkages between the limited health services provided by the schools and the health care system as a whole.

Federal Programs. At the federal level, the many programs to protect and promote the health of children and youth span all the fields of health service — preventive, therapeutic, and rehabilitative for both physical and mental conditions — and include all the functions in health service: planning, staffing, providing, financing, and evaluating care. The programs in five major departments, subdivisions of these departments, and independent agencies are so numerous that an Interdepartmental Committee on Children and Youth has been established to coordinate federal programs, many of which serve both infants and older children.

State Programs. Health services for children and youth involve substantially the same state departments as are involved in maternal and infant care, with the addition of the State Department of Education and the Office of Surplus Commodities. Within the Department of Education are its Divisions of Compensatory Education, Public School Administration, and Health Education, Physical Education, and Recreation, each of which has some impact on health service for children and youth. The five main departments involved in child health services — Public Health, Mental Hygiene, Health Care Services, Social Welfare, and Education — distribute federal-state funds for local services, set standards for programs, monitor services, maintain records and statistics, coordinate programs, furnish direct services in certain instances, and provide surveillance and intelligence on health needs and conditions in the state. Reflecting the multiplicity and complexity of administrative responsibilities at the state level is the finding that, for children with developmental handicaps in California, seven state departments administer 44 district programs providing a combination of special educational, clinical, rehabilitative, and social services to the handicapped.[38] These programs operate in addition to and largely apart from the system of regular health care.

Local Programs. The segmented programs of health and nutrition services for children and youth that originate at the federal level and are channeled through multiple state agencies find expression at the local level in services provided by public agencies under health, welfare, and educational sponsorships. Within the County of Los Angeles, public medical care for children and youth is provided by 23 districts of the County Health Department, two city health departments, three public general hospitals, several specialized hospitals, 11 medical aid districts, 20 family welfare service districts, 13 mental health areas, 96 public school districts, five community action agencies, and various demonstration projects, Compensatory Education Programs, and Children's Centers. Numerous services are also provided by free or part-pay clinics in private hospitals, by the vast array of voluntary agencies concerned with health problems of children, and by private providers.

Nearly every official agency in the health, welfare, and educational fields at the local level provides some services for children. The Health Department provides immunizations and tuberculin testing in the public schools, general school health services in the parochial schools, limited medical care in health officers' clinics, and dental treatment to children of specified ages who meet certain conditions, as mentioned. In the field of adolescent health, the Health Department has responded to the need for medical care acceptable to this age group by establishing a number of youth clinics, open mainly in the evenings. The youth clinics are well-attended, but they, too, provide categorical services for a specific age group and for limited conditions.[39]

Three general hospitals are the principal sources of ambulatory and inpatient medical care for children and youth from low-income families. The irrationality of concentrating medical care in a single pediatric outpatient department, where more than 10,000 children a month are seen, was revealed by a study conducted in the summer of 1967.[40] Not surprisingly, many of the families of the 3,058 randomly selected patients were found to use the hospital as their only source of medical care. Although 99 percent of the children needed, and received, the services of a physician, 73 percent of the cases were mild or not severe, 25 percent were chronic, and only five percent required hospitalization. More than half of the children had not been immunized. Thus, the study concluded that the vast majority of these children could have been served as well, if not better, by ambulatory care facilities in their own neighborhoods.

Many forces have contributed to efforts to provide public medical care in locations more convenient than distant county hospitals: the Medi–Cal program, the Model Cities projects, the demands of citizens, the protests against overcrowding of the main county hospital made by the interns and residents and carried forward through a legal suit against the county, and the recommendations of two expert groups on organization of health services in the county.[41] The merger of the county departments concerned with health is intended to integrate public resources for the provision of ambulatory and in-patient care, ending compartmentalization of services among several departments dealing with the same population. The folly of providing prevention without treatment and treatment without prevention can then be corrected.

Just as separate clinics have been established for adolescents, so services for specified handicapping conditions are segmented. The crippled children's services, a separate program under the Department of Hospitals in Los Angeles County, serves children with crippling conditions as defined by uniform state standards. This program provides high-quality, coordinated care, either through public or private providers, for the child's handicapping condition, but the program is separated from the general medical care of these children and from other specialized health services, such as those for the mentally retarded or those of the Health Department.

Mental health services for children and youth are the responsibility of another county agency. The County Department of Mental Health enters into contracts with nonprofit child guidance clinics, provides direct services in its own clinics, funds inpatient services, and offers psychiatric consultation to schools and other agencies (see Chapter 5). Although the 13 mental health regions are congruent with the boundaries of public health districts, services are not integrated to take advantage of· the opportunities for preventive mental health services or for early treatment that arise in the services of both the public health clinics and the hospital pediatric departments. The unified county health agency will, it is hoped, increase the capacity for such integration.

Another separate system provides services for the mentally retarded (see Chapter 5). Fortunately, the various public agencies in the health, welfare, and educational fields serving the retarded and the many voluntary and private agencies have been linked into a regional system with a single Regional Center for Mental Retardation. This structure, based on the concept of central, coordinated responsibility for diagnosis and evaluation and one-door entry to a wide array of decentralized services, is designed to improve accessibility of services for patients and their families. But it is limited to mental retardation services.

Still another constellation of general health services for children consists of school health services, with responsibility divided between educational and health agencies. In 1968-1969, more than $38 million was spent for health services by public educational agencies in California and another $3 million by local health departments, which included services to private schools.[42] Expenditures varied greatly among the 1,116 school districts and the 58 county education offices. They ranged from no expenditures for health services in 36 districts and 47 reporting county offices to more than $50 per child in other districts. Although no evaluation of quality of services was made, the following accounted for half of all costs of direct services: major and minor emergency care, vision and hearing screening, and health information.

Not only are school health services limited and highly variable, but they fail to assure adequate follow-up of defects found in the course of school health examinations. One study found that fewer than 60 percent of children even from families with some health insurance received care for health defects detected in school health programs and that these children were more likely to receive care than were children from noninsured families.[43] In the face of existing fragmentation of diagnostic and curative services, the study reached the limited conclusion that referral efforts of school health personnel should be concentrated on noninsured families, particularly those in low socio-economic groups.

Since it has not been within the jurisdiction of Boards of Education to provide treatment for conditions discovered by their physicians or dentists, and the resources for assuring follow-up are limited, the appropriateness of this expensive procedure within the schools is questionable. Nevertheless, 95 full-time equivalent physicians employed by the Los Angeles City School Districts reported spending 64 percent of their time on routine physical examinations and another 22.8 percent of their time on special referral examinations, with little assurance that the conditions diagnosed would be treated.[44] Similarly, with respect to dental services, the Los Angeles City School Districts provide only examinations and dental health education. This program has had the largest number of dentists in public employment, but they provide no dental treatment.[45]

Examinations and referrals in the schools are based on the assumption that the family has an available source of medical and dental care. The lack of such resources in poor communities and a ruling by the State Attorney General that school districts cannot, under the California Education Code, use school funds to provide medical and dental care led to establishment in 1946 of separately sponsored clinics for the treatment of school children. In cooperation with professional groups and with some staff from the school health services, the Parent Teachers' Association established medical and dental clinics for further diagnostic work-ups, limited eye services, some mental health care, and dental treatment. Despite the most valiant efforts, these clinics are restricted in the scope of services they may offer and in the numbers of children they can serve. In 1968, the Robert L. Taylor Dental Clinics, staffed by 13 full-time equivalent dentists, provided free or low-cost dental treatment to 7,500 children—about one percent of the school population; but 20 percent of the school population comes from families too poor to pay for dental care.[46]

The frustration that is felt by the mother when "the system" takes such pains to point out her child's pressing needs but is unable to take pains to provide the remedy may explain the policy of Head Start that "the only reason for tests and medical evaluations is to assure that every child who needs treatment gets it."[47] Until expanded resources are organized in poverty communities, the schools will continue to give tests without treatment and the newer preschool and day care programs will continue to arrange or purchase episodic, discontinuous health services.

Also under the jurisdiction of the Los Angeles City School District and 15 other school districts are the Children's Centers for children in need of special instruction, supervision, meals, and health services, such as speech therapy. Developmental Centers for Handicapped Minors and the compensatory education programs under the Elementary and Secondary Education Act are separate programs that are also operated by independent school districts or jointly in cooperation with the County Superintendent of Schools.

Nutrition services, mandated by programs at higher levels of government, are provided at the county and city levels by various agencies. The Department of Public Social Services and the educational system are responsible for food supplements and the school lunch program, respectively. The Health Department provides nutrition education, counseling, and consultation to other agencies. Voluntary organizations provide both food and special nutrition education. At the root of malnutrition, of course, is poverty. Granted that neither the health system nor the educational system is the primary vehicle for assuring provision of adequate food to children and their families, in the process of providing medical care opportunities are presented to detect chronic or potential malnourishment. At that stage, the health system should be equipped to intervene. Although food supplements through health programs can be deemed only an emergency measure, they should be readily available until basic reforms are made in both family assistance and food distribution programs.

Voluntary and Private Programs. Many health services for children are delivered by voluntary agencies and private providers. Numerous disease-specific agencies serve primarily children, for example the Crippled Children's Society and the Easter Seal Society, both providing services to handicapped children. Welfare, educational, professional, and fraternal organizations also are concerned with the physical or mental health of children. In response to the health needs of young people, "free clinics" and "hot lines" have emerged and received support from individuals and the local health department. Voluntary hospitals—both special children's hospitals and pediatric departments of general hospitals—provide care. In terms of magnitude of impact, voluntary health insurance programs are probably the most important agencies in the private sector for child health. Children are the principal dependent beneficiaries of health insurance policies held by employed adults.

ANOTHER EXAMPLE OF PERSON-SPECIFIC PROGRAMS: HEALTH CARE FOR THE AGED

Health services for many other categories of recipients reflect the same multiplicity of agencies, fragmentation of services, and lack of coordination as do maternal and child health services. Programs for the provision of health services exist at various levels of government for Indians, migrant workers and their families, the military, the poor, prisoners, rural people, veterans, workers, and the aged. For those categories for whom major responsibility is lodged at a single level of government, as for the military and veterans, fragmentation of care is minimized but still set apart from other community resources. For those categories for whom responsibility is shared by several levels of government and by both the public and private sectors, as for the poor, the resultant services are highly fragmented. Lest the story of fragmentation of health services for mothers and children be deemed a unique aberration, a brief account is presented of fragmentation in health services for persons at the other end of the life span.

Governmental Programs

The aged are served by a separate constellation of health programs, so segmented that in 1965 Congress enacted the Older Americans Act, established an Administration on Aging within the Department of Health, Education, and Welfare, designed, among other purposes, to serve as a clearinghouse for information related to problems of the aged, to administer grants for state and community programs on aging, to provide technical assistance to the states, and to stimulate improved use of resources and available services for the aged and the aging.[48] In 1969, Congress amended this statute to strengthen state agencies on aging and to establish new state plan requirements for the statewide planning, coordination, and evaluation of programs serving older people.[49] Areawide model projects on a statewide, regional, metropolitan area, county, or city basis were authorized. Interagency cooperation was mandated among the Department of Health, Education, and Welfare, the Office of Economic Opportunity, the Department of Labor, and many other federal agencies administering relevant projects, in order to achieve optimal coordination of all public and private programs. Congress thus expressed its intention not once but twice to bring about coordination of the many programs for the aged.

The reason is not hard to find. Following the defeat of national health insurance proposals in the late 1940s, increasing attention was devoted to proposals for underwriting medical care of the aged. This was accomplished in three incremental steps: through medical vendor payments for all aged persons on welfare enacted in 1950, through extension of medical benefits to the medically indigent aged in 1960, and finally, through enactment of Medicare and Medicaid in 1965. In addition, a number of categorical programs providing health-related services for the aged were initiated.

At the federal level, three major divisions of the Department of Health, Education, and Welfare are concerned with health services for the aged: the Social and Rehabilitation Service, the Health Services and Mental Health Administration, and the Social Security Administration. Within the Social and Rehabilitation Service are the Administration on Aging and five additional major programs related to the aged: the Assistance Payments Administration (payments of old age assistance cash benefits to dependent aged, including Aid to the Needy Blind and Aid to the Permanently and Totally Disabled); the Medical Services Administration (Medicaid payments for Old Age Assistance recipients and the indigent aged who are categorically linked); the Rehabilitation Services Administration (the federal arm of the federal-state vocational rehabilitation services, including physical and mental health services to the disabled and special projects); the Division of Research and Demonstration (pilot projects on rehabilitation and use of older workers); and the Community Services Administration (development of policy and programs for the needy aged and handicapped, including homemaker services, arrangements for and transportation to health care, and housing for the aged). Within the Health Services and Mental Health Administration (HSMHA) are the National Institutes of Mental Health and Child Health and Human Development, engaged in research on aging and its diseases, and at least six separate subdivisions of HSMHA concerned with community health services, chronic diseases, mental health, Regional Medical Programs, health services research and development, and health facilities planning and construction, all with significant impact on health services for the aged. The Social Security Administration is responsible for administering the vast program of Medicare, both the hospital insurance under Part A and the supplementary medical insurance under Part B for the 20 million Americans 65 years of age and older.

This proliferation of agencies and programs within a single federal department, accentuated by services provided for the aged by other federal departments and agencies, is repeated at the state level. Four departments of state government in California are involved in programs for the aged—the Departments of Health Care Services, Social Welfare, Public Health, and Rehabilitation—as well as the California Commission on Aging, which acts as a clearinghouse at the state level and provides consultation and guidance to local communities for development of programs for senior citizens. Numerous county departments, city agencies, and representatives of state and federal agencies are involved in providing services for the aged at the local level of government.

Voluntary and Private Programs

Many voluntary and private agencies — hospitals, nursing homes, home health agencies, private insurance companies, fiscal intermediaries, voluntary health organizations, professional groups, and educational institutions — are concerned with health care for the aged. Some of these voluntary organizations serve with governmental agencies on a 30-member Interagency Council on Health Needs of the Aged, established to coordinate services in the county. This council is able to reach the organized programs, but it is powerless to coordinate the services rendered by the many private physicians and other individual providers to the aged.

Significance of Categorical Programs and Services for the Aged

The life and death significance of multiple, uncoordinated public and private services for the aged in search of needed medical care has been documented in various Congressional hearings and reports. The patient who needs nursing home care but must be admitted for three days to a hospital to meet the federal eligibility requirements of Medicare for nursing home services — while the legislative intent is understandable — is often a victim of fragmented care.[50] The elderly who must travel to a union health center for an annual checkup, to an arthritis clinic, a heart clinic, or a diabetes clinic in various hospitals on different days for specialized care, to neighborhood doctors when too ill to travel, and who receive different medications and courses of treatment from several doctors are victims of fragmented care.[51] The 76-year-old man who would have to attend ten separate clinics to receive check-ups and treatments for several ailments is a victim of fragmented care.[52] The many elderly patients who are in mental hospitals because of a lack of more appropriate facilities are tragic victims of fragmented care.[53] The problems of fragmentation permeate the system and afflict persons of all income groups.[54] But the highest price for fragmentation is paid by the poor.

It is small wonder, therefore, that a Presidential Task Force on the Aging proposed as its top-priority recommendation a means for overcoming the lack of coordination among the "large number of units of the Federal Government (which) are engaged in a range of complex efforts which directly or indirectly affect the elderly in a variety of ways."[55] This Task Force said:

> No agency has authority to determine priorities, to settle conflicts, to eliminate duplication, to identify and assign responsibility, to search for gaps within and between agencies, to initiate concerted action, to keep Federal agencies constantly aware of how their programs affect the elderly. The Task Force is also concerned about the ways in which these problems become magnified at the State and local levels through Federal agency policies and grant programs.[56]

Recognizing the Congressional intent in establishing the Administration on Aging, the Presidential Task Force nevertheless concluded that interdepartmental coordination cannot be carried out by a unit of government subordinate to the units it is attempting to coordinate. The Task Force made numerous recommendations to improve services for the aged, but fundamental to all, in its view, was the need to establish an Office on Aging within the Executive Office of the President to develop national policy, to oversee planning and evaluation of all federal activities, to coordinate such activities, to recommend priorities, and to alert other government officials to the potential impact of their decisions on the interests of older persons. At the state and local levels of government, the need is equally urgent to combat the dispersion of responsibility among multiple programs and agencies for health care of the aged.

NOTES

1. Corsa, Leslie, Jr., M.D. and Bruce Jessup, M.D., "Tax-Supported Medical Care for California Children—Where Should It Be Going?" *Calif. Med.*, Vol. 96, p. 98 at 99, Feb. 1962.

2. *National Action to Combat Mental Retardation:* The President's Panel on Mental Retardation, U.S. Government Printing Office, Washington, D.C., 1962; *Proceedings of the National Conference for the Prevention of Mental Retardation through Improved Maternity Care* (Edwin M. Gold, M.D., Ed.), sponsored by New York Medical College, Department of Obstetrics and Gynecology and U.S. Department of Health, Education, and Welfare, Children's Bureau, Social and Rehabilitation Service, Washington, D.C., March 27-29, 1968.

3. See Rosen, George, M.D., *A History of Public Health*, MD Publications, New York, 1958. Much of the historical material in this chapter is drawn from this excellent source.

4. Eliot, Martha M., M.D., "The Fiftieth Anniversary of the Maternal and Child Health Section: Some Remarks on Background and Origin," *Am. J. Public Health*, Vol. 62, No. 7, p. 1018, July 1972.

5. Ibid. See also Schmidt, William M., M.D., "The Development of Health Services for Mothers and Children in the United States," *Am. J. Public Health*, Vol. 63, No. 5, p. 419 at 421, May 1973.

6. Rosen, supra note 3 at 364.

7. *Statistical Summary of Cases Served under Maternal and Child Health Programs of*

State and Local Health Departments, Fiscal Year 1969, U.S. Department of Health, Education, and Welfare, Social and Rehabilitation Service, National Center for Social Statistics, Tables 1, 2, 15, and 3.

8. U.S. Department of Health, Education, and Welfare, *1970 Annual Report,* p. 167, U.S. Government Printing Office, Washington, D.C., 1970.

9. Lesser, Arthur J., M.D., "Discussion," *Proceedings of the National Conference for the Prevention of Mental Retardation through Improved Maternity Care,* supra note 2, p. 205 at 206-208.

10. Wallace, Helen M., M.D., "Discussion," *Proceedings of the National Conference for the Prevention of Mental Retardation through Improved Maternity Care,* supra note 2, p. 215 at 217.

11. Breslow, Lester, M.D., "Proposals for Achieving More Adequate Health Care for Children and Youth," *Am. J. Public Health,* Supplement, Vol. 60, No. 4, p. 110, Apr. 1970.

12. *Report of the Child Health Services Committee,* Medical Assistance Advisory Council, p. 228, 1st draft, March 11, 1969.

13. Haggarty, Robert J., M.D., "Present Strengths and Weaknesses in Current Systems of Comprehensive Health Services for Children and Youth," *Am. J. Public Health,* Supplement, Vol. 60, No. 4, p. 89, Apr. 1970.

14. Information on matched medical birth records provided by the Epidemiological Unit, Bureau of Maternal and Child Health, California State Department of Public Health, 1967.

15. In this group, 22 patients manifested severe medical complications, and 10 perinatal deaths occurred. Information provided by the Los Angeles County-University of Southern California Medical Center to the Program Review of the Los Angeles County Health Department. See *Future Directions for Health Services, County of Los Angeles/1970,* Review of the Program of the Los Angeles County Health Department, undertaken at the request of the Los Angeles County Board of Supervisors, pp. 85-86, American Public Health Association, Community Health Action Planning Services (Malcolm H. Merrill, M.D., Director of Study), Los Angeles, 1970.

16. *Future Directions for Health Services, County of Los Angeles/1970,* supra note 15 at 85-86.

17. In a statement to the Senate Select Committee on Nutrition and Human Needs, the Director of the Los Angeles County Department of Public Social Services testified: "We find that approximately 53% of all families in Los Angeles County being aided under the State program (public assistance) are receiving less than what the State itself says they need to live on at a minimum level of efficiency and health." Hearings, Nutrition and Human Needs, 90th Cong., 2d Sess., and 91st Cong., 1st Sess., Part 9, p. 2803, May 1969.

18. During an eighteen-month period, the project reduced the perinatal death rates among its patients to 24.9%, compared with a rate of 37.7% for patients from the same socioeconomic background at the county hospital, and reduced the prematurity rate to 8.7% for MIC patients, compared with a rate of 11.2% for the hospital population. Morton, John H., M.D., "Experiences in a Maternal and Infant (MIC) Project," *Am. J. Obstet. Gynecol.,* Vol. 107, No. 3, p. 362, June 1, 1970.

19. Los Angeles County Health Services Planning Committee, *Report of the Study of Health Services of the County of Los Angeles,* 1970; *Future Directions for Health Services, County of Los Angeles/1970,* supra note 15 (both reports are contained in this volume).

20. *Need for Subsidized Family Planning Services: United States, Each State and County, 1969.* A Report by the Center for Family Planning Program Development, the Technical Assistance Division of Planned Parenthood-World Population for the Executive Office of the President, Office of Economic Opportunity, Office of Health Affairs, Family Planning Programs, p. 25.

21. Cunningham, George C., M.D., "Summary of the Development of Family Planning Programs in the State of California," presented to the Senate Committee on Health and Welfare, California Legislature, Jan. 12, 1972.

22. Los Angeles Regional Family Planning Council, *A Five-Year Plan to Provide Family Planning Services to Low-Income Families of Los Angeles County*, p. 11, Los Angeles, Oct. 1971.

23. Id. at 12.

24. Id. at 11.

25. *Future Directions for Health Services, County of Los Angeles/1970*, supra note 15 at 89.

26. Ibid. But *cf., Need for Subsidized Family Planning Services; United States, Each State and County, 1969*, supra note 20 at 174 that Los Angeles County had 125, 348 medically indigent women in need of family planning services in 1969.

27. *Keeping Children Healthy: Health Protection and Disease Prevention*, Report of Forum 10, 1970 White House Conference on Children, pp. 184-185.

28. See Stewart, W. H., M.D., "The Unmet Needs of Children," *Pediatrics*, Vol. 39, No. 2, pp. 157-160, Feb. 1967 and Richmond, Julius B., M.D. and Howard L. Weinberger, M.D., "Program Implications of New Knowledge Regarding the Physical, Intellectual, and Emotional Growth and Development and the Unmet Needs of Children and Youth," *Am. J. Public Health*, Supplement, Vol. 60, No. 4, p. 23 at 29, Apr. 1970.

29. Federal Interagency Day Care Requirements, pursuant to Sec. 522(d) of the Economic Opportunity Act, as approved by the U.S. Department of Health, Education, and Welfare, U.S. Office of Economic Opportunity and U.S. Department of Labor, Sept. 23, 1968. Requirement V.3 states that arrangements must be made for medical and dental care and other health related treatment for each child using existing community resources. In the absence of other financial resources, the operating or administering agency must provide, where authorized by law, such treatment with its own funds.

30. North, A. F., Jr., "Project Head Start and the Pediatrician," *Clin. Pediatr.*, Vol. 6, pp. 191-194, Apr. 1967.

31. U.S. Department of Health, Education, and Welfare, *1970 Annual Report*, p. 168, U.S. Government Printing Office, Washington, D.C., 1970.

32. Id. at 168-169.

33. Id. at 169.

34. California Legislature, Assembly Committee on Health and Welfare, *Malnutrition: One Key to the Poverty Cycle*, p. 8, Jan. 1970.

35. *Future Directions for Health Services, County of Los Angeles/1970*, supra note 15 at 92.

36. *The Child Health Conference in California*, Bureau of Maternal and Child Health, California State Department of Public Health, pp. 7-8, 1964.

37. National Committee on School Health Policies of NEA and AMA, *Suggested School Health Policies* (4th ed.), p. viii, American Medical Association, 1966.

38. Arthur Bolton Associates, *A Report to the Assembly Select Committee on Mentally Ill and Handicapped Children*, p. 14, Sacramento, Calif., March 1, 1970.

39. See *Future Directions for Health Services, County of Los Angeles/1970*, supra note 15 at 96 for recommendation that the performance of youth clinics be evaluated and their relationship to the comprehensive health service centers, when developed, be examined for possible incorporation in the comprehensive program.

40. Wingert, Willis, A., David B. Friedman, and William R. Larson, "The Demographical and Ecological Characteristics of a Large Urban Pediatric Outpatient Population and Implications for Improving Community Pediatric Care," *Am. J. Public Health*, Vol. 58, No. 5, p. 859, May 1968.

41. Supra note 19.

42. *A Report to the 1970 Legislature on Reimbursement of Public School Health Services in California*, pursuant to Chapter 995, Statutes of 1969 (S.B. 592), State of California, Human Relations Agency, Department of Public Health, Jan. 1970.

43. Cauffman, Joy G., Ph.D., Milton I. Roemer, M.D., and Carl S. Schultz, M.D., "The Impact of Health Insurance Coverage on Health Care of School Children," Public Health Reports, Vol. 82, No. 4, p. 323, Apr. 1967.

44. Wagner, Marsden, G., M.D., Carl S. Schultz, M.D., and Marian H. Heller, P.H.N., "A Study of School Physician Behavior," *Am. J. Public Health,* Vol. 53, No. 3, p. 517.

45. *Future Directions for Health Services, County of Los Angeles/1970,* supra note 15 at 121.

46. Id. at 122.

47. *Project Head Start, 2: Health Services, A Guide for Project Directors and Health Personnel,* Office of Economic Opportunity, Washington, D.C., 1967.

48. Older Americans Act, P.L. 89-73 (1965), amended by P.L. 90-42 (1967).

49. See Report of the Committee on Education and Labor on the Older Americans Act Amendments of 1969, Report No. 91-285, 91st Cong., 1st Sess., June 5, 1969.

50. *See Developments in Aging 1967,* A Report of the Special Committee on Aging, U.S. Senate pursuant to S. Res. 20, Feb. 17, 1967, Report No. 1098, p. 47, 90th Cong., 2d Sess., April 29, 1968.

51. Id. at 58.

52. Id. at 59.

53. Id. at 66 and testimony of Dr. Israel Zwerling, Director of the Bronx State Hospital, New York City, that the percentage of first mental hospital admissions accounted for by persons over 65 years of age is increasing more rapidly than is the total population over 65 years of age.

54. Roemer, Milton I., M.D., Statement on "Costs and Delivery of Health Services to Older Americans," Hearings before the Subcommittee on Health of the Elderly of the Special Committee on Aging, U.S. Senate, 90th Cong., 1st Sess., p. 80, 1967, quoted in *Developments in Aging 1967,* supra note 50 at 57-58.

55. *Toward a Brighter Future for the Elderly,* Report of the President's Task Force on the Aging, p. 12, U.S. Government Printing Office, Washington, D.C., Apr. 1970.

56. Ibid.

CHAPTER 5

Mental Health Services: Programs for Provision of Services for Specific Diseases

> But the current approaches to mental health seem to carry within them the seeds of isolation from other elements of the community. We are still too much invested in categorization: community mental health centers; mental retardation centers; separate and special services for children; for those with alcoholism, for drug-addicted or habituated people; for the suicidal. We are perpetuating fragmentation within the mental health sector as well as perpetuating the separatism of mental health from health in general and from helping agencies that are not in the health field. Government funding at all levels contributes to such perpetuation, by earmarking funds for special purposes. And there are always local groups with the dedication to some special subsector of the field, ready to develop yet another patch for the patchwork.[1]

Donald A. Schwartz, M.D.
Associate Professor of Psychiatry
School of Medicine
University of California,
Los Angeles, 1972

Mental health services in the United States constitute a system of care largely separate from the general health care system. Even the locale for treatment of mental illness is usually apart from the setting for care of physical ills. Moreover, mental health services tend to be separated from several other systems intimately concerned with mental health: the welfare, educational, vocational, and judicial systems. Isolation of mental health services from general health care on the one hand, and from welfare, educational, and other developmental programs on the other, is deep-rooted and may reflect the historical fact that care of the mentally ill, unlike most other fields of personal health service, has been largely a public function in the United States.

In mental health services, the public sector provides most of the financing and most of the care, in contrast to the dominance of the private sector in other health services. Of total spending for health in 1968, 37 percent was from public funds and 63 percent from private sources.[2] But of spending for mental health treatment and care during the same period, 65 percent was from public funds and 35 percent was private.[3] The bulk of general health services is furnished by private providers, but public agencies have, even after Medicare, Medicaid, and other federal funding programs offered new options, provided at least two-thirds of the care for mental illness. Thus, almost 90 percent of the $2.7 billion spent for care in psychiatric hospitals in 1968 was spent by and in public hospitals, less than 11 percent in private institutions.[4] Although private insurance is now providing more coverage for mental illness than in the past, public expenditures still vastly exceed private expenditures.[5] As a result of this assumption of the burden for mental illness by public institutions and programs, the relation between public and private sectors that characterizes the general health care system is reversed in the field of mental health.

Nevertheless, although public sponsorship of the majority of programs and resources should predispose toward coordination and integration, the same kinds of fragmentation exist within the mental health system as exist within the general health care system. Like the general health system, the mental health system is composed of categorical and segmented programs for special persons, diseases, and purposes. Divided among the several levels of government, the mental health programs vary in the contribution of each governmental level, depending on the views prevailing with respect to care of the mentally ill at the time each program was added. Differing financing mechanisms entail varied, often inconsistent, prescriptions.

The enormity and the gravity of mental problems are well known. Mental disturbance afflicts an estimated 10 percent of the population,[6] mental retardation 3 percent,[7] alcoholism almost 10 percent of the working population,[8] and drug dependence large proportions. Despite the magnitude of the problems, resources are not only sparse but dissipated because of splintered programs and uncoordinated, piecemeal efforts.

The following analysis of mental health programs follows the almost artificial fragmentation into separate entities that has grown up in the field: mental illness, mental retardation, alcoholism, and drug dependence. A chart of the many agencies and their functions at each level of government in these four fields is attached as Appendix II.

HISTORICAL BACKGROUND

In colonial America, the mentally ill and the mentally retarded were the responsibility of the family. Those who were poor were often thrust into jails and almshouses under appalling conditions. Many were kept hidden at home. In the mid-1700s, the work of Dr. Benjamin Rush initiated a more scientific and humane approach to the mentally ill than had existed before his time. Treatment, as distinguished from confinement, may be said to have begun in 1756, when two voluntary hospitals—Pennsylvania Hospital and New York Hospital—opened their doors to the mentally ill and accepted them in cells separated from the rest of the hospital. The first public hospital devoted entirely to the care of the mentally ill was established in Williamsburg, Virginia, in 1773.[9]

The Mentally Ill—State and Voluntary Efforts

In 1841, Dorothea Lynde Dix, horrified by the indiscriminate mingling of the insane with criminals, began her 40-year crusade for the creation of state institutions for the mentally ill, hospitals that cities and counties could not afford to build, maintain, and staff. By 1855, 32 mental hospitals had been built in the United States. In 1890, the New York Care Act formally established the principle of state financial responsibility for the care and maintenance of the mentally ill, as initiated by Dorothea Dix, impelling the transfer of mental patients from local jails and county poorhouses to special mental institutions.

The states thus assumed responsibility for the mentally ill. But mental hospital populations grew, and patients stayed for long periods, sometimes a lifetime. Overcrowding and miserable conditions were rife. The care provided in the large state institutions that developed between 1825 and 1850 was mainly custodial. In effect, the substandard conditions of local institutions came to be replicated in state mental hospitals.

The Mental Hygiene Movement.   In 1908, the year that Clifford Beers exposed conditions in state and private asylums in *A Mind That Found Itself,* the organized mental hygiene movement began in the United States.[10] Clifford Beers founded the Connecticut Society for Mental Hygiene

[t]o work for the conservation of mental health; help prevent nervous and mental disorders and mental defects; to help raise the standards of care . . .; to secure and disseminate reliable information. . . .[11]

Other state societies followed, and in 1909 the National Committee for Mental Hygiene was formed. Its early activities were addressed to obtaining laws to protect the mentally ill and to establishing minimum standards of care in institutions. It assisted the development of a uniform system of reporting on patients in institutions and of a standard terminology for the classification of mental disorders. In 1917, the Committee published its first annual statistical report, a function assumed in 1923 by the Bureau of the Census, when patients in mental institutions were first counted in the national census. The National Committee undertook a major role in establishing demonstration clinics in many American cities, with support from the Commonwealth Fund.

The National Committee for Mental Hygiene also conducted surveys of mental institutions, a function assumed in 1936 by the Mental Hospital Survey Committee, composed of eight professional and health organizations, including the American Psychiatric Association and the Public Health Service. In 1939, the Public Health Service assumed the survey function entirely. Modern state hospital licensure laws, enacted after 1946, applied to private mental facilities but generally exempted state mental hospitals. In 1948, the American Psychiatric Association established an inspection rating system for mental hospitals, and in 1958 the Joint Commission on Accreditation of Hospitals began to inspect and accredit mental as well as general hospitals.

Federal Role.   The federal government's role in mental health began to develop significantly only in the 1930's.[12] To be sure, certain federal facilities had been built earlier — St. Elizabeth's Hospital in the District of Columbia in 1855 and an Asylum for Insane Indians in South Dakota in 1903; in 1917 a division in the office of the Surgeon General of the Army undertook to screen recruits and to treat mentally ill service personnel. Following World War I, the Veterans Administration provided long-term care for veterans with psychiatric disabilities. Until the close of World War II, federal mental health programs were directed largely to special groups: the military, veterans, merchant seamen, Indians, and residents of the District of Columbia.

For the population as a whole, however, involvement of the federal government in psychiatric services began in a limited way in 1930, when the Public Health Service established a Division of Mental Hygiene, which evolved in 1949 into the National Institute of Mental Health. In the 1930s also, a notable contribution to mental health came through the spending by the Public Works Administration of some $140 million on state and local mental hospital construction, adding more than 60,000 mental beds.[13]

With the passage of the National Mental Health Act of 1946, the federal government "began to treat mental health as a general public health problem."[14] To a considerable degree, this law was a response to the high incidence of mental problems found through the 15 million examinations of Selective Service candidates in World War II. Of the 4,800,000 individuals rejected for service, nearly two million were rejected for neuropsychiatric disorders and mental and educational deficiencies. Mental illness accounted for 856,000 rejections, neurological conditions for 235,000, and mental deficiency for 676,000, making a total of 1,767,000 persons rejected for mental problems as of 1945.[15] These findings were particularly alarming in a young and presumably healthy group. Extrapolated to the general population, they spoke for the enactment of a vastly improved mental health program for the nation.

The new law was designed to widen the scope of mental health programs by expanding the direct involvement of the federal government in research, training, and technical assistance with respect to mental illness and mental retardation and by channeling federal funding to develop services for the mentally ill at the community level.[16] The use of National Mental Health Act funds was specifically prohibited for the support of traditional state activities in mental health. Federal funds under this program were earmarked instead for developing new kinds of services: expansion of central office facilities to enable mental health authorities to carry out basic functions, employment of trained personnel as consultants to or supervisors of state and local health and welfare agencies, development of community psychiatric clinics and preventive programs, training of personnel, and mental health education. In 1946, only 20 states had mental health programs other than state mental hospitals; twenty years later all but three states had developed such programs.[17]

Also in 1946, enactment of the Hill-Burton Hospital Survey and Construction Act provided federal funds for construction of mental facilities and initiated the first federal nationwide survey of hospital beds for the mentally ill.[18] In the 22 years from 1947 to 1969, some $78 million of federal funds aided the construction of 21,000 beds in mental institutions and psychiatric divisions of general hospitals.[19] This expenditure, however, represented little more than two percent of all Hill-Burton spending in that time span.

Community Care of the Mentally Ill. The postwar development of community mental health services took place largely under the aegis of state health departments because the National Mental Health Act of 1946 prohibited states from designating as their mental health authorities those agencies solely responsible for the administration of state mental hospitals, which "had shown little interest in community services."[20] This opportunity for the integration of mental health and public health programs, however, was short-lived. As state mental health departments sought increased visibility for and emphasis on mental health in state governments, the authority of mental health departments came to encompass community mental health services. The separation between public health and mental health became so marked that the New York State Legislature even established separate public health and mental health legislative committees. Thus, instead of combining public health and mental health activities in a unified delivery system, the trend has been to divorce community mental health services from public health services. The alternative route has been pursued of combining the administration of state mental hospitals and community mental health programs in a single mental health agency in an increasing number of states.[21]

While mental health services were thus developing in a system separate from general health services, bold steps were being taken to increase inter-governmental cooperation in mental health services. Programs of state-local community mental health services were enacted in New York State in 1954 and in California in 1957. Under this legislation, local communities were encouraged to develop preventive and therapeutic mental health programs with substantial state subvention, which increased in California from 50 percent in 1957, to 75 percent in 1963, to 90 percent in 1969.[22] As local mental health programs were expanded in California, the community psychiatric clinics operated directly by the State Department of Mental Hygiene were phased out.

Community mental health services would thus have been unified in a locally administered program in California with substantial state cost-sharing had it not been for the development of a new federal stream of activity in community care of the mentally ill. The acute shortcomings in mental health services identified by the Joint Commission on Mental Illness and Health in its 1961 report[23] led to the enactment in 1963 of the Mental Retardation Facilities and Community Mental Health Centers Construction Act, which authorized federal matching grants for the construction of community mental health centers; it was amended in 1965 to provide staffing assistance.[24] The federally funded Community Mental Health Centers were designed to provide comprehensive services in the community in order to prevent hospitalization. Generally sponsored by voluntary and private agencies, these centers were required to serve areas having populations between 75,000 and 200,000 — areas that did not necessarily coincide with other districts for health and welfare services.[25] Moreover, in Los Angeles County, but not in other counties, the federally funded centers were independent of the state-local program of community mental health services, and only one of the 11 centers was a county facility.[26] Thus evolved two separate systems of community mental health care — one deriving its principal funding from the federal government and the other supported by state and county contributions.

The movement for community care of the mentally ill, made possible by development of the tranquilizing and other psychotropic drugs, is an effort to treat mental illness in the same way as physical illness. Similarly, the provision in social insurance and medical assistance programs for some coverage of mental illness is a move, albeit limited,[27] in the same direction.

Mental Retardation Programs

The history of care for the mentally retarded reflects the same limited knowledge, neglect, and segregation that have afflicted the mentally ill until recent years. To the extent that services were developed, they were divided among special classes for the mentally handicapped within the public schools—begun in New Jersey in 1911—mental hygiene clinics serving school children, and state institutions for the care and training of the retarded, often called state schools for the mentally defective.[28]

Voluntary organizations early championed the cause of the retarded. The National Committee on Mental Hygiene formed a Division of Mental Retardation to oppose eugenic sterilization laws. In 1914, the Committee on Provision for the Feebleminded was established to promote residential institutions in place of asylums. After World War II, a national movement emerged as multiple organizations were founded: the American Association for Mental Deficiency, the National Association for Retarded Children, the Exceptional Children's Foundation, the Association for Neurologically Handicapped Children, and many local parents' and citizens' groups.

Protection of the mentally retarded benefited from the strengthening of mental health services following passage of the National Mental Health Act in 1946 and establishment of the National Institute of Mental Health in 1949. The Children's Bureau had long been concerned with the prevention of retardation and with services for the handicapped, but President Kennedy directed national efforts to "an intensive search for solutions to the problems of mental retardation."[29]

The first significant federal aid specifically for the mentally retarded was authorized in 1963 with the passage of the Mental Retardation Facilities and Community Mental Health Centers Construction Act, mentioned above. The Mental Retardation Amendments of 1967 provided staffing grants. Other programs—the hospital improvement program (HIP) and the hospital inservice training program (HIST)—were directed to meet the crisis in residential care for the retarded.[30]

Categorical assistance by the federal government explicitly for the mentally retarded is thus of recent origin. In a short time, however, the health, welfare, and training programs multiplied.[31] By 1969, the National Association of State Mental Health Directors labelled existing federal support of state and local mental retardation programs "fragmented, inflexible, competitive, ill-planned, and unrealistic" and "a mish-mash of competing schemes, dollars, and services."[32] Accordingly, in 1970, in an effort to strengthen and consolidate resources, Congress passed the Developmental Disabilities Services and Facilities Construction Amendments of 1970 providing broad grants for the integrated support of services, facilities, and training needed for the care and treatment of the mentally retarded.[33] This legislation to assist states in providing comprehensive services for the mentally retarded represented recognition that

. . . protective services do not protect when they are rendered by a multiplicity of agencies with ambiguously defined and often overlapping jurisdictions. In our researches, many instances were found in which effective help was denied, not because of failure to recognize need, or even lack of facilities, or of appropriate laws and regulations, but because of uncertainty as to which bureaucratic domain had decision-making authority.[34]

Integrated services for the mentally retarded have also been the goal of state and local governments in California. Faced with intractable waiting lists for the admission of retarded children to state institutions, the state had two choices: to expand its institutions for care of the retarded or to develop a system of community services.[35] In 1965, a legislative committee undertook an investigation of the waiting list problem and found that many mentally retarded persons were inappropriately hospitalized for lack of any alternative and that many families with retarded children desired community placement and facilities.[36] The result was a recommendation that "the state shift its responsibility from the time when the child enters the state hospital to the time when expert diagnosis establishes the fact that special care is needed that the family cannot provide."[37] In order to achieve this early intervention and flexible alternatives, regional diagnostic and counseling centers for the retarded were proposed.[38] Actually, as early as 1963 in Los Angeles County, the Departments of Health, Mental Health, Hospitals, and Public Social Services, the County Superintendent of Schools, and the City Unified School District had entered into a Joint Powers Agreement to form a Mental Retardation Services Board for planning and coordinating services for the retarded.[39] State legislation in 1965 created two pilot regional centers, then additional centers were funded, and the Mental Retardation Services Act of 1969 extended the principle of regional centers for the mentally retarded throughout the state.

Alcoholism Programs

The earliest attack on the problem of alcoholism came from the temperance movement.[40] The formation of Alcoholics Anonymous in the 1930s represented a new, nonmoralistic approach, characterized by mutual aid and self-help.[41] Scientific work began in the 1940s at the Yale Center of Alcohol Studies under the leadership of Dr. E. M. Jellinek, and the first alcohol treatment clinic was established in New Haven in the 1940s.[42] The Yale group helped to organize the National Council on Alcoholism, the leading voluntary organization in this field.

Special state programs on alcoholism were started in the 1940s in Connecticut, Oregon, New Hampshire, and the District of Columbia.[43] By 1967, 40 states had specifically designated programs, about one-fourth of which were organized under independent boards or commissions and the rest in state departments of public health or mental health.[44]

Federal aid for alcoholism programs was provided under several banners: under the 1963 legislation for support of Community Mental Health Centers, which provided treatment for problem drinkers, under the National Highway Safety Act of 1966, which required concern with the drunk driver, and under the Vocational Rehabilitation Act, which expanded its scope to permit inclusion of alcoholics in vocational rehabilitation programs. In 1970, the National Center for the Control of Alcoholism was established within the National Institute of Mental Health to coordinate and foster research and services related to alcoholism.[45]

At the state level, treatment of alcoholics has long been provided in governmental facilities, particularly state mental hospitals and general hospitals operated by local government. In 1970-71, 7,331 alcoholics were admitted to state mental institutions in California, for a total of 277,600 days of treatment.[46] During the same year, some 50,128 days of care were provided for alcoholics in local alcoholism programs under the aegis of the State Department of Mental Hygiene.[47] These were in addition to the alcoholics treated by the State Department of Rehabilitation under the so-called McAteer program mentioned below. In the major counties, admissions for alcoholism as a proportion of total admissions to state mental institutions in 1971 varied by county from a high of 52 percent to a low of 8.9 percent.[48]

Based on earlier local programs, the state outpatient alcoholic rehabilitation program of California began in 1954 with appointment of the California Alcoholic and Rehabilitation Commission.[49] Following its recommendations, a division of alcoholism was established within the State Department of Public Health in 1957. In 1961, this Division, in conjunction with the State Department of Mental Hygiene, developed the model of community-centered alcoholism rehabilitation programs that was to form the basis for subsequent services. A year-long study of the state's alcoholism work by the State Department of Public Health led to passage in 1965 of the McAteer-Rumford-Marks Act for support of a comprehensive state-local program to combat alcoholism. For four years the program operated on a year-to-year basis until in 1969 it was renewed by the Legislature without a terminal date.[50] At the state level, the program was administered at different times by the Departments of Public Health and Rehabilitation in order to qualify for maximum federal funding. At the local level, administrative responsibility for the operation of alcoholic rehabilitation clinics and for the coordination of all community efforts on alcoholism was assigned to county health departments.

Control of Drug Dependence

The early history of the control of drug dependence in the United States was shaped by stringent federal legislation regulating the production, sale, and prescription of narcotics.[51] The trust was punitive, not medical. Under the Harrison Narcotics Licensing Act, medical prescription of maintenance doses of narcotics for therapeutic purposes or even for research was effectively banned.[52] Consequently, treatment for drug addiction was largely hospital-based in facilities specially equipped and authorized to treat such cases.

In 1929, Congress established a Narcotics Division within the Public Health Service, provided aid to the states for the treatment of addicts, and authorized the construction of two federal treatment centers at Lexington, Kentucky and Fort Worth, Texas.[53] In 1944, Public Health Service hospitals were authorized to treat drug addicts. An Interdepartmental Committee on Narcotics, appointed by President Truman in 1951, stressed the need for control over narcotics distribution; and in response to a letter of President Eisenhower, two study committees of this Interdepartmental Committee in 1954 urged increased training for enforcement, development of hospital and related facilities by state and local governments, and revised commitment laws.[54]

In 1961, the voluntary American Social Health Association, in preparation for the White House Conference on Narcotic and Drug Abuse, found a total of 57 programs for treatment or rehabilitation conducted by governmental agencies, 42 programs conducted by nongovernmental agencies, and 33 states with no treatment or rehabilitation program of any kind.[55] In opening the White House Conference in 1962, President Kennedy stressed two objectives: elimination of illicit traffic in drugs and rehabilitation of the drug addict.[56] This conference marked the beginning of a new era, in which concern with treatment and rehabilitation of drug addicts would be at least as important as concern with law enforcement.

In 1966, Congress passed the Narcotics Addict Rehabilitation Act, which permitted addicts to apply for voluntary treatment and provided support for demonstrations of community treatment of drug addiction.[57] Six demonstration centers were authorized, with substantial federal funding for both construction and operation, to provide inpatient and outpatient services, emergency services, consultation, and education and to arrange for halfway houses. In 1970, the Comprehensive Drug Abuse Prevention and Control Act authorized vastly expanded programs of treatment and rehabilitation. In an unusual example of integrated programs, Congress directed the increased funding for community facilities for drug abuse, education on drug abuse, and rehabilitation projects not to some new agency but to the federal Community Mental Health Centers established under the 1963 legislation. A separate Drug Abuse Educational Act in 1970 provided for educational projects in the schools.

In 1972, the Drug Abuse Office and Treatment Act further expanded federal funding for prevention, treatment, and rehabilitation.[58] A Special Action Office for Drug Abuse Prevention in the executive office of the President was assigned authority to coordinate all federal programs, with the significant exception of those in the field of law enforcement. A National Advisory Council for Drug Abuse Prevention and a "comprehensive coordinated long-term federal strategy" for activities concerned with prevention of drug abuse and drug traffic were mandated. In the effort to increase access to services, the statute requires all states to include programs of drug abuse prevention and treatment in state public health plans.

MENTAL ILLNESS

Several factors have combined to produce fragmented programs to combat mental illness.

First are social attitudes. From time immemorial, the mentally ill have been ostracized and confined away from society. Although the mentally ill are no longer considered pariahs, this attitude persists in various endeavors and in public funding.

Second, the magnitude of the problem of mental illness leads to fragmented programs. An estimated 19 million persons in the United States — one in every ten — have some kind of mental or emotional disorder requiring psychiatric care.[59] Among children and youth under 25 years of age, 10 to 12 percent have major psychological problems; of these, an estimated 2 to 3 percent suffer from mental illness, including psychoses and severe disorders, and another 8 to 10 percent have serious emotional disabilities.[60] Such estimates tend to be paralyzing. They suggest that the large numbers of persons served by preventive, therapeutic, and rehabilitative programs may represent only the tip of the iceberg. The magnitude of the problem raises the critical question of how to define the public responsibility.

Third is the traditional separation of the care of the mentally ill from the care of the physically ill, in part because of the complex behavioral manifestations of mental illness. Insufficient knowledge of the causes of mental illness, lack of a demonstrable pathology, and many unknowns in therapeutics perpetuate this separation.[61] Moreover, the drive for specialization, which characterizes health services generally, has reinforced not only separation of the mental health field but separation of each subdivision of the mental health field from the others.

Fourth, mental illness has tangled behavioral and social components and consequences, which involve agencies outside the mental health or public health fields.[62] Social, educational, correctional, judicial, commercial, and religious organizations all participate. Each group has its separate mission and approach.

Fifth, as new needs are perceived or defects in old approaches uncovered, new programs are devised. New programs rarely build on old ones. They make a new place for themselves, create new administrative bureaucracies, and vie with old ones for scarce funds. This pattern characterizes all health services, but in the field of mental health it is compounded by differing and changing philosophies and purposes in care of the mentally ill. The pendulum has swung from confinement in local almshouses and jails for those who could not afford private care to state mental hospitals. As these turned into custodial institutions, isolated from society and providing minimal treatment, and with the revolution in treatment of the mentally ill made possible by the psychotropic drugs, the pendulum has swung back to care in the community but with massive federal funding. Each new phase has entailed a new set of programs superimposed upon the old or existing side by side.

Federal Programs

Federal programs for the care of the mentally ill may be divided into those providing direct services, those providing program development, and those providing payment for care. Programs for support of research and training of personnel have been discussed generally in Chapter 2.

Direct Services. Four separate departments or agencies provide direct mental health services to defined populations: the Veterans Administration, the Department of Defense, the Indian Health Service, and the Federal Health Programs Services.

The Veterans Administration provides a range of mental health services in its own facilities, including outpatient and emergency services, acute or rehabilitative psychiatric hospital services, long-term residential care, and social services for mentally and emotionally disabled veterans. Recently, the Veterans Administration has begun to substitute placement in community facilities for long-term psychiatric treatment in its own facilities, with counseling and social casework services provided on an outpatient basis by its own staff (see below under "Payment for Care").

The Department of Defense is also involved in treatment of mental illness through its network of base hospitals in the United States and abroad. Within the Department of Health, Education, and Welfare are two direct service programs. The Indian Health Service conducts programs for mental illness among Indians. The Federal Health Programs Service administers St. Elizabeth's Hospital and clinics in Washington, D.C., the two federal narcotics hospitals, the Public Health Service Hospitals that have provided treatment for the Coast Guard and others and may now become phased out, the preventive mental health programs for federal employees, including some diagnostic and therapeutic services in places where large numbers of federal employees work.

Program Development. Support for mental health programs, including planning, coordination, and funding, is provided by three federal departments. The Office of Economic Opportunity provides support for the care and treatment of the mentally ill in two ways: through support of its comprehensive neighborhood health centers, some of which have been transferred to the Department of Health, Education, and Welfare, and through its project grants for mental health in poverty communities. The Department of Housing and Urban Development supports mental health services through its Model Cities program. The guidelines of this program permit local projects related to teen-age and family counseling, drug dependence services, and alcoholism rehabilitation. Although mental health services have not been a priority for the Model Cities program nationally, some local communities have assigned priority to the mental health needs of low-income neighborhoods.

The largest and most varied programs for treatment and rehabilitation of the mentally ill emanate from the several major administrations of the Department of Health, Education, and Welfare. These include programs for Community Mental Health Centers, general local mental health services, improvements in state mental hospitals, child mental health services, and educational, welfare, and rehabilitation services of various kinds.

Within the Health Services and Mental Health Administration, the National Institute of Mental Health, aided by a 12-member National Advisory Mental Health Council, provides construction and staffing grants to the states, which have resulted in the establishment of 452 Community Mental Health Centers as of 1972. They may provide ten services, five of which are mandatory: outpatient care, inpatient care, partial hospitalization, emergency psychiatric services, and community education and consultation. The centers may be either public or nonprofit agencies, free-standing or hospital-based facilities. The majority are voluntary clinics and agencies.

The concept of Community Mental Health Centers was a significant step forward, and Congress channelled much of its support for various kinds of mental health services through the centers in a unified way. The 1970 amendments to the Mental Retardation and Community Mental Health Centers Construction Act of 1963 provided supplementary grants to the centers for specified child mental health services, and separate legislation provided grants to the centers for alcoholism and drug dependence programs. Jurisdictional problems developed, however, between the federally funded Community Mental Health Centers program, on the one hand, and other federal, state, and local mental health programs, on the other. These problems, which may be particularly pronounced in Los Angeles County, relate to the noncongruent geographic districts for services, defeating the best efforts at comprehensive services, and the differing philosophies and priorities of the federal, state, and local programs.[63]

Other community mental health services are supported by other federal programs. The Health Service Delivery Group of the National Institute of Mental Health within the Health Services and Mental Health Administration (HSMHA) administers 314(d) formula grants to the states under the Comprehensive Health Planning program. Under this legislation each state is required to allocate 15 percent of its total formula grant to mental health services. The Community Health Service of HSMHA administers 314(e) project grants for 55 comprehensive health service centers, 20 family health centers, and a number of migrant health centers, each of which provides some mental health services as part of its overall program. To the extent that mental health services are provided through these various kinds of centers, this effort tends to overcome fragmentation.

Other programs within the National Institute of Mental Health provide grants to improve services and staffing of state hospitals for the mentally ill and retarded. The Hospital Improvement Program (HIP) and the Hospital Inservice Training Program (HIST) are such programs.

Child mental health services are supported through a separate constellation of programs. The Maternal and Child Health Service, a separate agency within HSMHA, administers grants to the states for preventive maternal and child health services, comprehensive maternity and infant care projects (MIC) and children and youth projects (C and Y), and crippled children's services. The same unit has responsibility for the administration of special staffing grants, mentioned above, to the federal Community Mental Health Centers to strengthen child mental health services.

Three separate offices within the Department of Health, Education, and Welfare provide supportive services that contribute significantly to the mental health of children. The Office of Education administers a variety of programs for the mentally retarded, the mentally handicapped, and other children with behavioral disorders through the Bureau of Education for the Handicapped. These include formula grants to state educational agencies and special project grants for demonstration services. Other educational programs, such as the Elementary and Secondary Education Act (ESEA), provide supplementary support for low-income priority areas, including special educational services, facilities, and resources for mentally or behaviorally handicapped children. The Office of Child Development, which has assumed responsibility for the nonmedical programs of the former Children's Bureau, administers a number of programs that contribute to the mental health of children, such as Head Start, day care centers, and early education programs The Office of Juvenile Delinquency Programs and Prevention, although oriented toward the correctional system, administers programs to prevent juvenile delinquency, which include special counseling services and "rap" centers for adolescents.

In the field of rehabilitation of the mentally ill, the Social and Rehabilitation Service (SRS) of the Department of Health, Education, and Welfare operates separately from both the Health Services and Mental Health Administration, which administers most of the health care programs for the mentally ill, and from the Office of Education, which administers the educational programs. Within the SRS, the Rehabilitation Services Administration is responsible for specific programs for the mentally retarded, discussed below. In a rare example of integration, the same unit also administers grants to the states for the rehabilitation of a broad range of persons: the mentally retarded, the emotionally and socially handicapped, and also the physically handicapped.

Payment for Care. The major federal programs paying for care for mental illness are Medicare, administered by the Social Security Administration of the Department of Health, Education, and Welfare (HEW), Medicaid, administered by the Social and Rehabilitation Service of HEW, and the Civilian Health and Medical Program of the Uniformed Services (CHAMPUS), administered by the Department of Defense. In addition, programs that provide direct services may pay for care by other providers; other federal programs purchase care for special groups; and still other programs make welfare or disability payments that may be used to buy care.

In marked contrast to its treatment of physical illness, Medicare provides limited benefits for mental illness, both in hospitalization and in physician's services. Inpatient care in psychiatric hospitals is limited to 190 days during a person's lifetime in contrast to support for services in each benefit period for physical illness. A further fragmenting distinction is made between care for the mentally ill in psychiatric hospitals and in general hospitals. The 190-day lifetime limit does not apply to psychiatric care in general hospitals; the patient is entitled there to the same benefits as for physical illness. Under the Supplementary Medical Insurance for physician's services, Part B of Medicare, the mentally ill aged person is limited to $250 for psychiatric outpatient visits, but this limitation does not apply to inhospital psychiatric visits, thus encouraging hospitalization.

Only a minute fraction of Medicare funds goes for treating mental illness, and this largely in the hospital setting. In 1969, Medicare paid approximately $93 million for psychiatric care of the aged, 1.4 percent of its total expenditures of $6.6 billion in that year.[64] Of the $88 million spent for hospital care, 70 percent went to general hospitals and 30 percent to psychiatric hospitals. Only $5 million went for psychiatric services outside the hospital setting, and other services, including nursing home care, were negligible. Further, the requirement that a beneficiary, on completion of a benefit period of 90 days in a hospital, must be out of the hospital 60 continuous days before another hospital benefit period can begin "in practice would preclude extended inpatient psychiatric care under Medicare."[65] A reflection of the limited psychiatric outpatient care provided to the aged is the fact that in

1967 only 0.2 percent of enrollees — some 36,000 persons — received outpatient psychiatric services and total charges came to $2.6 million or about 0.3 percent of total Medicare reimbursements.[66]

Medicaid, although a highly fragmented program, furnishes more aid for mental illness of the aged than does Medicare. Medicaid is fragmented by federal and state jurisdictions and varies by state participation. It is divided by welfare categories and eligibility requirements, by income levels, and by divisions of services and benefits. In addition, under the Long Amendment to Title XIX of the Social Security Act, hospitalization in state mental hospitals and skilled nursing homes of mentally ill Medicaid beneficiaries is restricted to persons over 65. In no other medical service under Medicaid does this age discrimination occur. Further, only 35 states had adopted the Long Amendment by January 1, 1970, so that in the other states the Medicaid program does not reimburse state mental hospitals for care of Medicaid eligibles.[67]

Medicaid provides certain mental health services without regard to age: hospitalization in general hospitals, outpatient mental treatment in clinics sometimes including qualified Community Mental Health Centers, physician's services including psychiatric services, skilled nursing home care, services in free-standing clinics, and prescribed drugs out of hospital. These services are available, to varying degrees, according to state limitations, for treatment of the mentally ill, since Medicaid prohibits the states from differentiating or excluding services on the basis of diagnosis. But this general proscription does not prevent other state limitations and restrictions. Thus, in 1970, only 30 states provided payments for clinical services, including psychiatric services.[68] One state does not cover outpatient psychiatric care, one pays only for evaluation, and three set low monetary limits on psychiatric services. Alternatives to psychiatry, such as psychological services, psychiatric social work, and family, individual, or group therapy, are even more limited. Services of clinical psychologists are not covered in 42 states, and another three limit the services of psychologists to diagnosis and testing.[69] This variability of the Medicaid program means that in many states the mentally ill receive few, if any, benefits under the program. Enactment of P.L. 92-603 in 1972 permits payment for institutional care of mentally ill children up to age 21 but restricts length of stay for other mentally ill persons.

Under CHAMPUS, a program serving 2.3 million beneficiaries in 1970, the Department of Defense provides outpatient care and hospitalization for mentally ill dependents of military personnel and has a special program for mentally retarded and physically handicapped dependents. Long-term residential or institutional care and rehabilitation services are covered under a special benefit portion of this insurance program. Facilities of the Department of Defense generally do not provide these services. They are usually purchased by eligible families, with reimbursement through the appropriate fiscal intermediary. In 1968, the Department of Defense spent more than

$60,000,000 for mental health services under the CHAMPUS program, the bulk of it for services in general hospitals.[70]

Other federal programs purchase services for mental illness. The Indian Service purchases some care. In its effort on behalf of mentally ill veterans to purchase care in the community that meets its standards, the Veterans Administration functions as a separate mental health placement agency in competition with other agencies in the community for the limited number of approved facilities. Since the Veterans Administration is generally able to reimburse providers at a slightly higher rate than some other public agencies, the fragmented system creates inequities in residential care for the mentally ill.

In addition to programs that pay for care for mental illness, some federal programs provide pension disability or welfare benefits that are used by the beneficiary to finance care for mental illness. An estimated 160,000 noninstitutionalized veterans under 64 years of age were receiving veterans' disability pensions for mental illness in 1968.[71] Approximately 650,000 mentally ill persons were receiving disability benefits for mental illness under the federal Railroad Retirement, Civil Service, and Social Security Disability programs.[72] About 22 percent of the persons receiving Social Security Disability benefits—47 percent of those eligible for worker's disability and 15 percent of those receiving childhood disability benefits—qualify for these benefits on the basis of mental illness or mental retardation.[73] The proportion of these federal funds used to buy psychiatric treatment, nursing home care, or other services for mental illness, while undoubtedly high, is not known because the benefits are paid to the individual in cash for his own use.

A long-standing inequity of fragmentation has been partially corrected by the extension of the Medicare program in 1972 to cover the disabled.[74] Formerly, persons who received cash benefits for disability under the Social Security Disability program were not eligible for medical benefits, despite their demonstrated need, whereas the disabled covered by other federal programs were also eligible for medical benefits.

Welfare payments under the categorical aid programs—Aid to the Totally and Permanently Disabled (ATD), the Child Welfare Service and Aid to Families of Dependent Children (AFDC), Aid to the Blind (AB), and Old Age Security (OAS)—may also be used for mental health care. These programs are administered by state and local governments, but the Social and Rehabilitation Service of the Department of Health, Education, and Welfare is responsible for various aspects of the programs through two units. Its Community Services Administration (CSA) handles program development, setting of standards, and monitoring of services. Its Assistance Payments Administration (APA) handles the separate financial assistance program.

Although these programs are primarily social welfare rather than mental health programs, eligibility is determined in part by conditions that require mental health services. The aged may be eligible because of mental disabilities, particularly senility, and the permanently disabled because of mental, emotional, or neurological disabilities. Children may be eligible for out-of-home placement or social services because of mental or emotional disturbance or mental retardation. The financial assistance grants provided under these categorical welfare programs, however, are solely cash payments to eligible persons. These programs do not contain even the limited measures of quality control provided in the Medicare and Medicaid programs. Consequently, both the mentally disabled and the aged are placed and maintained in community facilities at governmental expense with minimal controls on the quality of care and, except in the child welfare services, with little guarantee of therapeutic or rehabilitative services.

State Programs

State programs for care of the mentally ill, like those at the federal level, are segmented, specialized, and administered by multiple agencies. In California, eight state departments and agencies share responsibility in this field. Merger of the major state departments concerned with health services in a single state agency in 1973 provides the opportunity for reducing this fragmentation.

The State Department of Mental Hygiene carries the main responsibility for mental health services. It operates the eight state mental hospitals and develops the State Plan for Mental Health. Funds designated for mental health services under the Comprehensive Health Planning program are allocated in accordance with priorities of the state plan. The Department reviews county plans as a basis for allocating funds. It reviews applications for the construction and staffing grants for federal Community Mental Health Centers and comments on their programs.

The Department of Mental Hygiene licenses certain psychiatric facilities: private mental hospitals, clinics, residential facilities, day care facilities, some board and care homes, and schools and homes for the mentally retarded. But licensing is fragmented. The Department of Public Health licenses general hospitals with psychiatric units, nursing homes, and alcoholism facilities. The Department of Social Welfare licenses still other facilities, including most board and care homes. Each of the three departments conducts its licensing function with emphasis on its own concerns. The standards of the three state departments also differ from criteria of other public agencies for approval of homes for placement of patients.

Most importantly, the State Department of Mental Hygiene administers an innovative program of community mental health services established under the Lanterman–Petris–Short Act of 1969. This legislation combines a new system of mental hospital admissions with a new program of local mental health services. It is designed to organize and finance community mental health services in every county through locally administered and locally controlled programs and to integrate state and community mental health programs into a single system with a uniform ratio of state and local financing.[75]

To carry out this cooperative state–local program, the legislation provides for a single state appropriation for state mental hospitals and community mental health programs, although separate budgets are maintained for certain purposes. Most importantly, community mental health services are financed 90 percent by the state and 10 percent by the county above patient fees and other revenues. Every county is required to participate in the program and to submit a plan for mental health services to the state; counties are then reimbursed for 90 percent of net costs of the approved plan. As part of this plan, counties assume financial responsibility for hospitalization of their indigent residents in state-operated facilities.

This imaginative program, designed to substitute active care in the community for long-term hospitalization, seems on the road to achieving its objective. In 1968–1969, community mental health programs accounted for less than one-third of the total budget for mental illness; in 1971–1972, more than half of the total budget of $275 million, or $140 million, was spent on community mental health programs.[76] In the three years since the program was launched, the census of California's state mental hospitals has declined from 16,116 on June 30, 1969, to 8,235 on June 30, 1972.[77]

Four jurisdictional consequences of this state–local mental health program are apparent. First, the shift of services from state mental hospitals to care in the community has imposed enormous strains on local resources and revealed serious inadequacies in numbers and kinds of alternatives to hospitalization.[78] Second, throughout the state, cities have endeavored, through their zoning regulations, to keep psychiatric facilities, either acute or long-term, out of residential areas, that is, out of the settings deemed vital for the rehabilitation and return to normal functioning of the mentally ill. As a result, in many counties and cities treatment facilities have been segregated in commercial or industrial areas, where recreational, educational, and social opportunities are limited.[79] Third, discrepancies in salary scales for psychiatrists and other personnel under state and county civil service systems have created competition for personnel.[80] Robbing Peter to pay Paul was a direct result of lack of integration. Fourth, despite the establishment of a single system of care for the mentally ill and uniform state financing of 90 percent of local mental health programs, persistence of local differences in attitudes towards mental health and in local tax bases results in wide disparity in the kinds of services available throughout the state. The difference is as much as

500 percent in per capita combined local and state budgets for mental health—from San Francisco's highest per capita of $26 to Orange County's lowest of $5.12 in 1969-1970.[81]

The State Department of Public Health also has significant responsibilities for mental health. Through its Bureau of Facility Planning and Construction, it administers funding for the construction of mental health facilities under the Hill-Burton program and the program for the construction of Community Mental Health Centers. Its Bureau of Health Facilities Licensing and Certification is responsible for licensure of hospitals (except psychiatric hospitals), nursing homes, intermediate care facilities, and other facilities such as day care centers for the mentally retarded. The need to incorporate psychiatric, psychological, and social considerations in the licensing standards of the Department of Public Health is heightened by the high percentage of patients admitted to general hospitals for psychiatric-related conditions[82] and the considerable payments under both Medicare and Medicaid to nursing homes for treatment of mental disorders.[83] Hopefully, the dichotomy between mental and physical illness embedded in the licensing standards for facilities will be remedied by the consolidated department of health.

Also within the Department of Public Health, the State Comprehensive Health Planning Council is required to approve construction of all facilities for mental illness licensed by the State Departments of Public Health and Mental Hygiene. The Council must also review the State Plan for Mental Health, developed by the Department of Mental Hygiene, and the plan for Community Mental Health Centers, developed by the Department of Public Health. Another separate program concerned with mental health within the Department of Public Health is the primary prevention work of the Bureau of Maternal and Child Health, which develops standards for preschool and infant day care centers and sponsors local prenatal, well-child, and family planning programs.

The State Department of Health Care Services provides limited reimbursement for private psychiatric services to eligible beneficiaries under the California Medicaid program. It also reimburses organized psychiatric services, such as Community Mental Health Centers, that meet its standards.

The State Department of Social Welfare has multiple responsibilities in the field of mental health, even though its former direct services for patients discharged from state mental hospitals have been transferred to the Alternate Care Services Unit of the Department of Mental Hygiene, which contracts with the counties. The Department of Social Welfare certifies family care, board and care, and other residential facilities used by recipients of federal disability payments. It develops standards and guidelines and monitors the categorical programs: Aid to the Totally Disabled, Old Age Security, Aid to Families with Dependent Children, Aid to the Blind, and the Child Welfare

Services programs. Administered by county welfare departments, these programs are financed by the federal and state governments with variable matching for services and for financial assistance.

The Department of Social Welfare has long licensed residential care boarding homes for the aged over 65 and a variety of residential and family care homes for children, including mentally retarded and disturbed children. In some instances, actual inspection and approval of facilities are delegated to county welfare departments. In 1970, legislation was passed requiring that residential care facilities for persons aged 16 to 64 be licensed. Closing this gap in the licensure of board and care facilities means that all mentally and physically disabled persons will be entitled to certain minimal standards in board and care facilities. These standards relate to physical requirements, safety, nutrition, and social, recreational, and religious resources. But if welfare assistance payments made by the various programs are inadequate to enable these facilities to meet the standards required for licensure, then unlicensed facilities will be used and the intent of the new licensing law will be thwarted.

The State Department of Rehabilitation prepares the State Plan for Rehabilitation Services and Facilities required for participation in the federal vocational rehabilitation services program. Adults who are disabled by mental or emotional disorders or mental retardation are eligible for evaluation, counseling, training, and rehabilitation provided by the Department through its district offices and special workshop facilities or through cooperative programs with some state mental hospitals. No overall policy has been established to enable clients of the Department of Rehabilitation to receive outpatient services from county mental health agencies, except insofar as individual rehabilitation counselors have personally established referral arrangements.

The State Department of Education is responsible for developing guidelines and assisting local districts with special education programs for mentally retarded and emotionally disturbed children. These programs may include separate schools or facilities, such as the Developmental Centers for Handicapped Minors, and special classes and courses of instruction, some provided at home and at hospitals. Like health programs, these education programs are financed through a variety of reimbursement mechanisms. School districts must arrange for diagnosis and evaluation of children for placement in these programs. Two State Diagnostic Schools for Neurologically Handicapped Children provide extensive evaluation as a specialized resource for local school districts.

The State Department of Corrections and the California Youth Authority also provide treatment for mental and emotional problems. Both agencies provide psychological evaluation, psychiatric treatment, and hospital care in their own facilities or, if necessary, wards can be sent to state mental hospitals for more thorough or specialized care. Both agencies also provide outpatient psychiatric and counseling services to parolees through purchase of services from community clinics and service centers.

Local Programs

Mental health services at the local level are a combination of programs sponsored and administered by local agencies—counties, cities, and school districts—and of public programs and private services, which may be provided or financed by higher levels of government. Although the following description of local programs for the treatment of mental illness concerns principally those programs that are locally sponsored and administered, the impact in a local area of federal and state programs must be mentioned for a true picture of total services available.

In Los Angeles County, the Veterans Hospital and its outpatient clinics provide services for mentally ill veterans, although the main psychiatric facility has reduced its inpatient census from 2,000 to 500 through a community placement drive. Similarly, Medicare, CHAMPUS, and other programs purchase services from local providers. Twelve federally assisted Community Mental Health Centers serve specified catchment areas. The State Department of Mental Hygiene operates state hospitals for local residents who are mentally ill and mentally retarded. The State Department of Education operates a Diagnostic School for the Neurologically Handicapped. The Neuropsychiatric Institute of the University of California provides highly specialized services in addition to its functions in research and training. The state also provides direct services within the county through local offices of the State Department of Rehabilitation, the Alternate Care Services Unit of the State Department of Mental Hygiene, the Parole and Community Services Division of the State Department of Corrections, and the California Youth Authority.

Approximately ten local governmental agencies are involved in some aspect of provision of services for the mentally ill (prior to formation of a consolidated county department of health services in September 1972). The County Department of Mental Health has the principal responsibility for planning and providing mental health services in the county. It prepares and administers the annual Plan for Mental Health Services, which is reviewed by the County Mental Health Advisory Board and approved by both the County Board of Supervisors and the State Department of Mental Hygiene. In accordance with the plan and its priorities, the County Department identifies, develops, and coordinates all public and private resources to provide ten basic services to the mentally disordered, mentally retarded, and persons afflicted with alcoholism. These services are (1) inpatient services, (2) outpatient services, (3) partial hospitalization, such as day care, night care, week-end care, (4) 24-hour emergency psychiatric services, (5) consultation and education for public and private agencies and information to the general public, (6) diagnostic services, (7) rehabilitative services, including vocational and educational programs, (8) precare and aftercare services in the community, including foster home placement, home visiting, and halfway houses, (9) training, and (10) research and evaluation.

The County Department of Mental Health carries out this large order through two main mechanisms — through contracts with public and private agencies and through direct provision of services. Initiated in 1962, county contracts with both public and private agencies cover a wide variety of mental health services. The Department contracts for 24-hour emergency psychiatric services, inpatient and outpatient care, partial hospitalization, and screening and diagnostic services with the County Department of Hospitals. It contracts with the County Probation Department for diagnostic and outpatient care and also for some residential care for juvenile wards. It contracts with state mental hospitals for inpatient care for residents of the county. Other basic community mental health services are provided by contract with the federally funded Community Mental Health Centers. Services are also provided by contracts with other voluntary and private agencies, including child guidance clinics. By 1970, the contract mechanism had become so widely used that some private agencies came to look upon public funding as their inalienable right.[84] Use of contract services involves fundamental issues, such as public accountability of private agencies operating under governmental contracts, difficulty of supervising services provided under contract, use of public funds to permit private agencies to hire personnel at rates higher than those public agencies are permitted to pay under civil service regulations, and lack of assurance that the persons in greatest need of care and unable to obtain it elsewhere will have priority.[85] In the effort to assure equity and public accountability in the provision of services, the Department has established certain principles that must govern future contracts.[86]

In recent years, also, in order to assure the availability of essential services to all county residents, the County Department of Mental Health has expanded direct provision of services. Outpatient psychiatric diagnosis, evaluation, treatment, counseling, emergency services, consultation to agencies, and public information and education are provided directly by clinics of the Department. Although services vary in accordance with community needs and availability of care from other providers, the Department requires that services be provided on a decentralized basis, that regional service boundaries be based on communities and neighborhoods, and that each region provide a combination of services, including prevention, treatment, community organization, and mental health education.[87] In its effort to achieve an integrated system of mental health and other personal health services, the Department emphasizes interagency relationships. From the start, the 12 mental health regions of the County Department of Mental Health were made congruent with the boundaries of local public health districts.

The County Department of Hospitals provides outpatient, inpatient, and emergency psychiatric services at three county general hospitals. In addition, the county operates a chronic disease hospital, where some care for mental illness is provided, and a rehabilitation center for long-term treatment and residential care of alcoholics and other mentally and physically disabled male patients referred by state and county agencies. These facilities serve as primary resources for the direct services provided by the county mental health regional offices. Financing for the services of the Department of Hospitals comes from the county budget, Medicare, Medi-Cal, private insurance, patient fees, and contracts with the County Department of Mental Health.

The County Health Department is concerned with mental health services on three levels.[88] On the level of primary prevention, the Health Department provides prenatal, well-child, family planning, health education, and nutritional services, all of which have significant potential for preventing and identifying mental problems. On the level of secondary prevention, public health nurses, social workers, and sanitarians are all involved in casefinding, referral, and provision of services. Tertiary prevention is conducted by 60 public health nurses who provide aftercare services for patients discharged from mental hospitals.[89] Cooperation with the County Department of Mental Health has been secured through an interagency committee on mental health, but a professional review of the program of the Health Department in 1969 recommended a number of measures to strengthen coordination between the two departments and to improve services.[90] Establishment of the unified County Department of Health Services will enhance the capability of assuring access to mental health services through a decentralized system of outpatient care.

The County Department of Public Social Services performs many functions related to mental health. It administers cash assistance for the mentally ill and retarded. It determines eligibility for the Medi-Cal and county general relief programs for persons who are mentally disabled. It places the mentally ill or retarded in board and care homes. Two units of the Department — Protective Services and Child Welfare Services — assist children who are neglected, battered, or in need of supportive care because of family instability or disability, as well as children who are mentally retarded or mentally handicapped who cannot be cared for adequately by the family. Another unit — Child Care Services — seeks to enforce through licensure of facilities a standard of care that will contribute to the mental, emotional, social, and intellectual development of all children placed in family care, foster care, day care, or other temporary out-of-home care. Social workers in the Aid to the Totally Disabled program provide essential casework assistance to mentally disabled or physically handicapped and dependent adults.

The Department also operates a Central Registry for Boarding Homes for the Aged and for other board and care facilities to aid social workers and the public in locating residential care facilities for the elderly and the disabled. The same facilities, including the recently licensed board and care homes for persons aged 16 to 64, are licensed largely by the State Department of Social Welfare. Neither the county registry nor state licensure requires even minimal mental health services in these facilities. Board and care homes are not required to assure access to psychiatric or psychological consultation nor to provide a therapeutic or rehabilitative program of any kind.[91] This gap in care may be partially explained by division of responsibility between welfare and health agencies.

Other county departments and agencies provide services for the mentally ill as well. The County Probation Department provides psychiatric and psychological evaluation and counseling for its wards. It places juveniles in family care homes or residential facilities, and it operates residential treatment institutions itself. The County Sheriff's Department authorizes emergency treatment and evaluation for involuntary patients. The Superior Court reviews hospitalization of involuntary patients, monitors the duration and appropriateness of treatment, and protects the rights of patients. The District Attorney's office provides representation for patients before the court. County mental health counselors assist both patients and the court. The County Public Administrator serves as guardian for some persons unable to handle their affairs. The Comprehensive Health Planning agency serving the county has a standing committee on mental health and mental retardation and participates in the review and approval of the construction of mental health facilities.

In addition to the local health, welfare, and law enforcement agencies involved in provision of services for the mentally ill, the county and city school systems provide child development services, especially for children with emotional and mental problems, and training for the mentally retarded. Both the County Superintendent of Schools and the City School Districts conduct special education classes for the handicapped, arrange counseling services for parents and children, provide consultation to teachers, and operate special facilities, such as Developmental Centers for Handicapped Minors. Actual treatment for mental and emotional problems is provided by community facilities.

Provision of mental health services to school children is thus divided between community agencies and the school system. Within the school system, special educational programs are the responsibility of independent school districts and may be operated by a single school district, jointly sponsored by two or more districts, provided through a contract with another district, or arranged through the Office of the County Superintendent of Schools. Thus, the scope, nature, and quality of child development, mental health, and mental retardation services vary greatly among the 96 school districts in Los Angeles County.[92] The trend toward additional state financing of education may help to correct this among other inequities in services associated with multiple local school districts.

Voluntary Agencies

Among the numerous voluntary agencies contributing to care of the mentally ill, the National Association for Mental Health, with its nearly 1,000 chapters throughout the country and more than a million volunteers, is the oldest and most powerful. It has four main functions: support of research on the causes, treatment, and prevention of mental illness, enactment of humane and sound legislation, education of professionals and the public about mental illness, and provision of services to patients with emphasis on community services and rehabilitation.

In California, other voluntary groups function at various levels. For example, the Citizens' Advisory Council is a voluntary organization established by the Legislature to advise and assist the State Department of Mental Hygiene on the development of the five-year state plan for mental health and on the system of priorities to be followed, to review all mental health services, to propose rules and regulations for administration of mental health services, and to encourage regional coordination of resources.[93] The California Conference of Local Mental Health Directors, also established by statute to advise the State Department of Mental Hygiene, consists of the directors and program chiefs of county and three city community mental health programs in California.[94]

At the local level, the Los Angeles County Mental Health Advisory Board has statutory authority to review the County Plan for Mental Health. In addition, the Mental Health Development Commission, created by the Los Angeles Welfare Planning Council and charged with responsibility for implementing recommendations of a major study of mental health services in Los Angeles County,[95] has functioned for more than a decade in the planning and development of mental health facilities and services. The Mental Health Association of Los Angeles County performs an important role in public education, development of mental health policy, and surveillance of services. In addition, other voluntary agencies such as United Way, the Council of Community Mental Health Centers, and family welfare organizations include mental health activities in their functions.

MENTAL RETARDATION

If one could select but a single field of health service to illustrate fragmentation, that field should be mental retardation, for two reasons. First, categorical programs are particularly marked, perhaps because mental retardation afflicts children and represents so painful a lifetime burden for families. Second, the problems of fragmented services for the mentally retarded have been singularly recognized, and efforts have been directed at all governmental levels toward coordination of services.

Federal Programs

Each of the three major administrations of the Department of Health, Education, and Welfare has numerous special programs for the prevention of mental retardation and for the care and rehabilitation of the mentally retarded. Within the Health Services and Mental Health Administration are maternal and child health and crippled children's programs, construction programs for mental retardation facilities, funding for improved institutional care, support of community care for the retarded, and special project grants, in addition to support of research and training. To the extent that some of these programs are organized on a functional basis and also serve the mentally ill, fragmentation is reduced. The Office of Education, through its Bureau of Education for the Handicapped, provides special educational assistance to the states for handicapped children. Its Vocational and Technical Education program provides formula grants to the states for vocational training of the handicapped. The Social and Rehabilitation Service, through its Division of Developmental Disabilities, provides funds for professional personnel in facilities for the mentally retarded, support for 19 university-affiliated research centers, and grants to the states for rehabilitation of the mentally retarded. Its Community Services Administration also provides grants for services to the totally and permanently mentally and emotionally disabled, including funds for day care and foster care for children in the Aid to Families with Dependent Children (AFDC) program.

The multiplicity of programs for the mentally retarded at the federal level has resulted in several coordinating committees. The President's Committee on Mental Retardation in the executive office of the President advises on policy and programs and coordinates the various activities of the departments concerned with mental retardation. The Secretary's Office of Mental Retardation Coordination coordinates the programs, policies, and activities of the Department of Health, Education, and Welfare and relates to the

President's Committee on Mental Retardation. Within this office are two other committees—a Steering Committee, responsible for advice and consultation, and a Mental Retardation Interagency Committee, composed of representatives of all the operating programs on mental retardation to provide a "means of communication, information exchange and program development for agency staff concerned with Federal mental retardation activities."[96] Similar interagency coordinating committees function on a regional basis within each of the ten regions of the Department of Health, Education, and Welfare. These national and regional coordinating committees attest to the multiplicity of programs that exists despite the enactment of the Developmental Disabilities Services and Construction Amendments of 1970, designed to integrate services for the mentally retarded.

State Programs

On the cover of a pamphlet describing the Lanterman Mental Retardation Services Act of 1969 is a picture of an appealing child made from pieces of a jigsaw puzzle. The picture symbolizes the intent of the Act to integrate services for the retarded:

> The State of California accepts a responsibility for its mentally retarded citizens and an obligation to them which it must discharge. Affecting hundreds of thousands of children and adults directly, and having an important impact on the lives of their families, neighbors, and whole communities, mental retardation presents social, medical, economic, and legal problems of extreme importance. The complexities of mental retardation require the services of many state departments as well as the community. Frequently there are gaps beyond the present duties and powers of departments in the development of state and community services. Services should be planned and provided as a part of a continuum. A pattern of facilities and eligibility should be established which is so complete as to meet the needs of each retarded person, regardless of age or degree of handicap, and at each stage of his life's development.[97]

The reasons for passage of this law read like a bill of particulars indicting the fragmented health service system, not merely care of the retarded. Among the problems that the legislation is designed to correct are lack of a single agency with responsibility and funds to assure services to those in need, lack of essential services in many parts of the state, excessive reliance on the state hospital system, and lack of coordination and planning at state and regional levels. The significance of these defects in the system for the mentally retarded and their families is set forth in a report to the California Legislature which found:

— —seven state departments administer 44 distinct programs serving the handicapped;

—— programs for the handicapped are financed by 21 separate funding mechanisms;

—— eligibility for state programs is governed by a total of 14 different age requirements, 14 different financial tests, 25 separate diagnostic categories, and a mass of miscellaneous requirements ranging from parental consent to prohibitions against "seeking alms";

—— responsibility for licensing residential facilities for the handicapped is divided among three state departments with jurisdictions based on inconsistent, overlapping categories;

—— only two programs for the handicapped out of 44 consistently evaluate their accomplishments;

—— of 44 state programs, 8 keep records consistent with programs of another department, and 4 of these 8 are cooperative programs of the Department of Rehabilitation.[98]

Understandably, therefore, the California Mental Retardation Services Act

seeks to join fragmented services, eliminate duplicated services, and provide services where none exist so that a parent may find help for a child at the earliest possible moment after mental retardation is suspected.[99]

Under this legislation, the state is divided into Mental Retardation Planning Areas. Areawide mental retardation program boards, composed of parents of the retarded, professionals who work with the retarded, and the general public, are responsible for planning and coordinating mental retardation services in their areas. The State Mental Retardation Plan is formed from the area plans. At the state level, the State Developmental Disabilities Council advises the State Health Planning Council, the Secretary of the Human Relations Agency, the Governor, and the Legislature on initiation, coordination, and implementation of projects for the mentally retarded.

In 1972, five state departments (Mental Hygiene, Public Health, Social Welfare, Rehabilitation, and Education) spent about $246 million in California on mental retardation activities under the aegis of the Office of Developmental Disabilities in the Health and Welfare Agency. A coordinating committee of 9 agencies involved in the provision of services for the retarded has been formed, including the 5 departments mentioned above plus Finance, Human Resources Development, the Youth Authority, and Health Care Services.[100] The cornerstone for the integrated system of care for the mentally retarded consists of a network of regional diagnostic, counseling, and service centers throughout the state and a single mental retardation program budget for all state agencies providing services. It is to these regional centers that state funds, previously allocated to other agencies for out-of-home prehospital, hospital, and posthospital care, are to be allocated to the fullest extent feasible for contracts with appropriate agencies for provision of out-of-home placements.[101]

Regional Programs

The 14 Regional Centers for the Mentally Retarded in various stages of development in California operate under contract with the State Department of Public Health. They provide direct services: medical diagnosis, psychological evaluation, individual and family counseling, community placement, guardianship, and state hospital placement. They purchase various kinds of care, including private residential care, medical services, nursery and preschool training and counseling, respite care, day care, and legal counseling. They locate community resources for education, recreation, and social adjustment training. In short, the regional centers are designed to provide a single entry point for the range of services any individual patient may need at any one time or at different times over the years as his needs change and his development calls for different services.

In addition to these functions in patient care, the regional centers for the mentally retarded are responsible for functional coordination of resources for the retarded within their respective geographic areas. The centers are required to identify unmet needs in community care and services, to define and interpret standards of care, to develop a plan for mental retardation services, and to stimulate development of community services. In this way, the regional centers are intended to bring to bear the resources of the community for service to individual patients and for community planning of overall services for the retarded, whether the resources emanate from federal, state, county, school district, voluntary, or private programs.

Local Programs

Governmental services for the mentally retarded are provided by local health, welfare, and educational agencies. Contracts with the regional center for the mentally retarded, which in Los Angeles is the voluntary Children's Hospital, may underwrite the cost of some of these services. The County Health Department provides diagnosis and evaluation for children under five years of age in mental retardation clinics in several health districts of the county. The largest county hospital, the Los Angeles County-University of Southern California Medical Center, examines large numbers of mentally retarded children for diagnosis, evaluation, and placement. The Department of Public Social Services arranges and supervises placement of mentally retarded persons in residential care. The Los Angeles County Superintendent of Schools and the Los Angeles City Unified School District develop curricula for special education programs for the educable and trainable retarded.

In 1965, a survey of resources for the mentally retarded examined the services provided by 335 agencies in Los Angeles County.[102] These services consisted of diagnostic and evaluation clinics, day care centers, preschool programs, compensatory education programs, Development Centers, classes for the trainable retarded, home training services, prevocational and vocational training programs, counseling services, and many others. The large number of programs is not necessarily a sign of adequate services. Rather, all these programs are multiple responses to the many facets of mental retardation and to tremendous needs. It is the services of these multiple agencies that the regional centers are empowered to coordinate.

Voluntary Programs

Many of the 335 programs surveyed in Los Angeles County are conducted by voluntary groups. More important than their numbers, however, is the role of voluntary organizations in behalf of the retarded. They have developed policy, pioneered new services, stimulated government to provide programs, filled gaps in services with their own programs, sponsored research, engaged in public education, and served as advocates of the retarded. The leading national voluntary organization is the National Association for Retarded Children. Its California chapter, the California Association for the Retarded, is represented on the coordinating committee of the state agencies concerned with mental retardation. The Exceptional Children's Foundation of Los Angeles County is engaged in many community activities, including provision of training for school-age mentally retarded children not accepted for special education by the public schools and development of a system of coordinated workshops for training the retarded throughout the county.[103]

ALCOHOLISM

Alcoholism has been called a medical–social problem

best dealt with within the state's system for the protection and advancement of mental and public health, with appropriate assistance from other care-giving instrumentalities, including the state's mental health, public health and social welfare systems.[104]

Current services are of four main types: (1) emergency medical care provided in various settings (medical and emergency services of general hospitals, psychiatric wards of general hospitals, special detoxification facilities, mental hospitals, and jails or other places of detention); (2) psychiatric inpatient care provided principally by state mental hospitals; (3) outpatient clinic care, which has expanded greatly in recent years; and (4) half-way houses and other residential facilities for problem drinkers.[105]

Estimates of the number of alcoholics in the United States range from 4 million to 30 million.[106] Since alcoholism strikes at the mental health and economic welfare of families of alcoholics, a conservative estimate is that 36 million Americans, or one in every six persons, is affected by this disease. In California, state hospital admissions for alcoholism rose from nearly 4,000 in 1963 to more than 6,500 in 1967.[107] Admissions for alcoholism increased from 16 to 21 percent of all admissions during this period. In Los Angeles County in 1969, 13 percent of admissions to the internal medicine department of the largest public hospital had alcoholism as a primary diagnosis; it has been estimated that at least one-fifth of the 100,000 total admissions annually are directly related to alcoholism.[108] Clearly, a problem of this magnitude requires many kinds and sources of service. The query is whether current organization of community services is adequate to meet the enormous needs.

Governmental Programs

As in the fields of mental illness and mental retardation, multiplicity of programs and agencies characterizes the field of alcoholism. Fragmentation of functions in alcoholism may be somewhat less marked than in the other fields described above simply because organized programs are relatively recent, but at each level of government the same or similar functions are split among numerous programs and agencies.

Recognition of the need for national policies and programs for an integrated attack designed to prevent, control, and treat alcoholism is expressed in the establishment in 1971 of the National Institute on Alcohol Abuse and Alcoholism within the National Institute of Mental Health. Designed to provide a focus for all work at the federal level on the many facets of alcoholism — health education, training of personnel, research, and program planning — the Institute implements the federal requirement for state plans for alcoholism and relates funding of alcoholism projects to the support of the federally funded Community Mental Health Centers. Despite this thrust toward unification, several federal agencies operate large, separate, and independent alcoholism programs. The Social and Rehabilitation Service of the Department of Health, Education, and Welfare provides grants to the states for the rehabilitation of alcoholics. The Office of Economic Opportunity provides project grants to communities for case-finding, treatment, and rehabilitation. Since alcoholism is a major factor in half of all auto-mobile accidents, the Department of Transportation funds a large-scale research program on alcoholism in relation to automobile accidents and administers grants for the development of comprehensive highway safety programs, in which control of alcoholism is a required element. All these programs, as well as direct services provided by the federal government to special populations for alcoholism, are largely separate from the Institute on Alcohol Abuse and Alcoholism.

At the state level, in fiscal year 1968-1969, 13 state agencies spent more than $54,000,000 for the prevention of alcoholism and for the treatment and rehabilitation of California's estimated 1,000,000 alcoholics.[109] The Departments of Mental Hygiene and Rehabilitation share statutory responsi-bility for the treatment and rehabilitation of alcoholics,[110] and other agencies are involved in specialized activities. The Department of Public Health is currently engaged in health education and in the licensure of alcoholic rehabilitation hospitals, clinics, and laboratories that test blood alcohol concentration levels. The Department of Education assists school districts with education on alcoholism. The Departments of Social Welfare and Health Care Services provide social services and medical care, respectively, to eligible alcoholics. The Department of Employment makes payments under the state disability insurance program for disability resulting from alcoholism. The Departments of Motor Vehicles and Highway Patrol are involved in programs to control drunk driving.

The basic fragmentation in the field of alcoholism derives from the segmented and partly overlapping responsibilities of the State Departments of Mental Hygiene and Rehabilitation. On the one hand, the Department of Mental Hygiene is responsible for inpatient care of alcoholics in state mental hospitals and for the development and funding of community mental health services, where alcoholics may receive treatment for mental and emotional problems. Services for alcoholics vary among the state hospitals and in the community mental health systems. None of the hospitals provides training, job placement, family support services, or follow-up. On the other hand, the Department of Rehabilitation is responsible for the federal-state program of outpatient clinics for the treatment and rehabilitation of alcoholics. Local health departments administer these clinics, although the State Department of Public Health is no longer involved because more favorable funding was available through the rehabilitation route.

As a result of this segmentation, an alcoholic patient may be served in any one of three separate systems of public ambulatory care, depending on the happenstance by which he gains access to care. He may be served in one of the eleven outpatient alcoholism clinics in California established under the federal-state alcoholism program. He may receive crisis care in a public or private mental health clinic funded by the state-local community mental health service program. He may occasionally be served in a federally funded Community Mental Health Center. To make these three streams of care available, the County Departments of Health, Hospitals, Mental Health, and Public Social Services share responsibilities for emergency, outpatient, inpatient, and rehabilitation services to varying degrees.

Although the federal initiative has increased the planning and fiscal role of the County Department of Mental Health in services for alcoholics, the scope of community mental health services has not yet been expanded to encompass the treatment of alcoholism. Mental health clinics generally refer alcoholics to community resources specialized in the treatment of alcoholics; only crisis intervention for alcoholics with mental problems is provided by mental health clinics. Of the 12 federally funded Community Mental Health Centers in Los Angeles County, only one has seen fit to apply for funding to provide outpatient and inpatient services for alcoholics. Thus, the jurisdictional division between alcoholism and mental health programs denies comprehensive care to alcoholic patients, who may also have underlying mental and emotional problems.

In 1969, a State Task Force on Alcoholism, appointed to study the need for the consolidation of health programs into a single department, found in the field of alcoholism control disparate, categorical programs for a problem requiring a broad spectrum of integrated services, lack of effective coordination, gaps in delivery of services, failure to use available resources for program development, and imbalance in preventive, therapeutic, and rehabilitative services.[111] On the basis of its recommendation for a "state-wide comprehensive delivery system . . . designed to encompass the broad spectrum of services required to deal with the physical, psychological and socio-economic dimensions of the problem,"[112] the Office of Alcohol Program Management was established under the Secretary of the Human Relations Agency, with authority to plan, provide technical assistance, and promote public health procedures for the treatment of alcoholics, to serve as a clearing house for information, and to coordinate state programs for alcoholics. Unified health agencies at the state and local levels have the potential to overcome fragmented services.

Voluntary and Private Programs

Many voluntary organizations at the national, state, and local levels contribute to the treatment of individuals afflicted with alcoholism and to the development of community services. In the category of organizations providing services to individuals are Alcoholics Anonymous (with more than 600 meetings a week in Greater Los Angeles), Al-Anon Family Groups of relatives and friends of alcoholics, Alateen for children of alcoholics, the Salvation Army, Applied Principles of Alcoholic Recovery (APOAR), an offshoot of Alcoholics Anonymous, and Counsellors on Alcoholism and Related Disorders (CARD), an organization of recovered alcoholics and others working with alcoholics.[113] Also serving alcoholics are the many voluntary social work agencies and individual professionals in medicine, social work, clinical psychology, and the clergy. Industrial medical services have been increasingly involved with alcoholism among employees. Their attention to alcoholism as a cause of industrial accidents is intensified by the new Occupational Safety and Health Act.

In the realm of community education, research, and program development, the leading voluntary organization is the National Council on Alcoholism and its local affiliates. These groups provide a wide range of services dedicated to prevention and elimination of alcoholism: public education, training of personnel, casefinding, information and referral, encouragement of industrial programs, coordination of services, and impetus for development of more and better services. In these efforts they are assisted by other organizations, such as the voluntary Welfare Planning Council and professional organizations of health personnel.

In Los Angeles County, more than 150 public and private clinics, mental health centers, hospitals, residential facilities, and community agencies provide varying kinds of treatment and services for alcoholics, Few of the facilities, however, provide comprehensive services. While alcoholism has achieved a high degree of visibility from these specialized, categorical efforts, this medical-social problem of enormous proportions has been set apart, in large measure, from community mental health programs and from general health care.

DRUG DEPENDENCE

Drug dependence has traditionally been treated separately from mental illness in an atmosphere with strong moral and criminal sanctions. Removal of legal obstacles to treatment by revision of the penalty structure and changed public attitudes might have fostered development of a therapeutic environment for control of drug dependence as part of the mental health system. But by 1970 the enormous proportions of the problem, and particularly its criminal aspects in large cities, called on the resources of many agencies equipped to provide particular services. In 1972, $190 million was spent on the treatment and rehabilitation of drug dependence, largely by six federal agencies, $65 million for education and training, and $56 million for research, planning, and coordination; spending for criminal enforcement totalled $164 million.[114]

Governmental Programs

Federal functions in the control of drug dependence are spread through 7 federal departments (Agriculture, Defense, Health, Education, and Welfare, Housing and Urban Development, Justice, State, and Treasury), 2 agencies (Veterans Administration and Office of Economic Opportunity), and other units, such as the National Advisory Council on Drug Abuse and Drug Dependence and the Intergovernmental Coordinating Council on Drug Abuse and Drug Dependence. Recognizing that multiple efforts are necessary but that their effectiveness could be heightened by coordination, Congress in 1970 established the Division of Narcotics Addiction and Drug Abuse within the National Institute of Mental Health.[115] Through this Division the Secretary of Health, Education, and Welfare is directed to coordinate all federal health, rehabilitation, and social programs related to drug dependence. New federal policy mandates state plans on the control of drug dependence and a single administrative agency as a condition for federal grants.

Similar efforts have been undertaken at the state level in California to coordinate activities of 12 separate correctional, health, educational, welfare, and rehabilitation agencies working on various aspects of drug dependence. In 1970, the State Office of Narcotics and Drug Abuse Coordination was established by executive order in the California Health and Welfare Agency. This Office shared responsibility for the coordination of all public and private efforts in the control of drug dependence with the California Interagency Council on Drug Abuse, designated in 1969 as advisory to the Governor on narcotics and dangerous drug abuse and funded jointly by the California Council on Criminal Justice and the California Medical Association. A third coordinating agency is the California Drug Abuse Information Project, established by the Legislature to collect and disseminate information on research and service projects in this field.[116]

At the county level in Los Angeles, the escalating incidence of drug dependence has led to a proliferation of governmental and voluntary efforts. Reflecting the many-pronged response to this crisis were newspaper headlines in 1972: "County Seeks to End Chaos in War on Drugs. Rivalries of Various Agencies Viewed as Most Vital Problem."[117] Responsibility for the development of the comprehensive county plan on drug abuse, required by state legislation,[118] is assigned to the County Department of Mental Health. Responsibility for development of the plan, however, is not tantamount to coordination of services. Prime adviser on development of the plan has been the Interdepartmental Drug Abuse Committee, composed of representatives of the main county departments concerned with drug dependence and other governmental and voluntary agencies, about 70 in all. These agencies are being called on to correct the findings of the Los Angeles County Grand Jury that "drug abuse programs remain fragmented, uncoordinated, inadequate and lost in a maze of bureaucracy and interdepartmental maneuvering."[119]

Voluntary and Private Agencies

Two groups of voluntary agencies are concerned with drug abuse. One group consists of the conventional voluntary and professional organizations, which address themselves to education, legislation, resources, and policies. The other, less traditional group consists of numerous local organizations formed to develop free clinics and special drug dependence resources to provide withdrawal services, counseling, group therapy, and halfway houses. The Narcotics Information Service in Los Angeles County, a voluntary organization, estimates that 175 to 200 such groups are working in Los Angeles County. The demand for community treatment has been increased by state legislation providing subsidies to county probation departments for community treatment in place of commitment to state correctional agencies and by judicial referrals of first offenders to community groups. These groups provide a unique service through the inspirational value of former drug users as counselors and other nontraditional approaches. Unfortunately, however, in many cases they suffer from being too small, too poorly funded, and too short-lived to meet the caseload. Moreover, linkages with other community resources are essential to provide the needed scope and continuum of services.

FRAGMENTATION OF MENTAL HEALTH SERVICES

In considering fragmentation between and within fields of mental health service, one must start with the premise that the needs for mental health services far exceed the resources currently devoted to these problems. As one wag has commented, "Everyone needs to be another's therapist; otherwise there are not enough to go around." The question is whether a non-categorical system of health services would allocate resources more equitably and more efficiently than does the current segmented system. No quantitative measures to answer that question emerge from this research, but the evidence assembled here suggests that the current system does not make equitable and efficient use of the resources currently allocated to mental health services. The barriers, gaps, and inadequacies in care are attributable to five principal features of the fragmented system: (1) the separation of the public and private sectors; (2) changing intergovernmental relations; (3) the division between health and nonhealth services; (4) the dichotomy between mental health services and general health services; and (5) the segmentation within the mental health system itself.

1. Separation of public and private sectors. The trend away from institutional care of the mentally ill toward care in the community has increased the involvement of the private and voluntary sector in the provision of mental health services. Despite allocation of increased responsibility to the private sector, it nevertheless remains relatively isolated from the total problem:

> Private practitioners, private and public clinics, family agencies operate in considerable isolation from each other. The private practitioner as an independent professional has his major ties not to clinics or agencies offering similar or related help but to his colleagues in the psychiatric profession and to his professional organizations. Clinics . . . tend to be oriented to specific populations and to take tasks they have carved out for themselves, without regard to either total needs or the ways in which private practitioners and other organizations do their work. . . . All this independent and unintegrated effort gives to the psychiatric out-patient system a diffuse and fragmented character which rules out concerted action, addressed to the "problem as a whole."[120]

An additional consequence of this isolation is that two-track care results. The private sector provides intensive therapy for those with ability to pay, thrusting an additional burden on the public sector for those who cannot pay.

2. Intergovernmental relations. In recent years, the emphasis on care in the community has led to increased responsibility by local governments and communities for the provision of care to the mentally ill. Although the state continues to provide the major portion of financial support, local communities vary in resources and preferences. As a result, the spectrum of care provided reveals great variability within any state.[121]

3. Division between health and nonhealth services. Mental health services are inextricably interwoven with the judicial, welfare, and educational systems. The role of the courts, the police, and the probation officers in prevention, early intervention, and treatment for mental illness, alcoholism, and drug dependence is critical, but the relationships with the medical care system are variable and generally unstructured. Care of patients on the caseloads of the State Department of Rehabilitation, the County Department of Public Social Services, or the County Department of Probation is paid for according to different funding ratios, related to the financial support of the particular agency, rather than to the medical-social needs of the patient. The role of the schools in preventing and detecting mental, emotional, and behavioral problems is largely separate from the mental health system. A person with an emotional or mental disorder receives a different range of services, depending on which agency—governmental or voluntary—first comes into contact with his need and accepts responsibility for his care, instead of the continuum of services required.

4. Dichotomy between mental health services and general health services. The patient faced with a mental health problem seeks care from a source different from that to which he turns for a physical ailment. Rarely are the two systems coordinated for the individual patient, despite deep inter-relationships of mental and physical conditions. Alcoholism and drug dependence, for example, have both physical and psychiatric aspects. Neither public nor private agencies have provided surveillance for the totality of care that may be required.

5. Segmentation within the mental health system. Mental health services are segmented by both specialty and by function. Some separation of mental health by categorical condition is understandable because of need for specialized services and need for visibility, but the current division allows virtually no sharing of resources. Systems within categorical fields are no substitute for an overall system.

As for segmented functions, licensing of facilities and placement of the mentally ill illustrate the problems of functional fragmentation. Three state agencies in California license facilities for the mentally ill. Each has a different set of criteria and a different emphasis. Placement agencies, both governmental and voluntary, require different kinds of facilities for their patients. Each of these, too, has a different orientation. Placement agencies are in competition with each other for appropriate facilities at a cost they can pay. In order to compensate for lack of facilities and perhaps for inappropriate licensed categories, placement agencies certify facilities for their own use. Thus, certification may undermine licensing standards. Lack of coordination between licensing and placement agencies means that placement agencies often cannot afford to meet the costs imposed by licensing standards, these standards are not enforced, and the quality of care is depressed.

Finally, categorical qualifications for the placement or treatment of the mentally ill mean that patients are not eligible for care until their condition is pronounced. Psychiatrists and social workers comment that they are less able to assist the marginally ill—those who would benefit most from treatment—than the severely disturbed. Without a specific policy to assure prevention and early treatment, categorical programs exact a high price for delayed treatment—increased use of personnel and facilities and increased human suffering.

A case in point is that of Steven A, a mentally retarded boy of 16, who was happy and progressing at his Farm Training School but needed foster home placement in the community because his divorced father could no longer provide proper supervision for him. Attempts by dedicated personnel at the Farm Training School to find funding for Steven A's placement resulted in fruitless contacts with 10 state and county agencies. The case record stops with Steven's residing in the home of one of the teachers at the Farm Training School and with the following comment:

> To place Steven in an institution, it would cost the State $4,000.00 plus a year. To keep Steven in a good program in a Mental Hygiene home in the community, it would cost the State approximately $2,500.00 a year. But there is something more important: Steven has made, and is making, excellent progress in his situation at the Farm School. This retarded youngster deserves a chance to meet his potential. Because the channels of communication are muddy and because no one seems to want to accept the responsibility for the funding of Steven's care, this boy remains in limbo while agencies pass the buck or throw up their hands in helpless gestures. The tragedy is not that these agencies are not doing their job—the tragedy is that the agencies do not seem to be aware of one another and certainly are not aware of each other's job. [Italics omitted.][122]

NOTES

1. Schwartz, Donald A., "Community Mental Health in 1972: An Assessment," *Progress in Community Mental Health* (Barten, Harvey H. and Leopold Bellak, Eds.), Vol. II. p. 23, Grune and Stratton, Inc., New York, 1972.

2. Rice, Dorothy P., Barbara S. Cooper, and Nancy, L. Worthington, "National Health Expenditures, 1929-1971," *Social Security Bull.*, Vol. 35, No. 1, p. 5, Jan. 1972.

3. Calculated from Conley, Ronald W., Margaret Conwell, and Shirley G. Willner, *The Cost of Mental Illness, 1968*, Statistical Note 30, Table 3, National Clearinghouse for Mental Health Information, Survey and Reports Section, Office of Program Planning and Evaluation, National Institute of Mental Health, Department of Health, Education, and Welfare, Oct. 1970.

4. *Financing Care of the Mentally Ill under Medicare and Medicaid*, Research Report No. 37. p. 10, Table 7, Office of Research and Statistics, Social Security Administration, U.S. Department of Health. Education, and Welfare, June 1971.

5. Id. at 10-12.

6. Id. at 1.

7. The President's Panel on Mental Retardation, *A Proposed Program for National Action*

to Combat Mental Retardation, pp. 1-2, U.S. Government Printing Office, Washington, D.C.. 1962.

8. *Departments of Labor and Health, Education, and Welfare Appropriations for 1973*, Hearings before a Subcommittee of the Committee on Appropriations, House of Representatives, 92nd Cong., 2d Sess., Part 1, p. 441, 1972. *See California State Plan for Comprehensive Alcohol Abuse and Alcoholism Prevention, Treatment, and Rehabilitation, 1972*, p. 1. Human Relations Agency, Office of Alcoholism, Sacramento, Calif. for the estimate that one out of every 12 adult Californians — over one million individuals — are alcoholics.

9. The historical account is derived from the following sources: Deutsch, Albert. *The Mentally Ill in America*, 2nd ed., Columbia University Press, New York, 1949; Abbe, Leslie Morgan and Anna Mae Baney, *The Nation's Health Facilities, Ten Years of the Hill-Burton Hospital and Medical Facilities Program, 1946-1956*, pp. 71-73, Public Health Service, U.S. Department of Health, Education, and Welfare, 1958; Ridenour, Nina, *Mental Health in the United States, A Fifty Year History*, published for the Commonwealth Fund by Harvard University Press, Cambridge, Mass., 1961; Rosen, George, *Madness in Society*, Routledge and Kegan Paul, London, 1968; and Connery, Robert H., Charles H. Backstrom, David R. Deener, Julian R. Friedman, Morton Kroll, Robert H. Marden, Clifton McCleskey, Peter Meekison, and John A. Morgan, Jr., *The Politics of Mental Health, Organizing Community Mental Health in Metropolitan Areas*, Columbia University Press, New York, 1968.

10. The summary of the mental hygiene movement is based on an unpublished manuscript by Pamela C. Krochalk, "The Mental Hygiene Movement in the United States." Grateful acknowledgment is made for its use.

11. Ridenour, supra note 9 at 1.

12. See Connery et al., supra note 9 at 15 ff.

13. *America Builds: The Record of PWA*, p. 147 and Table 12 at 280, Public Works Administration, Washington, D.C., 1939. Through 1939, the Public Works Administration. established by the New Deal, provided 121,760 beds in hospitals costing $368 million. More than half of these funds were spent on beds for mental illness.

14. Connery et al. supra note 9 at 15-16.

15. House Committee on Interstate and Foreign Commerce, Hearings on H.R. 2550. National Neuropsychiatric Institute Act, 79th Cong., 1st Sess., p. 36, 1945, discussed by Connery, supra note 9 at 16 and by Felix, Robert H., *Mental Illness, Progress and Prospects*, pp. 28-29, Columbia University Press, New York, 1967. From Dec. 7, 1941 through Dec. 1945, 42 percent of the 980,000 discharges of enlisted men from the army were for neuropsychiatric reasons. *National Neuropsychiatric Institute Act*, Hearings before a Subcommittee of the Committee on Education and Labor, U.S. Senate, 79th Cong., 2d Sess. on S. 1160, Statement of the Office of the Surgeon General, p. 137, March 1946.

16. See Connery et al., supra note 9 at 19.

17. Felix, supra note 15 at 52.

18. Ibid.

19. *Hill-Burton Program Progress Report, July 1, 1947-June 30, 1969*, Table H. p. 51. Health Facilities Planning and Construction Service, Health Services and Mental Health Administration, U.S. Department of Health, Education, and Welfare, PHS Pub. No. 930-F-3. 1969.

20. Connery et al., supra note 9 at 29.

21. Id. at 30.

22. See Brickman, Harry R., M.D., "California's Short-Doyle Program, The New Mental Health System, Changes in Procedure, Implications for Family Physicians," *Calif. Med.*, Vol. 109, p. 403, Nov. 1968.

23. Joint Commission on Mental Illness and Health, *Action for Mental Health*, Basic Books. N.Y., 1961.

24. P.L. 88-164 (1963); P.L. 89-105 (1965).

25. Schwartz, supra note 1 at 21.

26. Id. at 20; Brickman, Harry R., M.D., "Federal versus Local Community Mental Health Planning: A Plea for Conflict Resolution," *Am. J. Public Health*, Vol. 60, p. 2251 at 2253, Dec. 1970; *A Study of California's New Mental Health Law* (1969-1971), conducted by Enki Research Institute, p. 41, Enki Corporation, Los Angeles, 1972.

27. *Financing Care of the Mentally Ill under Medicare and Medicaid*, supra note 4 at 46.

28. See Deutsch, supra note 9 at 378-379.

29. Statement by President John F. Kennedy on the Need for a National Program to Combat Mental Retardation, Oct. 11, 1961, Public Papers of the Presidents, John F. Kennedy, 1961, p. 651, U.S. Government Printing Office, 1962.

30. Statement of Senator Edward Kennedy, "Introduction of a Bill to Provide Services and Facilities for Persons with Developmental Disabilities," *Mental Retardation and Other Developmental Disabilities, 1969*, Hearings before the Subcommittee on Health of the Committee on Labor and Public Welfare, U.S. Senate, 91st Cong., 1st Sess. on S. 2846, p. 28, Nov. 10, 1969.

31. The President's Panel on Mental Retardation, *Report of the Task Force on Law*, Washington, D.C., 1963.

32. *Mental Retardation and Other Developmental Disabilities, 1969*, Hearings supra note 30 at 270.

33. P.L. 91-517 (1970).

34. Allen, Richard C., "Legal Norms and Practices affecting the Mentally Deficient," paper presented to the First International Congress, International Association for the Scientific Study of Mental Deficiency, Montpellier, France, Sept. 18, 1967, Institute of Law, Psychiatry, and Criminology, The George Washington University, Washington, D.C.

35. See *A Proposal to Reorganize California's Fragmented System of Services for the Mentally Retarded*, p. i, Assembly Office of Research, California Legislature, Sacramento, March 1969.

36. *A Redefinition of State Responsibility for California's Mentally Retarded*, Assembly Interim Committee Reports, Vol. 21, No. 10, p. 12, Assembly Ways and Means Committee, Subcommittee on Mental Health Services, California Legislature, Sacramento, 1965.

37. Id. at 29.

38. Id. at 30.

39. Mooring, Ivy, Ph.D., *The Planning and Implementation of Comprehensive Services for the Mentally Retarded in Los Angeles County*, pp. 8-9, 83, Mental Retardation Services Board, Report of Activities Sept. 1, 1965-Oct. 1, 1968.

40. Meeker, Marchia, *The Inter-Relatedness and Impact of Alcoholism Programs in Los Angeles County 1967-1968, A Comprehensive Review and Analysis*, p. 7, prepared for the Los Angeles County Health Department under the staff direction of Alison K. Mauer and John C. Pixley, Welfare Planning Council, August 1968.

41. Plaut, Thomas F. A., *Alcohol Problems*, A Report to the Nation by the Cooperative Commission on the Study of Alcoholism, p. 25, Oxford University Press, N.Y., 1967.

42. Id. at 26.

43. Philp, John R., "What Has Happened in Other Parts of the United States?" in Second Los Angeles Conference on Alcoholism, Proceedings, p. 7, Welfare Planning Council, Los Angeles, 1967.

44. *Alcohol Problems*, supra note 41 at 26.

45. Philp, supra note 43 at 9.

46. *California 1972-73 Program Budget Supplement*, p. 720, Sacramento, 1972.

47. Ibid.

48. *California State Plan for Comprehensive Alcohol Abuse, Alcoholism Prevention, Treatment, and Rehabilitation, 1972*, p. 332, Table 2, California Human Relations Agency, Office of Alcoholism, Sacramento, 1972.

49. Meeker, supra note 40 at 7 ff.

50. Calif. Health & Safety Code, secs. 6990-6990.13 (1969).

51. For an excellent historical review, see Lewis, David C. and Norman E. Zinberg, "Narcotic Usage, A Historical Perspective on a Difficult Medical Problem," *New Engl. J. Med.*, Vol. 270, No. 20, p. 1046, May 14, 1964.

52. See, for example, *Treatment of Drug Addicts, A Survey of Existing Legislation*, pp. 36-42, World Health Organization, Geneva, 1962.

53. P.L. 70-672 (1929).

54. Executive Order No. 10302. Nov. 2, 1951, created an Interdepartmental Committee on Narcotics. In 1956, the Interdepartmental Committee issued a report with 14 recommendations for training, treatment, and enforcement, "Legislation on Narcotics, 1945-1964," *Congress and the Nation, 1945-1964*, Congressional Quarterly Service, pp. 1189-1190, 1966.

55. *Proceedings of the White House Conference on Narcotics and Drug Abuse*, p. 128, U.S. Government Printing Office, Washington, D.C., 1962.

56. *Congress and the Nation, 1945-1964*, supra note 54 at 1193.

57. Narcotics Addict Rehabilitation Act, P.L. 89-793 (1966).

58. Drug Abuse Office and Treatment Act, P.L. 92-255 (1972).

59. *Financing Care of the Mentally Ill under Medicare and Medicaid*, Research Report No. 37, p. 1, Office of Research and Statistics, Social Security Administration, U.S. Department of Health, Education, and Welfare, June 1971.

60. *Crisis in Child Mental Health: Challenge for the 1970's*, Report of the Joint Commission on Mental Health of Children, pp. 38, 150, Harper and Row Publishers, Inc., N.Y., 1969.

61. See statement of James V. Warren, M.D., Chairman, Council of Academic Societies, Association of American Medical Colleges, in *Departments of Labor, Health, Education, and Welfare Appropriations, for 1972*, Hearings before a Subcommittee of the Committee on Appropriations, House of Representatives, 92nd Cong., 1st Sess., Part 6, pp. 365-366, 1971: "We still lack the basic understanding of the origins and biological nature of mental disorder. In the absence of definitive therapeutics, we are solely dependent upon increasing scale in the management of the mentally ill and chemical suppression of the adverse manifestations of the disease."

62. Pasamanick, Benjamin, M. D., "What Is Mental Illness and How Can We Measure It?" paper presented at the Symposium on Definition and Measurement of Mental Health, sponsored by the U.S. National Center for Health Statistics, Washington, D.C., March 7, 1966.

63. See Schwartz, Donald A., "Community Mental Health in 1972: An Assessment," in *Progress in Community Mental Health* (Barten, Harvey H. and Leopold Bellak, Eds.), Vol. II, pp. 20-21, Grune and Stratton, Inc., N.Y., 1972; Enki Research Institute, supra note 26 at 27.

64. *Financing Care of the Mentally Ill under Medicare and Medicaid*, supra note 59 at 5, Table 5.

65. Id. at 16.

66. Id. at 26.

67. The Long Amendment was not obligatory on the states and further provided that the states must show maintenance of their own mental hospital efforts. By January 1970, only 35 states had adopted the mental health provisions of Medicaid. *Financing Care of the Mentally Ill under Medicare and Medicaid*, supra note 59 at 32-33 and Table 27.

68. *Financing Care of the Mentally Ill under Medicare and Medicaid*, supra note 59 at 34-35, Table 7.

69. See U.S. Department of Health, Education, and Welfare, Social and Rehabilitation Service, Assistance Payments Administration-Medical Services Administration, *Characteristics of State Medical Assistance Programs under Title XIX of the Social Security Act*, 1970.

70. *Fourteenth Annual Report, Civilian Health and Medical Program of the Uniformed Services in the United States, Canada, Mexico, and Puerto Rico*, Calendar Year 1970.

71. Conley, Ronald W., Margaret Conwell, and Shirley G. Willner, *The Cost of Mental Illness, 1968*, Statistical Note 30, p. 8, Table 1, Footnote B, National Clearinghouse for Mental Health Information, Survey and Reports Section, Office of Program Planning and Evaluation,

National Institute of Mental Health, Department of Health, Education, and Welfare, Oct. 1970.

72. Ibid.

73. *The Cost of Mental Illness, 1968*, supra note 71 at Tables 1 and 2 and footnotes.

74. P.L. 92-603 (1972).

75. See *California Mental Health Progress, LPS, 10 Services*, California State Department of Mental Hygiene, Oct. 1968.

76. See *State of California 1970-71 Budget*, p. 589 for 1968-1969 spending; *1972-1973 Program Budget Supplement*, p. 862 for 1971-1972 spending.

77. State of California, *1972-1973 Program Budget Supplement*, p. 859.

78. See *Analysis of the Budget Bill of the State of California for the Fiscal Year July 1, 1972 to June 30, 1973*, Report of the Legislative Budget Committee, p. 669 that savings in state mental hospitals were not being reflected in proportionate increases in community mental health care. Other groups, including the Citizens' Advisory Council to the State Department of Mental Hygiene and the California State Employees Association, representing some 16,000 employees in the state mental hospital system, deplored deficiencies in quantity and quality of community facilities for the mentally ill. *Los Angeles Times*, March 31, 1972 and Jan. 19, 1972. In 1970, inpatient hospitalization accounted for 71 percent of California's county mental health budgets, outpatient services for only 16 percent, partial hospitalization for 3.5 percent, and consultation for 3.1 percent. *California's Five Year Plan for Community Mental Health Services*, p. 6, submitted by the California State Department of Mental Hygiene to the Legislature on March 29, 1971.

79. A.B. 2406 was introduced in the California Legislature in 1970 to prevent local zoning ordinances from restricting use of licensed family care homes, foster homes, and group homes by physically or mentally handicapped individuals as a class. See also Seiler, Michael, "Showdown in Board-Care Controversy," *Los Angeles Times*, Part IV, p. 1, Feb. 13, 1973.

80. Testimony of Dr. Paul Williams, Los Angeles County Department of Mental Health at hearings on the operation of the California Community Mental Health Program before Assembly Ways and Means Committee, Subcommittee on Mental Health Services, California Legislature, Los Angeles, Nov. 10, 1970.

81. Schwartz, Donald A., M.D., "Community Mental Health Services Planning," *Selected Papers on Health Issues in California*, p. 646 at 652, State Office of Comprehensive Health Planning, California State Department of Public Health, Sacramento, May 1971.

82. The number of general hospitals with psychiatric units has been increasing steadily, particularly since Medicare and Medicaid, increasing by 39 percent from 1964 to 1967. Nearly 600,000 psychiatric patients were treated in general hospitals in 1965. Jost, Arthur, "The Private Hospital and Mental Health Services," *Selected Papers on Health Issues in California*, supra note 81 at 634.

83. *The Cost of Mental Illness, 1968*, supra note 71 at Table 3.

84. Testimony presented at Hearings of Assembly Ways and Means Committee, Subcommittee on Mental Health Services, supra note 80.

85. Los Angeles County Department of Mental Health, *Plan for Mental Health Services, 1971-1972, 1971-1976*, pp. 23-24, Oct. 1970.

86. Id. at 25-26.

87. Id. at 17-18.

88. For discussion of the role of the County Health Department in provision of mental health services, see *Future Directions for Health Services, County of Los Angeles/1970*, Review of the Program of the Los Angeles County Health Department, undertaken at the request of the Los Angeles County Board of Supervisors, p. 124, American Public Health Association (Malcolm H. Merrill, M.D., Director of Study), Los Angeles, 1970.

89. Id. at 125.

90. Id. at 126-7.

91. California Administrative Code, Tit. 22, Ch. 5, Minimum Standards for Residential Care Homes for Adults.

92. California State Department of Public Health, *A Report to the 1970 Legislature on Reimbursement of Public School Health Services in California,* p. 5, Jan. 1970.

93. Calif. Welfare and Institutions Code, secs. 5763-5764 (West 1972).

94. Calif. Welfare and Institutions Code, secs. 5757-5762 (West 1972).

95. *The Mental Health Survey of Los Angeles County, 1957-1959,* A Project of the Welfare Planning Council of the Los Angeles Region prepared under the direction of Wayne McMillen, Los Angeles, May 1960.

96. *Departments of Labor and Health, Education, and Welfare Appropriations for 1973,* Hearings before a Subcommittee of the Committee on Appropriations, House of Representatives, 92nd Cong., 2d Sess., Part 1, p. 291, 1972.

97. Calif. Health & Safety Code, sec. 38001 (Deering's Supp. 1972).

98. Arthur Bolton Associates, *A Report to the Assembly Select Committee on Mentally Ill and Handicapped Children,* Part I, Services for the Handicapped, pp. 7-8, March 1, 1970.

99. *Lanterman Mental Retardation Services Act* (pamphlet), p. 5, California Human Relations Agency, 1971.

100. Id. at 14.

101. Calif. Health & Safety Code, sec. 38250 (Deering Supp. 1972).

102. Mooring, I. and J. Currie, *The Mental Retardation Survey of Los Angeles County,* Welfare Planning Council, Los Angeles Region, 1965.

103. See Shushan, Robert D., *Coordination of Workshops for the Mentally Retarded in a Metropolitan and Suburban Area,* Exceptional Children's Foundation, Los Angeles, Calif., 1972.

104. Alcoholism and Intoxication Treatment Act, A Draft of a Model Act with Draftsman's Notes, prepared for the National Institute of Mental Health by the Legislative Drafting Fund, Columbia University, Frank P. Grad, Director, July 1969.

105. Plaut, Thomas F. A., *Some Major Issues in Developing Community Services for Persons with Drinking Problems,* Background paper prepared for Surgeon General's Conference with the Mental Health Authorities, pp. 6-10, U.S. Department of Health, Education, and Welfare, Dec. 1966.

106. Glasscote, Raymond M. et al., *The Treatment of Alcoholism, A Study of Programs and Problems,* p. 11, Joint Information Service of the American Psychiatric Association and the National Association for Mental Health, Washington, D.C., 1967.

107. *California's Alcoholism Program,* Report of Progress, Report to the Legislature under Sec. 427.11 of the Health and Safety Code, p. 31, California State Department of Public Health, Division of Alcoholism, May 1, 1969.

108. *Future Directions for Health Services, County of Los Angeles/1970,* supra note 88 at 128.

109. Assembly Office of Research, *Alcoholism Programs: A Need for Reform,* pp. 4, 12, California Legislature, March 1970.

110. Calif. Welfare and Institutions Code, sec. 5001 (West 1972).

111. *Report of the Task Force on Alcoholism,* Human Relations Agency, State of California, May 1969.

112. Id. at 25.

113. Meeker, Marchia, *The Inter-Relatedness and Impact of Alcoholism Programs in Los Angeles County, 1967-1968,* pp. 95-102, Welfare Planning Council, Los Angeles, California, 1968.

114. *Special Analyses, Budget of the United States Government, Fiscal Year 1974,* p. 286, Table R-2 and pp. 292-293, Table R-6.

115. P.L. 91-513 (1970).

116. Calif. Health & Safety Code, sec. 210 (1967). See Smith, David E., M.D., and David J.

Bentel, M. Crim., Third Annual Report to the Legislature, Drug Abuse Information Project, Dec. 1969.

117. *Los Angeles Times*, Part 1, p. 3, June 12, 1972.

118. Calif. Health & Safety Code, Ch. 9, sec. 1170 (1970).

119. *Los Angeles Times*, Part 1, p. 3 at 25, June 12, 1972.

120. Schwartz, Morris S., Charlotte Green Schwartz, et al., *Social Approaches to Mental Patient Care*, pp. 96-97, Columbia University Press, N.Y., 1964.

121. See *A Study of California's New Mental Health Law (1969-1971)*, conducted by Enki Research Institute, Enki Corporation, Los Angeles, 1972, for the variability of California's state-local system of mental health services in three major counties.

122. *A Proposal to Reorganize California's Fragmented System of Services for the Mentally Retarded*, A Staff Report prepared for the Assembly Ways and Means Committee, p. 1 at 3, Sacramento, March 1969.

CHAPTER 6

Emergency Medical Care: Programs for Provision of a Multi-Dimensional Service

I would reason that it is precisely because emergency medical services constitute an aggregation of separate and distinct efforts, each of which may be subject to separate professional, political and fiscal persuasions; and because we Americans are singularly poor at thinking in terms of totally integrated systems; that it should come as no surprise that, as a Nation, we have failed to mount a successful attack on the problem of emergency medical services.[1]

—Merlin K. DuVal, M.D.
Assistant Secretary
for Health and Scientific
Affairs, U.S. Department of
Health, Education, and Welfare, 1972

Of the 50 million Americans who suffer accidental injuries each year, some degree of disability results for nearly 11 million and death results for approximately 116,000.[2] More than 600,000 Americans die each year of coronary artery disease, and 50 to 60 percent of these victims die prior to reaching a hospital emergency room.[3] A substantial portion of the emergency medical cases that result in death could be prevented by appropriate application of currently known and available techniques. An estimated 60,000 premature deaths annually—and unmeasurable disability—result from inadequate emergency medical care.[4] The national mortality rate from accidents alone could be reduced by ten to twenty percent with proper care at the scene of the accident and en route to a hospital.[5] The magnitude of the problem of accidental death and disability has led to the multiplication of governmental and voluntary efforts to develop and deliver effective emergency medical services to all segments of the population.

Emergency medical services have traditionally been divided into two main kinds: (1) ambulance services and emergency pre-hospital care and (2) emergency medical care provided at hospitals. (A third type—disaster medical services—constitutes another, largely separate system and is not included here.) Each component of the emergency medical care system involves numerous official departments at all levels of government, voluntary agencies, and private organizations. Governmental programs have contributed to increased medical and technical sophistication in provision of first aid, transportation, communication, and treatment in hospital emergency rooms and intensive care units. These programs have established standards and developed resources in every phase of emergency care. The resulting capabilities, however, have not been translated into optimal emergency care readily and equally available to all.[6]

In part, the organizational deficiencies in delivery of emergency medical care may derive from the role of the fragmented private sector in providing services and the need to coordinate numerous, disparate organizations and facilities under different sponsorships. Although percentages are changing, 44 percent of ambulance services are operated by funeral homes, 14 percent by commercial firms, 24 percent by volunteer firemen or other independent groups, and only 13 percent by governmental agencies: fire, police, civil defense, city, or county units.[7] Hospitals operate only 3 percent of ambulance services, and 2 percent are operated by other and unspecified groups. Similarly, the majority of emergency room visits take place in voluntary hospitals because they are more numerous and widely dispersed than public hospitals. In 1968, 67 percent of all emergency room visits were made to voluntary hospitals, 30 percent to public hospitals and 3 percent to proprietary hospitals.[8] This mixture of public and private agencies in provision of emergency medical care has resulted in

... a remarkably intricate and intertwined system . . . crossing functional, jurisdictional, and political boundaries with impunity and leaving vital functions in the hands of non-communicating organizations both public and private.[9]

HISTORICAL BACKGROUND

Modern emergency medical care takes its origins from early ambulance services, pioneer efforts to develop training in first aid techniques, and emergency medical care provided at hospitals. At first designed to handle accidents and trauma cases, emergency rooms of hospitals have come to provide a large volume of ambulatory care for non-emergent conditions. The role of emergency rooms as round-the-clock sources of accessible ambulatory medical care is now as important as their role as trauma centers.[10]

Ambulance Services

Use of the ambulance on the battle fields of the Civil War was well established by 1862, and a century later the armed forces are still following many of the guidelines for coordination of ambulance services developed by the medical director of the Army of the Potomac.[11] At the close of the Civil War, hospitals became the main providers of ambulance services. The first hospital to operate an ambulance service was the Cincinnati General Hospital in 1865, and the first municipal service was established by Bellevue Hospital in New York City in 1870.[12] In urban areas, hospital ambulances were staffed by physicians, usually interns, who would come to the scene of the emergency to render immediate treatment and to accompany the victim to the hospital. In rural areas, where hospitals were remote, funeral directors increasingly became the providers of ambulance services. By 1931, more than half of the ambulance services in the country were operated by morticians, who generally had the only suitable vehicles available.[13]

With the advent of World War II, many hospitals terminated their ambulance services and turned them over to volunteer groups or to commercial companies capable of operating a transport vehicle.[14] In some places, city governments continued to operate ambulance services, but within the past 25 years an increasing number of private and commercial groups have undertaken this responsibility. In the decades following World War II, regulation of emergency medical transportation was minimal and thus

. . . it was entirely possible for an individual or an organization with a station wagon or other similar vehicle, to install red lights and a siren and initiate an ambulance service.[15]

In 1949, concern for the inadequacies of ambulance services prompted the American College of Surgeons, through its Committee on Trauma, to initiate nationwide surveys of facilities in 62 cities. Its 1953 report revealed that almost 30 percent of the cities surveyed had a fair to poor record for ambulance services.[16] Consequently, in 1956, the National Safety Council, a nonprofit organization of local and state safety agencies, institutions, and industries concerned with accident prevention, the American College of Surgeons, and the American Association for the Surgery of Trauma formed the Joint Action Program to "plan and oversee programs for . . . improving the transportation of sick and injured persons."[17] The Joint Action Program initiated still another survey, which confirmed the deficiencies and in-adequacies of ambulance services throughout the country, and in the early 1960s surveys by other groups yielded similar results. Hoping to develop an instrument that each state could adapt to its own use, the Joint Action Program in 1962 proposed a model ordinance for transportation of the injured.

In 1966, Congress enacted the National Traffic and Motor Vehicle Safety Act and the Highway Safety Act. The Department of Transportation, which was assigned responsibility for issuing standards to improve motor vehicle safety and driver performance, was specifically charged with developing a program of emergency medical services to save lives and lessen the severity of accidents. From 1966 to 1972, $33 million of federal funds and $94 million of state and local funds were spent on the emergency medical services program.[18]

Under the Highway Safety Act, the Department of Transportation has issued 16 standards for state programs of highway safety. Standard 11, issued in 1967, requires each state, in cooperation with local jurisdictions, to establish an emergency medical program that meets seven minimum require-ments, discussed below. Implementation of Standard 11 was assigned to the National Highway and Traffic Safety Administration of the Department of Transportation.

In 1970 the Occupational Safety and Health Act sought to coordinate and regulate the many diverse activities involved in the prevention and treatment of industrial accidents and disease, largely handled by private physicians and hospitals and the private emergency clinics found in industrial districts, as well as the medical and nursing staffs of larger industrial esta-blishments. But the Act set up a divided responsibility among federal and state labor and health agencies in carrying out the federal initiative.

In 1971, the President's Health Message placed renewed emphasis on emergency medical services. It stressed, particularly, the automobile and accident program of the Department of Transportation to prevent the annual toll of 50,000 highway deaths, half of which involve drivers or pedestrians under the influence of alcohol. In 1972, the State of the Union Message acknowledged emergency medical services as a national concern and proposed a major federal program to develop new ways of organizing emergency medical services.

Techniques of Care

Citizens' groups and professional organizations have played an important role in developing techniques of care. The American National Red Cross, a pioneer in training the public in first aid, undertook an educational program as early as 1909 to reduce accidents on highways, in homes, in schools, and in industries.[19] In 1935, the Red Cross established first aid stations on highways and later developed a widely utilized program for training law enforcement officers and operators of industrial and public service vehicles in use of first aid techniques and equipment. The National Safety Council, formed in 1913 for accident prevention, subsequently broadened its scope to include improvements in emergency medical care and transportation of the injured and to minimize the harmful effects of accidents. The International Rescue and First Aid Association, organized in 1948, has also developed mutual assistance and training for rescue and first aid workers. In some areas of the country, local volunteer fire departments have long provided emergency ambulance and rescue services.

Various professional organizations concerned with different aspects of trauma or emergency medical care have also contributed their expertise to development of techniques of care: the American College of Surgeons, the American Association for the Surgery of Trauma, the American Trauma Society, the American College of Emergency Physicians, the University Association for Emergency Medical Services, and the Emergency Nursing Services, among others. The National Academy of Sciences-National Research Council has provided a public forum of national experts to stimulate upgrading of emergency medical services, particularly with reference to techniques for training personnel; medical requirements for ambulance design, equipment, and personnel; emergency medical communications; and categorization of hospital emergency capabilities. In 1967, the American Medical Association's Commission on Emergency Medical Services was established. Composed of representatives of several medical specialties and of the United States Public Health Service, this Commission encouraged the formation of the National Registry of Ambulance Emergency Medical Technicians and the development of improved standards for emergency facilities.

Impetus for improved techniques for emergency medical care came from the creation of the federal Regional Medical Programs in 1965. The Commission on Heart Disease, Cancer, and Stroke, formed to recommend practical steps to reduce the toll of these three major killers through development of new scientific knowledge and better use of available life-saving medical techniques, recommended in 1964 the establishment of a national network of regional centers for patient care, research, and teaching in heart disease, cancer, and stroke.[20] Although the activities of the Regional Medical Programs have developed along paths different from those originally envisaged, the overall thrust has expanded the capability of hospitals with varying resources to improve pre-hospital and in-hospital emergency care for heart and stroke patients.

Hospital Emergency Medical Care

Prior to World War II, emergency facilities of hospitals consisted mainly of "accident rooms," which as the name indicates were used for accident cases and some seriously ill persons, usually charity victims of disease or injury.[21] At the close of World War II, growing demands for health services focused national attention on the need for additional hospital facilities. In 1946, enactment of the Hill-Burton Hospital Survey and Construction Act provided funds for construction and modernization of hospital emergency rooms. The 1949 amendments to the Act authorized grants for research, experiments, and demonstrations for the development, effective use, and coordination of hospital services and facilities, which included facilities for emergency services. Federal funding for emergency medical care, however, tended to be directed to the support of biomedical trauma research in laboratories and clinical research units of medical centers and selected hospitals, rather than to improvements in the quality and appropriateness of hospital emergency-room care.[22]

Since the 1950s, use of emergency medical facilities of hospitals has risen astronomically. From 1954 to 1969, the volume of emergency visits to all non-federal, short-term general and special hospitals rose by 314 percent, from 9,148,755 visits in 1954 to 38,770,409 in 1969.[23] Further, the proportion of all outpatient visits that were emergency room visits went from about 20 percent in 1954 to approximately 30 percent in 1969; in some hospitals, particularly in the smaller public institutions, emergency room services account for up to 43 percent of all visits.[24] In Southern California, the Hospital Council of Southern California reported in 1968 that the number of emergency outpatient visits to hospitals in the eight Southern California counties was increasing by 16.3 percent per year.[25] Nationally, the number of persons who come to emergency rooms is increasing by about 10 percent a year.[26]

Not all this increase is attributable to traumatic illness and injury, although the numbers of such cases are large and steadily increasing.[27] Much of this increase is explained by use of the hospital emergency room as a source of general ambulatory medical care. The hospital has come to be looked on "as a place for ambulatory care, not only for persons in outpatient departments but for patients of any social status in 'emergency rooms.' "[28] The picture described for one voluntary hospital is probably not atypical:

> At PCCH, some forty to fifty patients seek service in the "emergency room" each day. Most of these cases, however, are not life-threatening conditions in which delayed action might be fatal. There are estimated to be about four or five such urgent cases per week, but the great majority are simply patients of any income group

who come directly to the hospital because of a distressing symptom for which they cannot get quick help elsewhere. Most of these patients arrive between 3 p.m. and 10 p.m., and the workload increases on weekends when private physicians are less available.[29]

Thus, emergency medical services have come to fill the gap created by inadequate resources for general ambulatory medical care. By 1970, for every four visits to a physician's office there was one visit to an outpatient facility, whereas 25 years earlier the proportion was nine physician visits to one outpatient clinic visit.[30] Visits to the hospital emergency room account for a relatively small proportion of total visits in hospitals where outpatient clinic use is high; in hospitals with low outpatient clinic use, emergency visits constitute a large proportion of all ambulatory visits.[31] More than 60 percent of all cases entering the emergency rooms of Philadelphia hospitals were judged to be non-emergencies,[32] and about 75 percent of visits to the emergency services of large urban public hospitals in the United States were found to be for non-emergent conditions.[33]

Several factors have contributed to this considerable use of hospital emergency rooms for general ambulatory care: decreases in both the numbers and proportion of general practitioners, exodus of the private physician from inner city areas in which low-income groups are concentrated, lack of a regular family doctor because of mobility or inability to pay for medical care, decreasing availability of private physicians at nights and on weekends, increased health insurance coverage of emergency department treatment for insured groups, and increased public recognition and expectation of 24-hour availability of care at the hospital emergency room. As a result, many patients turn to the one available resource in the community that can provide care at any time — the emergency department of the local hospital. But even the highest quality emergency room, equipped to function as a trauma center, may be poorly staffed or organized to serve the full needs of its emergency room population.

AMBULANCE SERVICES AND EMERGENCY PRE-HOSPITAL CARE

The quality of ambulance services and emergency pre-hospital care involves both transportation and medical capabilities. This double thrust explains some division of responsibility; but, at all levels of government, parallel and duplicate functions, lodged in both transportation and health agencies, diffuse responsibility for services that may make the difference between life and death.

Federal Programs

Responsibility for emergency medical services for the civilian population at the federal level of government is divided between the Department of Transportation and the Department of Health, Education, and Welfare. The Department of Defense and the Veterans Administration provide emergency services for the military and their dependents and for veterans, respectively. The Department of Defense also participates with seven other federal departments in a program of assistance to civilian victims of traffic accidents and for other medical emergencies, known by the acronym MAST (Military Assistance to Safety and Traffic). Equipment from military units is used to transport civilian patients from the scene of an accident to an appropriate medical facility, to carry medical specialists and equipment, or to transfer critically ill patients from one hospital to another. The overall coordinating agency for emergency and disaster services is the Office of Emergency Preparedness in the Executive Office of the President.

Within the Department of Transportation, both the Federal Highway Administration and the National Highway and Traffic Safety Administration are engaged in numerous safety programs to reduce deaths and injuries resulting from accidents of all kinds. Under the Federal Highway Administration are programs concerned with standards for highways and vehicles and directed to improvement of highway design, vehicle safety, driver training and control, traffic control devices, and detection of road hazards. Some of the names of these programs are: TOPICS (Traffic Operations Programs to Increase Capacity and Safety, STEP (Selective Traffic Enforcement Program), YOUTHS (Youth Order United Toward Highway Safety), and the Motor Carrier and Highway Safety Program. Under the National Highway and Traffic Safety Administration are programs of the Highway Safety Act designed to promote safe driving, including the Alcohol Countermeasures Program, the Alcohol Safety Accidents Projects, Crash Survivability Programs, and the State and Community Highway Safety Program. Numerous specialized governmental boards and advisory groups are involved in these and related programs, including the National Transportation Safety Board, the National Highway Institute, the National Motor Vehicle Advisory Council, and the National Highway Advisory Council.

Most of the programs of the Department of Transportation have specific, categorical purposes, but one program has addressed itself to the development of standards for comprehensive emergency care systems. The State and Community Highway Safety Program of the National Highway and Traffic Safety Administration administers Standard 11 under the National Highway Safety Act, which requires each state to develop a program to ensure that persons involved in highway accidents receive prompt medical care. Minimum requirements of the program concern training and licensing of ambulance and rescue vehicle personnel, including first-aid training and refresher courses; types, numbers, and equipment of emergency vehicles; coordination of ambulances and other emergency care systems; two-way communications systems; procedures for summoning and dispatching aid; and development of a comprehensive plan for medical services. This comprehensive plan is required to cover facilities and equipment, definition of areas of responsibility, agreements for mutual support, and communications systems.[34] Failure of a state to comply with Standard 11 can entail a 10 percent reduction in federal highway funds, but the Act does not expressly provide that if a state fails to comply with the required standards funds must be withheld.[35] Thus far, provisional approval of state programs has prevented imposition of this sanction.[36]

Within the Department of Health, Education, and Welfare and distributed throughout every major administration of the Department are numerous programs designed to promote improved ambulance services and sophisticated emergency pre-hospital care. The National Institutes of Health contain special projects and programs for biomedical research and training in specialized aspects of trauma care. For example, the National Heart and Lung Institute provides research and training grants for laboratory and clinical research for diagnosis and treatment of heart and pulmonary disease through the establishment of Special Centers of Research (SCORs) at universities and hospitals. It supports the Blood Resource Program for improvement of the quality and quantity of blood available for emergency transfusions. It promotes the Myocardial Infarction Program. The National Institute of Neurological Diseases and Stroke provides grants for development of research centers on acute spinal cord injury. The National Institute of General Medical Sciences also supports research centers on trauma. The new National Institute for Occupational Safety and Health will contribute studies in this field.

The Food and Drug Administration, through the Bureau of Product Safety, is responsible for implementation of nationally uniform requirements for adequate packaging and labelling of hazardous substances sold in interstate commerce.[37] Many of these products are suitable for household use and are a common cause of accidental injury and death, particularly among young children.[38] The Poison Control Branch of the Bureau of Product Safety also provides toxicity information on household products and medicines, publishes national summaries and statistics on accidental poisoning deaths and ingestions, and sponsors National Poison Prevention Week to alert the public to methods of preventing accidental poisoning. These activities are conducted through the National Clearinghouse for Poison Control Centers, which receives statistical data from a network of 580 local poison control centers throughout the United States. The Division of

Biological Standards, now within the Food and Drug Administration, inspects and controls the production and distribution of blood and blood plasma so essential to emergency care.

Within the Health Services and Mental Health Administration, 16 programs are related to improved capability for emergency medical care.[39] The National Center for Health Statistics collects, analyzes, and releases statistics on critical illnesses and injuries essential for the planning and evaluation of emergency medical care programs. Within the Community Health Service, the Comprehensive Health Planning program provides grants to the states which may be channelled to areawide health planning agencies for assessment of community needs for ambulance services and for projects on emergency medical care. The Regional Medical Programs Service is specifically concerned with ambulances, emergency pre-hospital care, and improved design for intensive care for heart disease and stroke patients. Through funding of biomedical research, support of training projects for ambulance personnel, and promotion of cooperative planning by university medical centers, by voluntary agencies, and by private providers of emergency medical care, the Regional Medical Programs have encouraged strengthened capabilities for emergency medical care. The Federal Health Programs Service, through its Division of Emergency Health Services and its ten regional program offices, supports emergency care programs of the states. In July 1971, this Division developed a set of "Recommended Standards for the Development of Emergency Medical Services Systems," in consultation with national authorities.[40] These standards cover all aspects of emergency medical care, including those required by Standard 11 under the National Highway Act: ambulance design and equipment, personnel, emergency facilities and communication, and supportive community action for emergency care. The Division has also supported the development of medical requirements for ambulance design and equipment and guidelines for training of ambulance personnel, matters partly within the province of the Department of Transportation as well.

Within the Social and Rehabilitation Service, the Medicaid program finances ambulance services for categorical recipients and the medically needy and establishes standards for facilities to qualify for payment. Within the Social Security Administration, the Medicare program under Part B pays for emergency ambulance transportation to a hospital, provided that ambulance services are necessary to protect the patient's health, that transportation by other means could endanger the patient's health, and that the patient is taken to the nearest institution equipped to provide appropriate care. For reimbursement as a provider under Medicare, ambulances must carry certain equipment, and attendants must meet specific training requirements. But these standards are lower than those required for vehicle design, equipment, and personnel training by the National Highway Traffic

Safety Administration and by the Division of Emergency Health Services in the Department of Health, Education, and Welfare.[41]

Recent Congressional hearings have revealed that no state has complied more than partially with various federal requirements for emergency medical services.[42] Although elaborate, cooperative relationships have been developed between transportation and health agencies at the federal, regional, and state levels of government,[43] perhaps there is an inherent weakness in attempting to effect an improvement in a medical service, such as ambulance care, through efforts of transportation agencies which have other priorities.[44] As mentioned, the Department of Transportation has a powerful sanction available to achieve enforcement of federal standards governing emergency medical services, but it has not exercised its option to withhold federal funds for highway construction as long as the states are making "reasonable progress in implementing their total programs."[45] Recognition of this dichotomy between the transportation and medical aspects of emergency medical services, and of its consequences for the quality of care, has resulted in the introduction of federal legislation to establish an Emergency Medical Services Administration within the Department of Health, Education, and Welfare, with responsibility for all aspects of emergency medical services. But many other independent departments and agencies are involved in emergency services: the Departments of Transportation, Labor, Housing and Urban Development, the Office of Economic Opportunity, the Office of Science and Technology, as well as the Veterans Administration and the Department of Defense. The varied activities of these agencies can scarcely be encompassed in a new coordinating agency solely within the Department of Health, Education, and Welfare.

State Programs

As at the federal level, state programs for ambulance services and emergency pre-hospital care are divided between transportation and health agencies. Standard 11 of the National Highway Safety Act requires each state to assign to its state health agency the responsibility and authority necessary to ensure prompt and effective emergency medical care. In California, the state health agency is authorized by statute to "maintain a program of accidental injury study and control" and to assist county Emergency Medical Care Committees throughout the state.[46] At the same time, the Office of Traffic Safety of the State Business and Transportation Agency is responsible for developing the state traffic safety program and for coordinating all highway safety activities, which include ambulance and emergency medical services.[47] In fact, ". . . there are involved in California, 2,400 separate entities in traffic safety, all of whom are working ostensibly toward the same goal. And these include eight major agencies . . ."[48] at the state level and several thousand at the local level as well as in the private sector, with diffused responsibilities.

Multiple agencies share responsibility for the same function in provision of emergency medical services. Standards for ambulance vehicles and equipment are established by the California Highway Patrol of the Business and Transportation Agency, which licenses all publicly and privately owned and operated ambulances annually. But consultation is required with the State Department of Public Health, which is authorized to make recommendations on the health and safety aspects of regulation of ambulances and to establish recommended standards for emergency medical services.[49]

Criteria for training of ambulance personnel, similarly, are the province of several agencies. The Department of Motor Vehicles of the Business and Transportation Agency certifies ambulance drivers, requiring them to pass a special driving test before they may operate an ambulance. Almost 40 percent of ambulance drivers in California, however, do not have an ambulance driver's license because they are exempt as police or firemen.[50] Since all law enforcement officers are required to have first aid training and periodic refresher courses, the California Highway Patrol has its own program for training its officers. Additionally, the Commission on Peace Officers' Standards and Training in the office of the Governor establishes criteria for recruiting and training local peace officers. The State Department of Education has separate authority and its own criteria for first aid training for school bus drivers. Finally, the Bureau of Emergency Medical Services of the State Department of Public Health has established minimal training criteria for professional and nonprofessional personnel engaged in emergency medical care and approves training programs offered by community colleges.[51]

The main state agency responsible for regulating the equipment and safety of ambulance vehicles is the California Highway Patrol. It is required to investigate all traffic accidents involving deaths or injury on freeways and on roadways in unincorporated areas of the state. Patrol officers are usually the first to arrive at the scene of an accident and are responsible for placing appropriate calls for emergency ambulance services. Because coordination of ambulances is determined largely by cooperative agreements between agencies on a city, county, or areawide basis, officers of the California Highway Patrol must coordinate and delegate calls for assistance to local law enforcement officers. The State Department of Public Works within the Business and Transportation Agency also provides immediate assistance to injured persons on six toll bridges in the state through its Maintenance and Operations program and operates electronic surveillance devices and radio communications systems to expedite aid to injured motorists. Reimbursement for Medi-Cal beneficiaries who use emergency ambulance services is made by the State Department of Health Care Services.

As a result of divided authority for virtually every function in emergency medical services, no single state agency has clear responsibility for assuring the availability and quality of emergency services. A 1969 report to the California Legislature noted the inconsistent levels of service, varying types and amount of emergency equipment, variable training of personnel, and different systems of record-keeping, and it concluded:

> There is no statewide coordinated Emergency Medical Plan in effect in California at the present time. No agency has been assigned the responsibility for planning and coordinating a statewide program.[52]

This report led to an interagency agreement between the Business and Transportation Agency and the State Department of Public Health to conduct an inventory and survey of state ambulance services. The survey recommended a number of measures to improve California's emergency medical services and specifically recommended that the State Department of Public Health be funded to carry out the emergency medical care activities required by Standard 11 of the National Highway Safety Act.[53] In 1970, the Governor's Automobile Accident Study Commission agreed that a critical problem was "absence of strong, adequately funded coordinating agencies at the state and county level with the authority and responsibility for planning and coordinating a statewide emergency medical services program.[54] The Bureau of Emergency Medical Services of the State Department of Public Health has related the problems of inadequate and variable emergency medical services to

> the present diffuse responsibility for initial aid which is allocated among a number of state agencies currently with inadequate quality control.[55]

In five states, demonstration programs have been established for total emergency medical services systems.[56]

Regional Programs

Action on a regional level to assure effective ambulance and pre-hospital care has emanated from three sources. The Comprehensive Health Planning program, the Regional Medical Programs, and the State Department of Public Health have all undertaken activities in this field on a regional basis.

Each of the nine areawide Comprehensive Health Planning agencies in California has participated in planning for emergency ambulance services for its geographic area, but none has as yet achieved a regional system. In the nine areas of the California Regional Medical Programs, areas not congruent with those of the Comprehensive Health Planning program, efforts have likewise been directed toward encouraging planning and cooperative arrangements among public and private emergency ambulance services. The Regional Medical Programs have also supported many specialized projects for training personnel in mobile intensive care techniques.

Efforts to integrate resources on a regional basis have made progress in Los Angeles County, where three areas of the Regional Medical Programs combined to seek funding for two purposes: first, to support a training program in community colleges and hospitals to upgrade all ambulance personnel to the level of Emergency Medical Technician-1 and, second, to develop a Los Angeles County Emergency Medical Services Community Coordinating Council.[57] The Hospital Council of Southern California, an organization of community hospitals, has been designated to coordinate this training program and has already initiated pilot training programs for Emergency Medical Technicians-1 in ten member hospitals and community colleges.

The proposed regional emergency medical services coordinating council is to be composed of representatives from all the public and private agencies involved in emergency medical services. Its immediate aim is to develop "specific plans for a countywide emergency care system which allows for local flexibility and the necessary sub-systems."[58] A preliminary conference addressed the means for improving and coordinating emergency medical care in Los Angeles County.[59]

The Bureau of Emergency Medical Services of the California State Department of Public Health has also furthered the concept of "functional Regional Emergency Medical Service Area Centers," particularly in rural areas. These would consolidate and categorize existing rural hospital emergency capacity, unify communications through fixed and mobile units, amalgamate ambulance resources into transport networks, and provide standardized and uniform training of nonprofessional emergency medical personnel, as well as augmenting the medical capabilities of existing facilities. A 30,000-square-mile area crossing political boundaries is envisaged as the appropriate geographic area for such a regional system.[60] The concept awaits realization.

Local Programs

The seven million residents of the 4,083 square miles of Los Angeles County are served by 46 ambulance services operated by commercial companies or provided by various departments of state, county, and city government.[61] To summon aid for a victim of trauma in Los Angeles County, depending upon where in the county the emergency arises, one must select one of 54 telephone numbers from which an ambulance may be dispatched.[62]

The cornerstone of the county system of emergency medical services is the Emergency Aid Program (EAP), administered by the County Department of Hospitals, currently merged into the unified County Department of Health Services. Designed to assure emergency ambulance transportation and medical facility care, the program reimburses providers of ambulance services for indigents in 69 of the 77 municipalities within the county and in the county's unincorporated areas. Of the 69 municipalities in the program, 10 use their own fire department ambulances. Established in 1947 under the County Sheriff's Department to assure ambulance coverage to cities unable to afford their own ambulance service, the Emergency Aid Program was transferred in 1951 to the Department of Hospitals, although the Sheriff's Department still retains responsibility for expediting the movement of ambulances.

The Emergency Aid Program involves two kinds of contracts: (1) contracts between the county and cities within the county, whereby the cities agree to pay the county for emergency ambulance services to their residents or in connection with emergencies occurring within their boundaries and the county undertakes to provide these services for all and to pay for them for indigent patients; and (2) contracts between the county and private ambulance companies and community hospitals to provide emergency services. The county currently has contracts with 25 private ambulance companies, which maintain facilities in 67 locations throughout the county, and with 76 community hospitals for emergency medical care.[63] The Department of Hospitals also operates its own fleet of 40 ambulances for inter-hospital transfer of emergency patients, usually from a community hospital to a county hospital. The Emergency Aid Program is thus both a system of transport and a system of payment. Under its auspices, public and private agencies join in a complex set of relationships to provide emergency ambulance services.

Supplementing the Emergency Aid Program, other local official agencies may provide ambulance or emergency pre-hospital care. In 29 cities and unincorporated areas, the County Sheriff's Department screens telephone calls for aid and dispatches ambulances from 14 Sheriff's stations in the county. The County Department of Forestry and Fires provides emergency ambulance rescue services but does not transport patients. In addition, ambulances are dispatched for emergency care in 8 municipalities by fire departments, in 18 by police departments, and in 14 by both fire and police departments.[64]

For emergency psychiatric care, the County Department of Mental Health sponsors psychiatric emergency teams. These operate, however, only from 8 a.m. to 4.30 p.m. and provide emergency psychiatric evaluation and transportation only for voluntary patients. Transportation of involuntary mental patients is provided by the County Sheriff's Department. In cities served by the Emergency Aid Program, local police or fire departments may call the County Sheriff's Department to authorize an ambulance for a mental patient. No single source of evaluation and transportation exists for psychiatric emergencies.

Within the City of Los Angeles—the largest of the 77 cities in the county—ambulance services are under the jurisdiction of the City Fire Department. Its fleet of 27 operational ambulances and 5 supplementary ambulances, with resuscitation equipment located at various fire stations, respond generally to calls for service, but in two areas of the city and for additional ambulance service the Fire Department contracts with private companies to provide ambulance service. The City Receiving Hospital provides initial emergency transport for city employees, particularly for policemen and firemen injured in the line of duty, and for certain kinds of custody cases, such as victims of gunshot wounds, stabbings, fractures, or major lacerations. Responsibility for ambulance and emergency hospital care are split between the city and the county within city limits.

Several measures have been undertaken in Los Angeles County in the effort to unify the network of agencies involved in provision of emergency care and to improve the quality of service, but each of these measures has had to contend with multiple and variable providers, services, and reimbursement arrangements. The Hospital Council of Southern California has developed an emergency radio communications network, called HEAR, which links 140 community hospitals in Southern California with ambulance vehicles and county departments;[65] but not all the Emergency Aid Program contract facilities have joined the HEAR network, and different agencies continue to use different radio channels. Although radio HEAR networks have been budgeted for the County Health Department, the Department of Forestry and Fires, the Sheriff's Department, and the City Receiving Hospitals, the network is not available in the city of Los Angeles for ambulance-to-hospital communications because of frequency crowding. In the City of Los Angeles, its use is limited to inter-hospital communication.

The County Department of Communications, which is responsible for planning design, approving quality and standards, and maintaining all communications equipment and services in county departments, serves as the technical communications support for the large radio systems of the county Sheriff's Department, the Department of Forestry and Fires, and the Department of Hospitals. Its authority, however, does not extend to private ambulance companies and community hospitals participating in the emergency care program. An increasingly popular proposal for establishing an effective system of access to the many agencies providing emergency ambulance and facility care is implementation of the Universal Emergency Telephone Number. State legislation has been proposed to speed adoption of the 911 emergency number throughout California, but in the Los Angeles area adoption of the 911 system will require cooperation from more than 77 jurisdictions. A single emergency telephone number, however, is only the entry point to a needed, unified system of emergency services.

Another mechanism for improving the quality of emergency medical care is the development of a trained paramedic service to staff the ambu-

lances. State legislation authorizes the training of mobile intensive care para-
medics in programs approved by the county health officer or director of
hospitals.[66] The county government provides training for firemen–para-
medics both for county firemen and for those from some cities; the Los
Angeles City Council has approved a plan to replace the emergency
ambulance personnel of the City Fire Department with a highly trained
civilian paramedic service. The proliferation of training programs in
hospitals and community colleges receives some surveillance from the Ad Hoc
Committee on Emergency Medical Technician Training of the Hospital
Council of Southern California and from the Los Angeles County Emergency
Medical Care Committee.[67]

Fundamental problems related to the multiplicity of ambulance and
transportation services persist. In some areas of the county, the response time
of ambulances is as much as 45 minutes. Absence of adequate facilities for
drug and alcohol overdose cases in voluntary hospitals requires that these
patients be transferred to county hospitals. The ambulance service of the
Department of Hospitals has been criticized for slowness in responding to
requests for transfers, but the delays may be caused by poor communication
or incorrect evaluation by the transferring hospital. Providers of emergency
services are permitted to avoid the obligation of serving certain difficult or
undesirable kinds of emergency patients because no sanctions are imposed by
the Medi-Cal, Medicare, or Emergency Aid programs and because no
payment to private physicians is authorized for their care.

At the same time, the many agencies involved in emergency ambulance
services result in a diffusion of responsibility for prompt emergency treatment. The lack of interagency communications and overlapping jurisdictional responsibility are epitomized in the testimony of a representative of
the County Fire Department to the Los Angeles County Emergency Medical
Care Committee:

The Sheriff's Department responds to every Fire Department call. As soon as the
call is received the Fire Department and the Sheriff's Department respond simultaneously. We do not evaluate, both simply go. The organizations settle any differences after the emergency has been taken care of.[68]

Coordination of different agencies and services is all the more possible and
practical today through the application of modern computer technology and
management techniques to ambulance services and pre-hospital care of
emergencies. A single computerized referral system containing all the available categorized resources, training in preliminary triage and referral, a
single dispatching system linked to the strategic location of ambulance
services throughout the county based on probability and forecasting models,
and the use of innovative mobile emergency-room vans[69] are within the grasp
of any modern metropolitan community. The elements exist; the tools are

available. What seem to be lacking are the organizational framework and appropriate use of financial incentives to coordinate disparate elements.

Multiple programs of emergency medical services might function satisfactorily if they were required by an effective regulatory system to provide uniform and equally responsive services everywhere for every emergency. In Los Angeles County, however, responsibility for standards governing various aspects of ambulance services is divided among a number of agencies: the County Board of Supervisors, the Board of Public Utilities of the City of Los Angeles, and the California Highway Patrol, as well as a number of cities within the county. In addition, regulation of ambulances also involves the County Tax Collector, the County Mechanical Services Departments, and the County Department of Hospitals, as well as the County Emergency Medical Care Committee. A significant omission from the list of county agencies with regulatory authority over ambulances is the County Health Department. Its Health Facilities Service Division, which performs a variety of functions connected with licensure of approximately 750 health facilities in the county, has no authority to develop or enforce standards governing sanitary conditions or medical care in ambulances.[70]

EMERGENCY HOSPITAL CARE

The core element in emergency services is the hospital emergency room. Although a uniform national survey of hospital emergency capability is lacking, surveys in 22 states, as of March 1971, revealed major deficiencies:

The majority of the hospitals have no emergency department where the emergency service has equal status with the other departments of the hospital. What this demonstrates is a low level visibility and, consequently, low level priority of emergency medical care planning and service in many of the hospitals in the United States. . . .

In the 22 surveys an average of 17% of the hospitals surveyed had 24 hour coverage by a licensed physician on duty in the emergency department or on call within the hospital. However, it must be noted that without looking at a hospital as a part of a regional system of emergency medical care, it is for the most part impossible to make judgments as to the reasonableness of this percentage. The need indicated by these statistics is one of planning for and implementing emergency medical care on a regional basis. . . .

Communications— The hospital emergency department is part of the emergency medical services system, along with other components, such as ambulances. The 22 States which were evaluated showed that only 6.6% of the ambulances had radio communications with hospital emergency departments.[71]

If to these deficiencies is added the estimate by the American College of Emergency Physicians of the need for another 15,000 physicians trained in emergency room procedures, it is apparent that the hospital emergency room is in serious straits.[72]

Many of the same programs and agencies that are concerned with ambulance and emergency pre-hospital care are also concerned with provision of emergency hospital care. Assigning responsibility for both pre-hospital and in-hospital emergency care to the Health Services and Mental Health Administration of the U.S. Department of Health, Education, and Welfare, to the Bureau of Emergency Medical Services of the State Department of Public Health, and to the County Department of Hospitals tends to encourage a continuum of services for the patient. Nevertheless, this integrated responsibility at top echelons of government is not sufficient to overcome the effects at the level of delivery of services of the multiple, categorical programs — both public and private — involved in planning, providing, financing, and regulating emergency room services for different populations and in different geographic areas. In addition, the modern emergency room suffers from the legacy of being an undesirable assignment for the physician and a last resort for entrance into the health care system for the patient.

Federal Programs

The current federal focus is on emergency medical services as part of a community's total health care system and composed of the inpatient facilities, ambulatory care, and preventive services that constitute the overall system of health care.[73] At cross-purpose with this goal of an integrated system, however, is the multiplicity of federal programs, concerned in different and uncoordinated ways with each function in development of emergency hospital care.

The principal agency involved in the planning and development of improved hospital emergency capabilities is the Division of Emergency Health Services. It has developed recommended standards for hospital emergency facilities, provides limited assistance to states and local areas for improved emergency care potential in hospitals and health departments, and sponsors conferences on emergency medical services at the national, state, and local levels. At the same time, the Regional Medical Programs Service and the Comprehensive Health Planning Service have both given strong emphasis to development of hospital emergency services through financial and technical support. The Regional Medical Programs Service has provided funds to the American Heart Association to establish an Inter-Society Commission on Heart Disease Resources. The Commission has developed guidelines for and defined resources necessary for emergency hospital treatment of patients with cardiovascular diseases. The Regional Medical Programs Service has also provided funds to establish a Joint Committee for Stroke Facilities, administered by the National Institute of Neurological Diseases and Stroke for development of guidelines for different aspects of stroke facilities. The Comprehensive Health Planning program has supported projects for improved planning and provision of emergency medical care. Outside the federal health agency, the Office of Economic Opportunity has funded neighborhood health centers. Impelled by the need for comprehensive ambulatory care in local neighborhoods, these centers have been used and welcomed both as a source of emergency medical care for trauma cases and for general medical care around the clock.

The activities of these agencies have achieved considerable visibility, but the fundamental program for planning emergency medical facility care is the Hill-Burton program, administered by the Health Facilities Planning and Construction Service of HSMHA (see Chapter 7). The 1970 amendments to the Hospital and Medical Facilities Construction Act authorized $20 million annually for three years for modernization and construction of hospital emergency rooms, thus reflecting the importance of emergency and outpatient services as alternatives to inpatient hospital care.[74] Since 1970, the Hill-Burton program has collaborated with many other federal programs and professional organizations in the effort to develop standards for emergency medical facilities, including the Division of Emergency Medical Services of HSMHA, the National Academy of Sciences-National Research Council, the National Highway and Traffic Safety Administration, the training branch of the National Institutes of Health, the Committee on Trauma of the American College of Surgeons, and the Commission on Emergency Medical Services of the American Medical Association. The subjects of common concern include categorization of the capabilities of hospitals to provide trauma services, staffing requirements for 24-hour coverage, minimum training requirements for emergency medical technicians, ambulance design and equipment, and two-way radio communication and telemetry.[75] This emphasis of the Hill-Burton program provides a framework for a more comprehensive approach to planning and development of emergency facilities and services than has existed in the past, but it affects only those hospitals in the Hill-Burton program.

In addition to programs for planning and setting standards for emergency room capabilities, numerous federal programs support biomedical research and training for specialized facilities and for specific categories of trauma conditions. For example, the National Institute of Neurological Diseases and Stroke provides grants for development of emergency room diagnostic techniques for acute stroke units. The National Heart and Lung Institute supports research and treatment projects for cardiovascular disorders through its Intramural Research Program and its clinical center for applied research and specialized patient care. The Maternal and Child Health Service provides funds for training personnel and developing specialized facilities for intensive care of high-risk infants. Through its Manpower Development and Training Program, the Office of Education of the Department of Health, Education, and Welfare provides assistance in training hospital emergency technicians, whereas the Division of Emergency Health Services and Mental Health Administration of the same federal department supports several hospital disaster programs for training physicians, nurses, and paramedical personnel. A program to train orthopedic assistants for work in hospital emergency rooms and operating rooms is jointly funded by the Departments of Labor and Health, Education, and Welfare. Within the National Institute of Mental Health, specialized training and research activities prepare personnel for emergency care of patients with psychiatric, drug, and alcohol problems. Still other programs furnish grants for construction, initial operation, and staffing of facilities that provide emergency services for mental illness, drug dependence, or alcoholism.

Federal programs providing direct emergency medical services or reimbursing providers are categorical programs for certain conditions or services or for particular segments of the population. The Federal Health Programs Service provides emergency medical care to active and retired members of the armed forces and their dependents, Public Health Service officers, and federal employees with job-related injuries and illnesses. The Indian Health Service provides emergency care to Indian and Alaskan Native populations and plans to provide emergency services in Indian Health Service facilities for the non-Indian and non-Alaskan Native populations in those areas where other services are not available — a significant step toward combating fragmentation at the community level. Similarly, emergency and outpatient services formerly provided by the Veterans Administration only for service-connected conditions are currently being expanded. The new National Health Service Corps provides emergency care in a small number of medically under-served areas. Medicare, Medicaid, and CHAMPUS reimburse hospitals and physicians for emergency medical care.

Although many governmental and voluntary agencies set standards for different kinds of emergency medical services, implementation of these standards is largely voluntary. The main mechanism of the federal government for regulating the quality of emergency medical care is certification of the facility as a provider under Medicare. Since accreditation by the Joint Commission on Accreditation of Hospitals satisfies the Conditions for Participation for certification as a provider under Medicare, the effective standards for regulating the quality of emergency care are those set by the Joint Commission. Its standards, revised in 1970, require a well-defined plan for emergency care based on community need and the capability of the hospital; proper organization, direction, and integration of emergency services with other departments of the hospital; certain facilities, equipment, and resources; written policies; and official medical records on all patients. The basic requirement of the Joint Commission is that every ill or injured person who presents himself for emergency treatment should receive at least an assessment of his condition and referral to an appropriate facility.[76] The 1970 standards reflect increased concern with the organization and operation of hospital emergency services; but hospitals are not required to maintain an emergency department,[77] and, if they do, the standards are so general that they allow a wide range of services as compliance.

Moreover, failure of a hospital to be certified under Medicare only prevents the hospital from participating in Medicare; it does not affect the hospital's acceptance of emergency patients. Hospitals not certified can still be reimbursed for emergency services if the hospitals are in rural or isolated areas where alternative sources of emergency care are non-existent or limited.[78] Thus, despite the many standards and guidelines established for emergency hospital care, no program of the federal government requires state or local implementation of uniform standards to assure access to and adequacy of emergency medical care. In the effort to strengthen currently deficient mechanisms for assuring an acceptable standard of emergency medical care, proposed federal legislation would provide substantial funding to the states for coordination and improvement of emergency medical care.[79]

State Programs

In 1972, the California state program of emergency medical services involved 20 state agencies in various functions related directly or indirectly to emergency care. Statewide planning for emergency medical facilities is the responsibility of the State Departments of Public Health, Mental Hygiene, and Rehabilitation. The 1971 State Plan for Health sets forth the goal of "development and enforcement of suitable minimum standards to insure uniform quality and availability of emergency services."[80] Three units within the Department of Public Health—the Office of Comprehensive Health Planning, the Bureau of Emergency Medical Services, and the Bureau of Health Facilities Planning and Construction—are involved in aspects of planning emergency medical care. The Departments of Mental Hygiene and Rehabilitation have developed state plans for construction of facilities that provide emergency medical care for the mentally ill and the alcoholic, respectively. In addition, the Department of Health Care Services, which administers the California Medicaid program, has established standards for the quality of care provided by health facilities, including emergency services.

California's largest public program financing ambulatory and hospital emergency care is its Medicaid program. Emergency services are defined by the Department of Health Care Services as "those services required for alleviation of severe pain or immediate diagnosis and treatment of unforeseen medical conditions, which, if not immediately diagnosed and treated, would lead to disability or death." This definition was adopted as a fiscal device to cut costs.[81] Evaluation or additional diagnosis to determine whether or not a patient has a heart attack is not covered by the Medi-Cal program unless the patient in fact has had the attack.[82] This definition of emergency care is thus not the same as the definition of emergency care used by physicians in the hospital emergency room.

Other state agencies provide or finance emergency medical care for certain categories of disease. The Department of Mental Hygiene provides grants to counties for emergency medical care for mental illness. The Department of Rehabilitation supports local alcoholism programs, including emergency detoxification.

Regulation of facilities providing emergency medical care is the responsibility of three state agencies. The Bureau of Health Facilities Licensing and Certification of the State Department of Public Health licenses annually all hospitals in the state, certifies facilities for participation in Medicare, and approves facilities for receipt of Medi-Cal funds. Its inspections of emergency rooms usually focus more on physical, safety, and sanitation aspects than on operation of the facility's services, adequacy of staffing, patients' rights, and other aspects of quality of care. Standards for participation of facilities in Medi-Cal and reimbursement rates are set by the Department of Health Care Services. The Department of Mental Hygiene licenses psychiatric hospitals and sets standards for other mental health facilities providing emergency care.

Legal requirements for hospital emergency departments in California are governed by the state hospital licensing law, as mentioned, and by a statute which requires emergency services to be provided to persons requesting such care, or for whom such care is requested, for life-threatening conditions or serious injury or illness at any licensed hospital

that maintains and operates an emergency department to provide emergency services to the public where such hospital has appropriate facilities and qualified personnel available to provide such services or care.[83]

Under this statute, however, no hospital is required to maintain an emergency department nor an emergency department of specified capability, nor to equip itself with facilities or personnel for the provision of such care to the community it serves. No standards are required for the facilities, equipment, personnel, or quality of emergency care provided.

Although a survey in 1969 of the 459 California hospitals providing some form of service for vehicular trauma found that 63 percent met minimum standards of emergency care established by the California Hospital Association and the California Medical Association,[84] no generalization can be made from these statistics as to the quality or availability of emergency medical care. Concerning deployment of emergency care facilities, it has been pointed out that

> . . . without an evaluation for capacity for care per institution caution must be exercised also in concluding that an over-supply or under-supply of emergency care facilities exists within a given area.[85]

No agency in California is responsible for compiling and maintaining an up-to-date directory of existing capabilities for all emergency facilities in the state or in a region of the state, although specialized trauma units are inventoried by the State Department of Public Health, as mentioned below. In the absence of a single agency or combination of agencies with authority for regular inspection and monitoring of emergency facilities on the basis of medical quality and level of service capability, effective planning for improved availability of emergency facilities or services to increased numbers of patients becomes difficult, if not impossible.

Regional Programs

The 1971 California State Plan for Health stressed the need for regional planning of emergency facilities to achieve the state's objective of an integrated statewide system for emergency medical care. It recommended:

> Within the regional concept each locality begin planning for unification and consolidation of existing facilities that there may evolve a coordinated effort to utilize appropriate existing and planned medical resources and that all medical care facilities within the locality have the proper ties to the emergency medical care systems portals of entry.[86]

Regionalization permits the development of an efficient and economical system of specialized trauma units — burn centers, intensive coronary care centers, poison control centers, and crisis intervention centers for psychiatric emergencies — each organized according to its capacity for treatment and level of capability. The Bureau of Emergency Medical Services of the State Department of Public Health distributes up-to-date information on specialized trauma control and suicide prevention centers. In some places, emergency facilities providing specialized emergency treatment and care have been designated as regional or area centers for a particular type of service. For example, Children's Hospital in Los Angeles is designated as a poison information center for the county, and certain county-operated hospitals are specialized in the provision of various services for drug detoxification and treatment of alcoholism.

The main regional agencies concerned with emergency hospital care are the areawide Comprehensive Health Planning organizations, the Regional Medical Programs, and the Hospital Council of Southern California. Their functions include planning, financing, regulation, and support of demonstrations and research in the field of emergency hospital facilities and services.

The areawide Comprehensive Health Planning agencies have a role in planning and developing emergency facilities and services through their statutory authority to review and approve all new construction and alteration of hospital facilities. Approval by the areawide agency is required for licensure of the emergency facility; thus the planning agency has some power to influence the distribution of emergency facilities of varied capabilities. The Regional Medical Programs have sponsored projects for planning and developing emergency medical care, especially pre-hospital management of trauma patients and conditions. They have been instrumental in furthering planning of an integrated, countywide system for Los Angeles.

The Hospital Council of Southern California, the voluntary association of hospitals in the region, has made an important contribution to regional planning of and regional responsibility for emergency facilities and services. As early as 1960, the member hospitals adopted a regional concept:

> . . . since it is not possible within the limits of available . . . resources to duplicate comprehensive emergency services in every hospital, reason dictates that there be developed a system of shared community responsibility . . . a system of specifically designated emergency facilities, each having an emergency service area . . . (such a) system . . . may be organized by individual hospitals as in the Santa Monica system or by government as in the Los Angeles City Contract System. . . .[87]

The Council has classified its member hospitals according to five categories of capability: Referral Service, First Aid Room and Referral Service, Stand-by Emergency Service, Intermediate 24-hour Emergency Service, and Comprehensive 24-hour Emergency Service. Approximately 200 hospitals provide one or more of these five levels of emergency services, and each hospital presumably meets the minimal requirements specified by the Hospital Council for that category of service. In assigning levels of capability to member hospitals, however, the Council accepts the facility's own rating of its emergency capacity.[88] In Philadelphia and Detroit, emergency facilities and capabilities of hospitals were rated and classified through independent, on-site visits and observations of care delivered.[89]

Despite trends in the direction of regionalization and efforts by the State Department of Public Health to regionalize emergency services in rural areas, as mentioned, a statewide plan for regionalization of emergency facilities and services has not yet been developed. The critical barrier in California, as in many other states, is not the absence of capabilities in specialized aspects of trauma services, facilities, equipment, or personnel but rather inability of agencies at various levels of government and in the private sector to organize existing resources and to implement a system of categorization.

A hopeful demonstration of planning and implementation of regionalized trauma facilities and services is now in progress in Illinois, where government has taken the lead in securing the cooperation of voluntary organizations and local medical societies with public agencies, in disbursing funds to build a regionalized system, and in developing administrative guidelines directed at comprehensive management of trauma patients.[90] If resources can be organized to achieve an effective regional system of care for trauma patients, who constitute about 10 percent of the emergency care problem, then it may be possible to expand the system to serve all critically injured or ill patients who require effective emergency medical services.

Local Programs

Functions performed at the local level of government to plan, provide, and regulate emergency hospital facilities and services are divided among numerous county and municipal departments and between government and the private sector. Emergency medical care derives a special priority and emphasis, among the fields of health service, from the involvement of the elected officials of county government in its problems. The County Board of Supervisors and the County Administrative Officer have assumed direct responsibility for planning emergency medical facilities and services and for approving contracts with hospitals. The Los Angeles County Emergency Medical Care Committee assists the Board of Supervisors and the County Administrative Officer through its reports and recommendations on matters of policy.

Fundamental to the planning, provision, and regulation of emergency hospital services is an agreed-upon set of standards. In the past, no such standards governed the award of county contracts to community hospitals for emergency care. Although the Los Angeles County Emergency Medical Care Committee had recommended in 1969 that the Department of Hospitals consider for the Emergency Aid Program only applicant facilities with a Class 1 or Class 2 designation, according to the capability rating of the Hospital Council of Southern California,[91] it was not until 1972 that this recommendation for use of a standard classification of hospitals was adopted. The Department currently classifies each of the county's contract facilities according to the five categories of the Hospital Council, and specialty services contractually provided by each facility are categorized by the medical consultant newly assigned to the Emergency Aid Program. The standards used as a basis for award of contracts under the program generally include designation of Class 1 or 2 level of capability, approval by either the Joint Commission on Accreditation of Hospitals or the California Medical Association Staff Survey Program, described below, and determination of the need for an emergency facility in the particular geographic area.

Planning. The Department of Hospitals has major responsibility for assessment of local needs in planning for the county's emergency facilities and services under the Emergency Aid Program. The assessment is based on the judgment of law enforcement departments and private ambulance companies and particularly on the reports and recommendations of the County Sheriff's Department, considered by many to be the most accurate, first-hand source of information about the adequacy of emergency treatment and facilities for patients served by the Emergency Aid Program.

Separate planning is required for specific kinds of emergencies or categories of patient. The County Plan for Mental Health Services, developed by the County Department of Mental Health, concerns emergency psychiatric services provided by the Departments of Hospitals and Mental Health and by Community Mental Health Centers and other clinics. Planning emergency services for alcoholism and drug abuse involves the Departments of Hospitals, Health, and Mental Health, now combined in a single Department of Health Services. Finally, increased capacity of hospital emergency facilities, including applications for state and federal grants, are subject to review and approval by the Los Angeles County Comprehensive Health Planning Association.

Another dimension was added to planning of emergency hospital care when the City of Los Angeles joined the County Emergency Aid Program on July 1, 1971. A participation agreement gave the city considerable voice in advising the County Department of Hospitals, the Board of Supervisors, and the Los Angeles County Emergency Medical Care Committee on addition of emergency facilities, resources, and staff. Prior to the recent implementation of standards for contracts with facilities under the Emergency Aid Program, the City's Medical Advisory Council, appointed by the Mayor and responsible to the City Council, had developed separate standards for emergency facilities within the city that sought contracts under the Emergency Aid Program. Adoption by the county of substantially the same standards has eliminated a serious jurisdictional disparity.

Despite improved planning for emergency facility care, improper utilization and overloading of contract hospitals persist. As a consequence, a 30-minute delay was the average within the hospital emergency room before victims of serious accidents were seen. Or, out of a total of 70 minutes between the time that an accident occurred and treatment was provided — including delay in notification, travel of ambulance to and from the scene, and time at the scene — more than two fifths of the total delay before the patient was seen by a doctor took place within the hospitals' emergency rooms.[92] These problems result in part from lack of communication and coordination among the various hospitals, ambulance services, and law enforcement agencies. As the 1971 report of the Los Angeles County Emergency Medical Care Committee noted,

> Ambulance service, Sheriff, and Fire Department dispatchers should be alerted to temporary overuse of specific emergency facilities so that patients may be directed to adjoining emergency rooms.[93]

In part, this problem of improper use of facilities stems from a dichotomy between planning and providing services. While planning for emergency care is based on the facility's capability, in practice the Emergency Aid Program directs that the victim be taken to the nearest contract hospital, which may have only limited capabilities.

Providing Services. Just as provision of ambulance and pre-hospital services is organized under the county Emergency Aid Program, so the bulk of emergency hospital care is provided under this same program, administered by the County Department of Hospitals. Contracts between the county and 76 community hospitals in 69 municipalities and direct emergency services furnished by three county hospitals provide coverage of the total population. Service areas for emergency facilities are established by the Emergency Aid Program in accordance with the boundaries for the stations of the County Sheriff's Department, which have jurisdiction over dispatch of ambulances.

The Department of Hospitals may enter into three types of contracts for emergency hospital care: (1) contracts with municipalities to enter the program; (2) contracts with community hospitals for provision of emergency care, including all hospital services necessary for treatment during the initial 24-hour period of hospitalization; and (3) so-called "Z" contracts with community hospitals for inpatient emergency services necessary after the initial 24-hour period. Although the "Z" contract guarantees county reimbursement of hospital costs for indigent patients who cannot be removed to county facilities after 24 hours, these contracts do not cover physician's services rendered in the hospital. For this reason, most patients are transferred from contract hospitals to county facilities, often without prior notice or proper records. This practice by voluntary hospitals of "dumping" patients on overcrowded county facilities led interns and residents at the largest county hospital in Los Angeles to bring suit against the county in the effort to alleviate overcrowding and assure adequate patient care.

Other county departments administer additional programs that authorize emergency care for specific conditions or groups of persons. The Department of Mental Health provides and contracts for emergency outpatient and inpatient psychiatric care in county and voluntary hospitals. Federally funded Community Mental Health Centers also provide emergency care to the mentally ill in their separate catchment areas. For alcoholic patients, emergency care is arranged by the Department of Hospitals at the Los Angeles County-University of Southern California Medical Center and at three other county hospitals. The Occupational Health Service of the County Personnel Department provides emergency medical care for county employees with physical or emotional problems, including alcoholism. For drug overdose victims, emergency care and detoxification are provided by the Department of Hospitals at three county hospitals.

Within the City of Los Angeles, a separate program of emergency care is layered over the county system, in spite of the integrated planning, mentioned above. The Medical Services Division of the City Department of Personnel provides emergency facility care for city employees and police custody cases. The city until recently operated two receiving hospitals. It has contracts with 22 community hospitals to render emergency services, particularly for police and firemen and also assumes some responsibility for the emergency care of walk-in patients unable to pay for care. The city's emergency care program is restricted to "first care" for the initial 24 hours of treatment. Patients with more serious conditions are generally transferred to county-operated hospitals or to hospitals under the Emergency Aid Program of the county.

Regulation. In Los Angeles County, the principal regulatory authority over emergency hospital care rests with the Health Facilities Services Division of the County Health Department, which is responsible for hospital licensing by contract with the state. The Division also certifies hospitals for participation in Medicare and approves them for Medi-Cal reimbursement. Licensing of specialized emergency facilities, such as those providing care for the mentally ill or retarded, is also performed by the same Division through a separate agreement with the State Department of Mental Hygiene.

Under the Emergency Aid Program, the Medical Consultant of the Department of Hospitals makes both scheduled and unscheduled visits to emergency facilities under contract with the county to observe the handling of patients and to monitor billing and utilization. The Department enlists aid from the Los Angeles County Emergency Medical Care Committee, which has established task forces to conduct site visits to facilities providing services under the Emergency Aid Program and to other emergency facilities. A task force on emergency psychiatric facilities and services has also been formed. The practice has been adopted under the Emergency Aid Program of reviewing facilities and services periodically and prior to renewal of contracts.[94]

In the City of Los Angeles, the Medical Advisory Council has been delegated authority under the Emergency Aid Program to review and recommend to the County Department of Hospitals and the Board of Supervisors award of contracts to applicant city hospitals. The Council also advises the Emergency Medical Care Committee of the county on all matters pertaining to emergency medical care in the city.

Recent revision by the Department of Hospitals of policies and procedures in the Emergency Aid Program has been an encouraging indication of the program's potential for crossing geographic and political boundaries to achieve improved standards and services. Nevertheless, serious deficiencies remain. Some geographic areas are inadequately covered by emergency care facilities. No department or program coordinates specialized functions in emergency care nor assures appropriate use of existing facilities by developing other resources for general ambulatory care. No single, authoritative mechanism has been established nor financing provided for regulating the availability and quality of emergency medical facility care in the county, despite assumption of part of the responsibility by several governmental agencies and despite efforts by various local, private, and professional groups to make improvements on a more or less ad hoc basis.

Voluntary Programs

The dramatic problems in providing adequate emergency medical care have enlisted the efforts of numerous professional and voluntary organizations. The categorization of emergency hospital facilities according to their capabilities, accomplished by the California Hospital Association, is a basic contribution to rational use of resources for emergency hospital care. But to date there has been little effort to upgrade those emergency rooms that lack adequate capability for emergency care and to fit hospitals into a more rational scheme according to capability. Development of a system may mean dropping some hospitals and enlarging the capability of others, as suggested by the Philadelphia experience.[95] The Staff Survey Program of the California Medical Association is a statewide, voluntary accreditation program of hospitals, including emergency services, based on peer evaluation of medical staff activities. It is designed to supplement accreditation by the Joint Commission on Accreditation of Hospitals and state licensing requirements.[96]

Many national, state, and local professional groups have an impact on the quality of emergency medical care. For example, insurance companies and the National Safety Council have initiated preventive activities, particularly to reduce work and driving accidents. Standards for various aspects of emergency care have been developed by a number of professional organizations with expertise in this field, including the American College of Surgeons, the Committee on Acute Medicine of the American Society of Anesthesiologists, the Committee on Injuries of the American Academy of Orthopedic Surgeons, the Committee on Emergency Medical Services of the American Medical Association, the American College of Emergency Physicians, and the Inter-Society Commission for Heart Disease Resources. The multiplicity of agencies in the public sector is not to be outdone by that in the private sector.

APPROACHES TO INTEGRATION

The central problem in emergency services concerns coordination of the disparate and fragmented entities that now provide those services, in order to render quality care and stabilize the condition of the patient quickly. If proper care were given immediately by correction of outstanding deficiencies, it is estimated that 18,000 lives of the 115,000 lost in accidents could be saved, 350,000 pre-hospital coronary deaths could be prevented, and 5,000 deaths from poisonings, drownings, obstetrical complications, and other causes could be prevented.[97]

The approach to coordination or integration is at two levels, national and local. Two basic approaches at the national level have been proposed.

In its bare outlines, one approach would establish an emergency medical services administration within the Department of Health, Education, and Welfare to set standards for operation of ambulance-related services, provide financial assistance for operation of local ambulance equipment, transfer certain highway safety functions to the Department of Health, Education, and Welfare, and appropriate funds to support these activities.[98] The essence of this proposal, and of its variants, is integration in a single federal health agency of the various functions related to emergency medical services now divided among about 25 federal agencies,[99] with a trickle-down effect to bring about emphasis and coordination of efforts at the community level.

Another approach, espoused by the Department of Health, Education, and Welfare, is based on the premise that emergency medical services should not be separated from the rest of the health service system. This approach would organize existing resources so as to develop local emergency medical systems on a regionalized basis.[100] Achievement of this objective would require consolidation of federal functions under the leadership of a health agency and reorganization of community resources, first in demonstration communities and later throughout the nation.

To accomplish either of these approaches requires a new legislative directive that, in effect, would be superimposed on the 130 current legislative directives that affect emergency room and transportation services and the 156 directives or statutory citations that affect emergency services.[101] This new legislative directive should use governmental financing to create appropriate incentives for achieving a coordinated system of services in this vital field.

Whatever form integration takes at the national level, integration at the local level, where services are delivered, is even more urgent. Local initiative cannot and need not wait on national directives. A systems analyst who has made a careful study of emergency services in the Los Angeles area describes it in the following telling words:

> . . . the present so-called emergency medical "system" is in fact more of a loosely knit "network" of activities carried out by differentiated, specialized organizations. . . . Agreement on objectives and such coordination as exists is far too frequently based on political considerations which tend to insure the continuation of the existence of the subunit. . . . There are numerous gaps and mismatches in emergency medical care because of its fractionation. There tends to be poor matching of the needs of victims to the most appropriate sources of care. . . . Fractionation of the care system can at best only produce sub-optimization of performance of both the units and total system, accompanied by waste of resources. . . .[102]

Within this fractionated "system" are all the elements necessary to transform it, through appropriate organizational and financing mechanisms and application of modern communication technology and systems analysis, into an integrated system that would yield savings in costs and lives. The folly of fragmentation has been amply demonstrated in other health services. In this field, where life and death hang on minutes saved, it is worse than folly. It is this urgency that is moving many localities into integrating and regionalizing their systems of emergency care, even risking the aforementioned "political considerations."

Faced with the facts that "maybe 15 percent (of accredited hospitals) can adequately handle the medical emergencies and psychiatric emergencies, in the sense of truly adequate capability,"[103] that ambulance services are often outdated, lack adequate equipment, and do not have two-way communication with capable hospital centers, that physicians may not be trained for emergency work, that public agencies often work at cross-purposes or duplicate each other's efforts, faced with these facts in emergency services, community after community across the nation is moving into more integrative patterns. Perhaps the current attack on fragmentation of functions in emergency medical services may provide experience leading to a more rational system of health services generally.

NOTES

1. Duval, Merlin K., M.D., "The Hidden Crisis in Health Care," *Proceedings Second National Conference on Emergency Health Services*, p. 3 at 6, Division of Emergency Health Services, Health Services and Mental Health Administration, Department of Health, Education, and Welfare, Pub. No. DEHS-16, Jan. 1972.

2. Artz, Curtis P., M.D., "Emergency Care for Trauma," *Proceedings*, supra note 1 at 14 (based on figures compiled by the National Safety Council).

3. Conn, Robert D., M.D., "The Prehospital Care of Medical Emergencies," *Proceedings*, supra note 1 at 17.

4. Huntley, Henry C., M.D., "National Status of Emergency Health Services," *Proceedings*, supra note 1, p. 8 at 12-13.

5. This is a conservative estimate. See statement of Dr. Merlin K. Duval in *Emergency Medical Services Act of 1972*, Hearings before the Subcommittee on Public Health and Environment of the Committee on Interstate and Foreign Commerce, House of Representatives, 92nd Cong., 2d Sess., p. 50 at 51, June 13, 1972, that "[s]urgeons estimate that 20 percent of the more than 50,000 dying from highway accidents annually could be saved if proper care could be given at the scene and during transport to a medical facility."

6. Hampton, Oscar P., Jr., M.D., "Opening Remarks," *Proceedings*, supra note 1 at 1.

7. *Ambulance Services and Hospital Emergency Departments*, Digest of Surveys Conducted 1965 to March 1971, p. 5, Division of Emergency Health Services, Health Services and Mental Health Administration, Department of Health, Education, and Welfare, Pub. No. DEHS-11, May 1971.

8. Piore, Nora, Deborah Lewis, and Jeannie Seeliger, *A Statistical Profile of Hospital Outpatient Services in the United States: Present Scope and Potential Role*, pp. 120-121, Association for the Aid of Crippled Children, New York, 1971.

9. Nahum, Alan M., M.D., "Analysis of Emergency Medical Care Systems," *Selected Papers on Health Issues In California*, p. 467 at 471, State Office of Comprehensive Health Planning, California State Department of Public Health, Sacramento, 1971.

10. Taubenhaus, Leon J., "Emergency Services," *Hospitals*, Vol. 47, No. 7, p. 81, Apr. 1, 1972.

11. Weisberg, Carole, "Health Law Project Memo on Ambulances," *Preliminary Materials on Health Law*, Sec. 3, p. 216, Health Law Project, University of Pennsylvania Law School in conjunction with the National Legal Program on Health Problems of the Poor, University of California, Los Angeles, Summer 1971.

12. Ibid.

13. Ibid.

14. Duval, supra note 1 at 4.

15. Id. at 5.

16. Spencer, James H., "American College of Surgeons Committee on Trauma," *Immediate Care and Transport of the Injured* (George J. Curry, Ed.), pp. 11-12, Thomas Books, Chicago, 1965.

17. Pyle, Howard, "The National Safety Council," *Immediate Care and Transport of the Injured*, supra note 16 at 156.

18. *Emergency Medical Services Act of 1972*, Hearings, supra note 5 at 88.

19. Oswald, Robert M., "American National Red Cross," *Immediate Care and Transport of the Injured*, supra note 16 at 145.

20. The President's Commission on Heart Disease, Cancer and Stroke, *A National Program to Conquer Heart Disease, Cancer and Stroke*, Vol. I, p. 29, U.S. Government Printing Office, Washington, D.C., 1964.

21. Division of Medical Sciences, National Academy of Sciences-National Research Council, *Accidental Death and Disability: The Neglected Disease of Modern Society*, p. 18. Division of Emergency Medical Services, Health Services and Mental Health Administration, U.S. Department of Health, Education, and Welfare, PHS Pub. No. 1071-A-13, Sixth Printing, 1970.

22. See Duval, supra note 1 at 5 and *Accidental Death and Disability*, supra note 21 at 32-33.

23. Gibson, Geoffrey, Ph.D., "Status of Urban Services-1, Emergency Services," *Hospitals*, Vol. 45, p. 49, Dec. 16, 1971.

24. Piore, supra note 8 at 67-8.

25. Hospital Council of Southern California, "Responsibility to the Community in the Provision of Hospital Emergency Outpatient Services," p. 2, processed 1968.

26. *Emergency Medical Services Act of 1972*, Hearings, supra note 5 at 84.

27. Gibson, supra note 23 at 50.

28. Roemer, Milton I. and Jay W. Friedman, *Doctors in Hospitals*, p. 47, Johns Hopkins Press, Baltimore, 1971.

29. Id. at 132-133.

30. Piore, supra note 8 at 21.

31. Id. at 178-179.

32. Hamilton, William F., Ph.D., and Joanne E. Finley, M.D., "Planning for Urban Emergency Medical Services," p. 14, paper presented at 100th Anniversary meeting of the American Public Health Association, Atlantic City, N.J., Nov., 1972 and *Report of the Emergency Medical Services Task Force of the Philadelphia Department of Public Health*, p. 46, Philadelphia, Feb. 1972.

33. Cooney, James P., Jr., Ph.D., Milton I. Roemer, M.D., and Martin B. Ross, M.P.H., *The Contemporary Status of Large Urban Public Hospitals—Ambulatory Services*, Summary Report, Large Urban Public Hospitals, Ambulatory Services Project, p. 71, School of Public Health, University of California, Los Angeles, Nov. 1971.

34. Hearings, supra note 5 at 89.

35. Id. at 96.

36. Alexander, Susan G., "The State of Emergency Medical Services under the Highway Safety Act or Don't Be Caught Dead in an Ambulance," *Clearinghouse Review*, Vol. 5, No. 2, p. 72, June 1971.

37. These requirements have been established by the Federal Hazardous Substances Act of 1960 and the Poison Prevention Packaging Act of 1970, 15 U.S.C. sec. 1261 (Supp. 1971), 7 U.S.C. sec. 135 (Supp. 1972).

38. *Consumer Programs*, Hearings before the Subcommittee on Agriculture, Environmental and Consumer Protection of the Committee on Appropriations, House of Representatives, 92nd Cong., 2d Sess., Part 4, p. 184, 1972. The Public Health Service estimates that approximately 600,000 children swallow household aids each year.

39. DuVal, supra note 5 at 56.

40. Division of Emergency Health Services, *Recommended Standards for the Development of Emergency Medical Services*, Pub. No. DEHS-4, U.S. Department of Health, Education, and Welfare, July 1971.

41. Hearings, supra note 5 at 32-33.

42. Id. at 100 ff. showing current status of each state's compliance with the 1966 standards.

43. Id. at 78-79.

44. Id. at 32-33.

45. Id. at 96.

46. Calif. Health & Safety Code, secs. 405, 1750 (Deering Supp. 1971).

47. Calif. Vehicle Code, secs. 2900-2910 (Deering 1972).

48. Frankland, Bramford, "California's Traffic Safety Programs," *Proceedings of the Governor's Automobile Accident Study Commission*, p. 607, May 28, 1970.

49. Calif. Vehicle Code, sec, 2512 (Deering 1972).

50. California State Department of Public Health, *California Ambulance Survey*, Final Report, p. 15, May 1970.

51. Farr, Lee E., M.D. and Florence R. Weiner, R.N., "Emergency Medical Services: State Strives for Uniform Readiness, Availability," *California's Health*, p. 4 at 5, Oct. 1972.

52. *California Highway Safety Program*, EMS-311, Report to the California Legislature, p. 57, Jan. 10, 1969.

53. *California Abulance Survey*, supra note 50 at 28.

54. Governor's Automobile Accident Study Commission, *Final Report*, Vol. 1, p. 39, Dec. 1970.

55. Farr, Lee E., M.D., "Emergency Medical Services, A Resumé for the State Health Planning Council," EMS 70-212.1, p. 9, July 1970.

56. Hanlon, John J., M.D., M.P.H., "Emergency Medical Services, New Program for Old Problem," *Health Services Reports*, Vol. 88, No. 3, p. 205, March 1973.

57. California Regional Medical Programs, Areas IX, IV, and V, "Los Angeles County Emergency Medical Services System Development Project," Application for an Operational Grant Award, submitted to the California Regional Medical Program Technical Review Panel, Apr. 1972.

58. Id. at 48-49.

59. *Proceedings, EMS, Countywide Conference on Emergency Medical Services*, Los Angeles, June 1972.

60. Farr and Weiner, supra note 51 at 4-5.

61. *California Ambulance Survey*, supra note 50 at 197.

62. Weil, Max Harry, "The Present System of Emergency Medical Services in Los Angeles County," *Proceedings*, supra note 59 at 30.

63. Ibid.

64. *Proceedings*, supra note 59 at 30.

65. Los Angeles County Committee on Emergency Medical Care, *Annual Report for 1970-1971*, p. 27, Los Angeles, 1971. See Workshop Report on Communications, *Proceedings*, supra note 59 at 87.

66. Calif. Health & Safety Code, Secs. 1480-1485 (Deering Supp. 1971).

67. Workshop Report on Manpower Training, *Proceedings*, supra note 59 at 141.

68. Los Angeles County Committee on Emergency Medical Care, *Annual Report for 1969-1970*, p. 5, Los Angeles, 1970. See "Paramedic Program Spreading across Nation," *Los Angeles Times*, Sept. 25, 1972, for account of rivalry between private ambulance crews and firemen-paramedic teams.

69. Holloway, Ronald M., M.D. and Julius E. Stolfi, M.D., "Mobile Vans as Disaster Scene Emergency Rooms," *Hospitals*, Vol. 46, No. 23, p. 43, Dec. 1, 1972.

70. See *Future Directions for Health Services, County of Los Angeles/1970*, Review of the Program of the Los Angeles County Health Department, undertaken at the request of the Los Angeles County Board of Supervisors, p. 157, American Public Health Association, Community Health Action Planning Services (Malcolm H. Merrill, M.D., Director of study), Los Angeles, 1970.

71. *Emergency Medical Services Act of 1972*, Hearings before the Subcommittee on Public Health and Environment, Committee on Interstate and Foreign Commerce, House of Representatives, 92nd Cong., 2d Sess., Part 1, pp. 83-84, June 13, 14, and 15, 1972.

72. Id. at 197.

73. Statement of Dr. Merlin K. DuVal, Assistant Secretary for Health and Scientific Affairs, U.S. Department of Health, Education, and Welfare, Hearings, supra note 71 at 50 ff.

74. U.S. Department of Health, Education, and Welfare, *1970 Annual Report,* pp. 161-162, U.S. Government Printing Office, Washington, D.C., Dec. 1970.

75. *Departments of Labor and Health, Education, and Welfare Appropriations for 1972,* Hearings before a Subcommittee of the Committee on Appropriations, House of Representatives, 92nd Cong., 1st Sess., Part 2, p. 682, Apr. 1971.

76. Joint Commission on Accreditation of Hospitals, *Accreditation Manual for Hospitals,* Standards on Emergency Services, Dec. 1970.

77. Porterfield, John D., III, M.D., "Accreditation Problems," *Hospitals,* Vol. 45, No. 10, p. 38, May 16, 1971.

78. 20 C.F.R., sec. 405.1010 (1970).

79. See Hearings, supra note 71.

80. Task Force for the Development of the State Plan for Health, *California State Plan for Health 1971,* p. 210, State Office of Comprehensive Health Planning, California State Department of Public Health, Sacramento, 1971.

81. Workshop Report on Emergency Services, Third Party Payment Mechanism, *Proceedings, EMS, Countywide Conference on Emergency Medical Services,* supra note 59 at 125.

82. Ibid.

83. Calif. Health & Safety Code, sec. 1407.5 (Deering Supp. 1971).

84. California Hospital Association and California Medical Association, *Survey of Emergency and Disaster Medical Services* (Analysis of Data by the Bureau of Research and Planning CMA Division of Socio-Economics and Research), San Francisco, Dec. 1969.

85. Duffey, Kenneth E., M.D., "Emergency Medical Care and Care Systems in California — Motor Vehicle Accidents," *Calif. Med.,* Vol. 166, p. 30 at 33-34, Feb. 1972.

86. *California State Plan for Health 1971,* supra note 80 at 211.

87. Hospital Council of Southern California, "Responsibility to the Community in the Provision of Hospital Emergency Outpatient Services," p. 2, July 1968.

88. Information provided by the Emergency Aid Program, Los Angeles County Department of Hospitals.

89. *Report of the Emergency Medical Services Task Force of the Philadelphia Department of Public Health,* pp. 50-51, Philadelphia, Feb. 1972; Cranshaw, Thomas M., "Regionalizing Emergency Health Care in Detroit," paper presented at the American Public Health Association Annual Meeting, p. 3, Atlantic City, N.J., Nov. 13, 1972.

90. *The Critically Injured Patient Concept and the Illinois Statewide Plan for Trauma Centers,* Illinois Department of Public Health, Division of Emergency Medical Services and Highway Safety, May 1972; Flashner, Bruce A., M.D. and David R. Boyd, M.D.C.M., "The Critically Injured Patient: A Plan for the Organization of a Statewide System of Trauma Facilities," *Ill. Med. J.,* March 1971.

91. County of Los Angeles Committee on Emergency Medical Care, *Annual Report* for 1969-1970, p. 11, Los Angeles, 1970.

92. "How Traffic Safety Relates to the Emergency Medical Services System," Report on Workshop XIV, *Proceedings, EMS, Countywide Conference on Emergency Medical Services,* p. 198, Los Angeles, June 1972.

93. County of Los Angeles Committee on Emergency Medical Care, *Annual Report for 1970-1971,* p. 22, Los Angeles, 1971.

94. Ibid.

95. *Report of the Emergency Medical Services Task Force of the Philadelphia Department of Public Health,* supra note 89 at 83 ff.

96. Halter, Bert, "Emergency Care Facilities in California," Proceedings of the Governor's Automobile Accident Study Commission, p. 10, Sacramento, March 1970.

97. Testimony of Dr. James D. Mills, President, American College of Emergency Physicians, Hearings, supra note 71 at 187, 190.

98. H.R. 12787, a bill to establish an emergency medical services administration within the Department of Health, Education, and Welfare to assist communities in providing professional emergency medical care, Hearings, supra note 71 at 11, 28-29.

99. See testimony of Representative Robert F. Drinan, Hearings, supra note 71 at 49.

100. Hearings, supra note 71 at 55.

101. Id. at 73-74.

102. Andrews, Robert B., "The Systems Approach to the Improvement of Emergency Medical Services," *Proceedings,* supra note 92 at 47.

103. Statement of Dr. Merlin K. DuVal, Hearings, supra note 71 at 82.

CHAPTER 7

Construction, Planning, and Regulation of Health Facilities: Programs for Resource Production and Social Controls

> *Surveys and reports indicate that hospitals in many communities have tended to operate in splendid isolation, perhaps because they saw themselves as self-sufficient in the medical talent and the mechanical technology necessary to serve most of the needs of most patients. This attitude is changing dramatically and, if the hospital continues to look outside its windows into the doors of other agencies, it can become the facility, the place of reference for much of a community's medical service. Viewed in this light, the future general hospital, providing comprehensive medical services in the acute, chronic, and psychiatric fields, while emphasizing prevention, care, and rehabilitation, can become an integrating factor in community health care facilities.*[1]

> —National Commission on
> Community Health Services, 1966

The medley of functions necessary to plan, construct, and provide surveillance for the many kinds of health facilities is described for three reasons. First, health facilities, particularly hospitals, are the principal sites of health care. In the words of Anne Somers, "it is difficult to exaggerate the importance of the hospital in contemporary society."[2] Hospitals, together with nursing homes, account for the largest proportion of expenditures for health care. Second, these three functions—planning, construction, and regulation of facilities—uncover the separate and diverse, but nevertheless related, roles of the public, voluntary, and private sectors in health services. Third, social controls over health facilities illustrate the multiple and ambivalent roles of government. Health facilities are planned, sponsored, built, operated, and regulated by both public and private agencies. The public agencies include all levels of government. The private agencies are both nonprofit and for-profit entities.

Description of construction, planning, and regulation of health facilities will illustrate the complex interrelationships that follow from the categorical approach and its implications for the availability, appropriateness, quality, and cost of health care. The multiple programs involved in discharging these three functions are considered separately, and their interrelationships are shown in a brief history of the California experience with hospital planning and construction.

HISTORICAL BACKGROUND

Hospitals have existed for centuries, but governmental and voluntary programs to construct, plan, and regulate hospitals and other health facilities in an organized way are relatively recent. Over the years, three separate systems of hospitals and other health facilities have evolved. One system is public, consisting of city- and county-operated hospitals mainly for the poor; state-operated mental, tubercular, and other specialized hospitals; and federal hospitals—Public Health Service hospitals, including those serving Indians, military hospitals, and veterans' facilities. The second system consists of not-for-profit general and specialized hospitals, most frequently organized by community and philanthropic groups, many church-related, operating under self-governing boards, staffed by physicians in private practice and some on salary, raising their own funds, setting their own standards, and with few relations to the system of governmental hospitals. In California, district hospitals, although sponsored by local governmental units, generally fit the same pattern as the not-for-profit facilities. A third system consists of the growing numbers of private, for-profit hospitals.

Of the 7,600 hospitals with some 1.6 million beds in the United States in 1970, 412 were federal hospitals with 161,000 beds, 2,300 were state and local hospitals with some 780,000 beds, and the rest were 4,360 non-governmental hospitals with some 670,000 beds. Most of the state hospitals are long-term, psychiatric facilities; most of the local government hospitals are short-term, general hospitals. Of the 6,800 general medical and surgical hospitals with almost a million beds in 1970, 1,700 with more than 200,000 beds were state and local government hospitals. The prevailing community general hospital is the voluntary hospital, of which there were 3,400 with 592,000 beds in 1970. For-profit, short-term general, and other special hospitals had grown to 770 in 1970 with 53,000 beds. In addition, there are now some 19,000 providing nursing and personal care, with more than 700,000 beds. Most of these facilities are proprietary. Some 450,000 handicapped, disturbed, or mentally retarded persons are served annually by 4,300 other inpatient facilities.[3]

Public regulation of non-governmental hospitals began indirectly with state requirements for the qualifications of physicians. The oldest form of public control of hospitals in the United States is to be found in the state licensure laws for physicians and other health personnel.[4] Minimum qualifications for medical practice were enacted as early as 1760 in New York, but most of the state medical licensing laws were passed in the late 19th and early 20th centuries. They indirectly set a floor for the level of hospital care because regulation of the quality of personnel who worked in hospitals inevitably affected the care provided there. In 1910, the Flexner report recommended sweeping changes in medical education. Implementation of these recommendations extended beyond medical schools proper to teaching hospitals and to the practice of the clinical specialties, closely associated with hospitals.[5]

The main voluntary mechanism for regulation of facilities — accreditation by the Joint Commission on Accreditation of Hospitals — is an outgrowth of earlier efforts by the American College of Surgeons to assure appropriate specialty qualifications.[6] In 1913, the Council on Medical Education and Hospitals of the American Medical Association began inspecting hospitals, with the cooperation of state and city hospital committees appointed by state medical societies. In 1914, the American Medical Association published its first list of hospitals approved for training interns and, in 1927, a list of those approved for resident training. In 1918, the American College of Surgeons adopted its Minimum Standards for Hospitals relating to medical staff, clinical conferences, medical records, laboratory and X-ray facilities, and elimination of fee-splitting.[7] For more than 30 years, this program of hospital approval was conducted by the American College of Surgeons through annual surveys of hospitals. Not until 1952 did four sponsoring organizations — the American College of Surgeons, the American Medical Association, the American Hospital Association, and the American College of Physicians — combine to provide broader sponsorship and increased financing through the Joint Commission on Accreditation of Hospitals.[8]

The cornerstone of public regulation of health facilities is the relatively recent state licensing of hospitals, now expanded to include virtually all kinds of facilities. An early form of inspection and licensing was that conducted for maternity units of hospitals on a state or city basis.[9] Antecedents of hospital licensing can also be found in federal standards set by maternal and child health programs and crippled children's services for providers of care under their programs.[10] Comprehensive state licensing laws, however, were not enacted until after the passage in 1946 of the Hill-Burton Hospital Survey and Construction Act, which required states to specify minimum standards for facilities receiving federal subsidy.[11] When the Act was passed, only ten states had licensing laws for hospitals, most of them quite limited; since 1946, all states have enacted hospital licensing laws.[12]

CONSTRUCTION OF FACILITIES

Private funding has dominated recent construction of health facilities. In 1972, private funds for construction of facilities amounted to $2.7 billion; public funds amounted to $1.4 billion, $350 million of which supported construction of private facilities.[13] Public programs have been influential in providing a much-needed source of funds for private construction, particularly in the long period when hospital construction by the private sector was deficient. Moreover, public programs have guided the development of needed facilities in under-served areas.

The Hill-Burton Program

The Hill-Burton Hospital Survey and Construction program, enacted in 1946, represents a great divide in the development of health facilities in the United States. By providing funds for both private and public construction, it set in motion a deepening involvement of public and private sectors in the production of resources. It inaugurated organized planning of health facilities. It set standards, required licensing of facilities, and affected the quality of care by helping to modernize facilities and improve their distribution. Over the years, it provided widening aid to planned development and strengthened regulation of facilities. Basic support for construction of hospitals, funds for planning, and requirements for standards were supplemented by support of new types of facilities, new kinds of aid, broadened purposes, and increased social control of health facilities in a remarkable example of an integrated program.[14]

   The Hill-Burton program was a departure in federal aid for health service, in that it gave grants not only to state and local government but to non-governmental institutions as well. The extreme shortage of hospital beds and other facilities, particularly in rural areas, and the unsuitability of many older facilities, aggravated by years of depression and wartime belt-tightening, contributed to its enactment. Voluntary hospitals had suffered during the depression, many had failed, private philanthropic funds for construction had dried up, and virtually no building had occurred during the war years. By the end of World War II, the number of hospital beds had fallen more than 40 percent below estimated requirements.

The Hill–Burton program has been in force for more than a quarter-century. In the period from 1947, when funds were first made available, to 1970, the program helped to provide 460,316 inpatient care beds in hospitals and nursing homes.[15] A major share of the funds went to 5,130 projects in voluntary nonprofit institutions, contributing to the building of 262,000 beds. In addition, some 1,600 long-term care projects were supported in general hospitals, chronic disease hospitals, and nursing homes. Assistance was provided to 195 mental hospitals and 80 tuberculosis hospitals; some 500 rehabilitation centers were established. Support was given to 640 projects in state-owned facilities with 39,500 beds and 4,400 projects in other public facilities with 142,000 beds; help was provided to build 40 state health laboratories and 1,233 public health centers. The program contributed significantly to the growth of outpatient departments of hospitals through its support of more than 1,000 diagnostic and treatment centers,[16] now called outpatient facilities.

By the early 1960s, the Hill–Burton program had not only gone a long way toward erasing the deficit in hospital beds in small towns and rural areas but had helped redress the imbalance in ratios of hospital beds to population between the richer and poorer states.[17] Emphasis began to shift toward the urgent needs of the inner cities and to modernization of facilities rather than new construction. By 1970, more than 90 percent of Hill–Burton funds had been allocated for additions to, or replacement of, existing facilities, and for rehabilitation of obsolescent facilities. While some loans had been available in earlier years, particularly for religious-sponsored hospitals that refused grants, in 1970 a three-year extension of the program launched an explicit policy to provide loans, loan guarantees, and interest subsidies for construction and modernization of not-for-profit facilities in place of grants. An effect of this emphasis on loans is to shift the major cost of repayment of both principal and interest on loans to patients through higher daily charges.

A signal contribution of the Hill–Burton program has been its generative role. Although its $3.5 billion contribution of federal funds represents little more than 11.6 percent of the total $30 billion spent on construction of health facilities since 1945, it generated another $9 billion in state, local, and private funds. Hence, Hill–Burton funds, together with the funds it stimulated, amounted to some $12.3 billion and accounted for two-fifths of all spending for health facilities in this period. Moreover, it reached into 3,800 communities in the nation, directly aiding a majority of voluntary hospitals by constructing some 270,000 beds — almost half the total beds in voluntary hospitals. While the Hill–Burton program stimulated the private sector, the substantial private investment in construction of health facilities has, until recently, been largely removed from and independent of community or area-wide planning for expansion and location of health facilities.

Other Federal Programs

In addition to the Hill-Burton program, other federal aids to construction accentuate the fragmentation in construction of health facilities. These include (1) federal aid to public and private facilities similar to but quite separate from the Hill-Burton program; (2) construction of federally operated facilities, also divorced from overall construction policy; (3) indirect federal assistance through payments for medical care; and (4) the aggregation of federal subsidies and tax incentives to construction.

1. In addition to the Health Facilities Planning and Construction Service, which administers the Hill-Burton program, many other divisions of the Department of Health, Education, and Welfare provide support for construction of facilities. The National Institute of Mental Health provides grants for construction of community mental health facilities and alcoholic and drug abuse facilities. The National Institute of Child Health and Human Development provides grants for child mental health treatment facilities. The Rehabilitation Services Administration provides construction and remodeling grants for rehabilitation centers; its Division of Mental Retardation provides grants for construction of special facilities for diagnosis, training, education, treatment, or care of the mentally retarded. Each of these programs is designed to support public and nonprofit agencies and facilities but with varying purposes, standards, and requirements. For example, some grants are solely for construction, and some may be applied also to modernization. Some include staffing or equipment; others do not. Each agency plans for the kind of facility that it is authorized to fund, apart from the overall state planning required by the Hill-Burton program.

Other direct support of construction is provided by the Department of Health, Education, and Welfare through programs for construction of schools or training facilities for the health professions and occupations. Three major programs are authorized: construction grants for schools of medicine, osteopathy, public health, pharmacy, podiatry, optometry, and teaching hospitals affiliated with medical and osteopathic schools; construction or remodeling grants for collegiate, associate degree, and diploma schools of nursing; and construction grants (not funded) for qualified training institutions for allied health manpower.[18]

In addition, numerous non-health agencies and programs provide support for construction of health facilities, quite distinct in policy and purpose from those of the Department of Health, Education, and Welfare.

The most important of these is the Department of Housing and Urban Development, which spent $155 million in 1972 for construction of health facilities through at least four separate programs. Its Federal Housing Administration in one program insures mortgages made by private lenders to finance construction or rehabilitation of for-profit and nonprofit hospitals, nursing homes, and group medical practice facilities; in another program, provides mortgage insurance for rental housing with special facilities for the aged and handicapped; and, in still another program, provides direct loans for health facilities. Its Model Cities program provides construction grants for comprehensive health centers.

The Office of Economic Opportunity has made construction and staffing grants to public and nonprofit organizations to establish community-based neighborhood health centers. The Department of Commerce, through its Economic Development Agency, provides up to 50 percent of the cost of projects for construction and rebuilding of hospitals in economically depressed areas, as local matching funds for the Hill-Burton program. Through its Small Business Administration, it makes loans and loan guarantees to construct and equip primarily for-profit hospitals with no more than 150 beds, nursing homes with receipts not exceeding $1 million, and medical and dental laboratories. Part of the aid to poverty areas served by Regional Commissions, such as the Appalachian Regional Commission, consists of the financing of hospitals, diagnostic and treatment centers, and other facilities. None of these programs has operated within a single framework of policy for construction of health facilities, but each operates within its own mandate.

2. The federal government maintains sizeable and distinct programs of construction and renovation for its own facilities. In 1972, for example, the Veterans Administration spent $124 million for modernization of the 169 Veterans hospitals, some built more than 50 years ago. In the same year, the Department of Defense spent $100 million to construct or remodel its many health facilities. Smaller sums were spent on construction by the Departments of Justice and Interior and by the Agency for International Development.[19]

3. The federal government also contributes significantly to support of facility construction through purchase of services under a variety of programs. The Indian Health Service not only operates a system of 51 hospitals and 70 health centers but purchases care from non-governmental hospitals. More than 200 private and community hospitals have contracts with the Indian Health Service to provide care and to receive reimbursement for their costs, which covers depreciation of facilities.[20] Similarly, purchase of private nursing home services covers depreciation costs.

More important in dollar amounts are the sums paid by the Medicare, Medicaid, CHAMPUS, and Federal Employees Health Benefits programs, which reimburse hospitals and nursing homes on a reasonable cost basis. Costs include interest on loans paid by the facility and a factor for depreciation. In 1971, of payments to hospitals under the Medicare and Medicaid programs, an estimated $600,000,000 represented reimbursement for depreciation.[21] These substantial payments for depreciation may be considered federal support of future facility construction, and yet they are not subject to the standards established in any of the several programs for planning and direct support of construction of health facilities.

4. A number of federal subsidies and tax incentives provide support for construction of medical facilities. Many hospitals participate in research and training programs subsidized by federal grants and contracts, which contain an overhead factor that covers depreciation of facilities. Voluntary hospitals are granted tax-exempt status under the Internal Revenue Code; gifts to voluntary hospitals are also tax deductible.

Each of the many federal agencies involved in supporting construction determines its own needs, sets its own standards, and fixes its own locations, with no overall policy. As the National Advisory Commission on Health Facilities found in 1968,

> [A]lthough there are certain agreements in effect between some agencies concerned with the support of health facilities construction, each Federal program differs in its particular requirements for project eligibility. This often leads to duplication of effort, difficulties in establishing consistency at State, regional and area or local levels, and often makes it difficult to accomplish the proper planning for all health facilities in a given subdivision within desired time limitations.[22]

State Programs

State assistance to construction exhibits divisions of responsibility and relatively unrelated activities similar to those found at the federal level: direct aid for construction funds for state-operated institutions, and indirect funding of construction through medical care payments. In California, the Departments of Public Health, Mental Hygiene, Health Care Services, Rehabilitation, Corrections, the Youth Authority, Veterans Affairs, and the University of California all have some concern, to a greater or lesser degree, with support of the construction of health facilities. Within the State Department of Public Health, the Bureau of Health Facilities Planning and Construction administers the Hill-Burton funding, which includes both federal funds and the matching state funds provided until recently by California. State support has now shifted largely to loans and loan guarantees. The same bureau is responsible for approving plans for construction of various kinds of facilities: hospitals, extended care facilities, community mental health centers, facilities for the mentally retarded, and others.

Other departments of state government operate separately and on totally different bases from the facility construction programs administered by the State Department of Public Health. The Department of Mental

Hygiene is responsible for modernization and construction of state mental hospitals and clinics. Other state departments concerned with specialized inmate populations—the Department of Corrections and the Youth Authority—undertake construction and renovation programs for health care of their populations. The Department of Rehabilitation makes grants to local rehabilitation agencies to cover the costs of a wide range of rehabilitation facilities. These agencies carry out their responsibilities on construction in accordance with varying federal and state prescriptions and with variable amounts of federal aid for which they may qualify under different federal construction programs. In general, their activities in construction of facilities are independent of both the state Hill–Burton program and the areawide comprehensive health planning efforts.[23]

Contributions to the bricks and mortar of health facilities that are subject to little or no controls are payments by the State Department of Health Care Services to hospitals and nursing homes under the Medi-Cal program. These payments include a sum for depreciation as part of costs. In 1970-1971, California hospitals were paid $333 million by the Medi-Cal program, and nursing homes were paid about $219 million, of which six percent, or about $31 million, was for depreciation and therefore indirectly for construction.[24]

Finally, the University of California undertakes construction and modification of health science centers, which are not subject to any state planning control. These costs are funded by bond issues that require voter approval.

Local Programs

Programs at the county and city level, whether public or private, are largely concerned with construction of their own facilities. At the county and city levels, the governmental agencies involved with the construction of facilities are the County Departments of Hospitals, Health, and Mental Health, which are responsible for construction and modernization of county-operated hospitals, public health centers, and a variety of other health facilities. Federal aid from the Hill–Burton and other programs has been an important factor in this county construction. Local contributions to these efforts are derived from local property taxes or from bond issues authorized by the electorate. In the event that a facility is to serve more than one city or area, the Los Angeles County Health Facilities Authority, created in 1971, is empowered to issue bonds for construction or remodeling of facilities.

"Hospital districts" are a form of special governmental district established to finance, build, and operate community hospitals in areas not served by county-operated or voluntary hospitals. Within Los Angeles County, only two such hospital districts have been formed, but there are 63 hospital districts in the state. These districts constitute an independent, separate governmental entity involved in hospital construction.

In fiscal year 1970, Los Angeles County government spent less than $4 million for construction of hospitals and health facilities. In the same year, within the county $3.4 million of Hill-Burton funds were allotted for construction of facilities, primarily voluntary, costing $14.6 million.[25] Construction permits for health facilities in the county in the same calendar year came to $66 million,[26] of which a considerable amount was for private nursing homes. The major share of financing thus comes from private sources — banks, insurance and mortgage companies, other investors, and philanthropy — that have underwritten the development of private hospitals, nursing homes, and other facilities, subject only to review by the areawide comprehensive health planning agency.

PLANNING OF HEALTH FACILITIES AND SERVICES

The Hill-Burton program is as significant for its contribution to the growth of planning as it is for its aid to construction. The full name of the statute was the Hospital Survey and Construction Act. It not only required development of annual state plans by a single state agency but provided funds to establish planning groups within each state to make the necessary surveys. Moreover, by relating planning to distribution of construction funds, the planning process became more than an academic exercise or a formal requirement. The annual Hill-Burton state plan became the critical instrument for determining allocation of construction funds. Although the concept of tying planning to construction was far-seeing, in actual practice the amount and quality of planning of facilities varied greatly. As Fry pointed out in his now classic work, *The Operation of State Hospital Planning and Licensing Programs,*

> Planning is relative; it can be done in large or small amounts. . . . Unfortunately, the minimal amount of planning will suffice for the purposes of federal approval of the statewide Hill-Burton plans. . . . when it is necessary to reduce costs of the program, the aspect of the program most easily cut back is one of the most important ones: the planning that goes into the placing of the proper facility in the proper place.[27]

Variability in the amount and quality of planning of facilities and services is compounded by division between the public and private sectors and dispersion among numerous programs and agencies, with underlying differences in objectives. A basic dichotomy exists between planning for facilities and planning for services. Recognition of this dichotomy led to the expanded authority under the Hill-Harris Amendments of 1964 to plan for both area-wide health facilities and areawide health services. In 1966 this authority was transferred to the Comprehensive Health Planning agencies. The categorical development first of a hospital construction and planning program under the Hill-Burton Act and much later of a comprehensive health planning program has raised problems in interrelationships still unresolved.

Federal Planning

At least eight major federal agencies and a number of minor ones attest to the fragmentation of planning for facilities at the federal level. Each agency and sub-agency conducts its own planning, as it does its construction, in accord with its own legislative mandate and administrative direction, with little relation to the planning of other agencies. Certainly, the Office of Management and Budget in the Executive Office of the President exerts some influence over planning by agencies through its controls over annual budgets and rates of spending. It provides, however, no central planning for the overall, disparate construction activities funded by the federal government.

Planning for construction by the Veterans Administration and the Department of Defense, as well as by the Departments of Justice and Commerce and other agencies, takes place within the requirements of each agency. The Office of Economic Opportunity conducted extensive planning of facilities and of networks of services for the poor.

Major planning efforts within the Department of Health, Education, and Welfare proceed in separate compartments, so that Hill-Burton planning is separate from Comprehensive Health Planning, although both are within the purview of the Health Services and Mental Health Administration. Hill-Burton planning is conducted by the Health Facilities Planning and Construction Service, which reviews state plans, while Comprehensive Health Planning is administered by the Community Health Services, assisted by a National Advisory Council on Comprehensive Health Care Planning and Services.

Other agencies within the Department of Health, Education, and Welfare conduct their own planning for facilities. The Regional Medical Programs Service funds projects for development of services and facilities within its province. The National Institute of Mental Health and the Social and Rehabilitation Service require and review state plans for special facilities for the mentally ill and retarded and the aged. Other agencies plan facilities for mothers and children, the disabled, Indians, migrants, and the poor.[28]

Five other agencies within the Department of Health, Education, and

Welfare supplement direct planning and therefore provide some degree of coordination. The Office of the Assistant Secretary for Community and Field Services coordinates activities in planning of community facilities. An Assistant Secretary for Planning and Evaluation carries on evaluation and analytical studies of particular programs, including construction. Within the Office of the Secretary, the Facilities Engineering and Construction Agency provides advisory services on engineering, architectural, and technical problems in construction of facilities, particularly for the Hill-Burton program. The National Center for Health Statistics gathers data on services and facilities essential for all planning. Finally, the National Center for Health Services Research and Development sponsors research related to the planning of services but with no mandate over planning itself.

This multiple planning activity for health facilities and services is overlaid by numerous programs concerned with promoting general social planning, often on a regional basis, which has some impact on health facility planning. Several federal departments have significant impact on health planning, besides the Department of Health, Education, and Welfare. For example, the Department of Housing and Urban Development provides funds for metropolitan and regional agencies to encourage cooperation of governmental units; under the Model Cities program, it provides comprehensive areawide planning for selected metropolitan areas. The Appalachian Regional Commission and five other Regional Commissions are funded to promote the economic and social development of these geographic areas, including support of planning of health services.

State Planning

At the state level, responsibility for planning health facilities and services is lodged in three departments of state government and several independent agencies. Within the State Department of Public Health, planning under the Hill-Burton and Comprehensive Health Planning programs are separated, reflecting the dichotomy at the federal level. The Bureau of Health Facilities Planning and Construction is responsible for developing and implementing the State Plan for Health Facilities, the plan with the most precise legislative sanctions but only over facilities which apply for Hill-Burton funds. The Office of Comprehensive Health Planning is concerned with the planning of health services, including facilities. The State Health Planning Council is officially responsible for advising the Department in developing the State Plan for Health Facilities. It is also responsible for establishing the criteria for planning by the areawide Comprehensive Health Planning agencies, which have authority to approve or disapprove all new construction, whether Hill-Burton funded or not. Planning for other kinds of facilities, such as board and care homes, is the responsibility of the State Departments of Mental Hygiene and Social Welfare.

Despite these extensive resources devoted to planning of various kinds of health facilities, concern with health services as distinguished from health facilities, and particularly with deployment of highly specialized services, has only just begun. The state health department has directed some attention to provision of emergency services and to assurance of kidney dialysis on a state-wide basis, but no consistent, overall planning has yet been undertaken for the total spectrum of specialized services, including coronary care units, cancer therapy units, open-heart surgery, and brain surgery. Planning for these expensive components of health facilities is still the prerogative of individual facilities without regard to community needs or resources.

Formation of a single state health agency provides a framework in which planning for different kinds of health facilities for different groups and conditions can be related. It will also facilitate planning for services. But even when a single state health agency merges the planning functions now performed by several state departments, general planning functions will still remain apart. In the Governor's Office is the Office of Planning and Research, which prepares and updates reports on statewide land use and population growth, evaluates progress of state agencies on environmental matters, and provides surveillance for expenditure of federal grants. The Council on Intergovernmental Relations, representing the cities, counties, school districts, special districts, regional agencies, and the state, is charged with the responsibility for developing long-range policies to assist the state and local agencies in meeting problems of growth and for coordinating the functions of various levels of government with respect to development and regional planning.[29] Although these agencies are concerned with health facilities and services only peripherally, their activities may have a significant impact on the planning of health resources.

The current multiplicity of state agencies engaged in planning health facilities evolved from 25 years of experience on the part of governmental and voluntary agencies. A review of the development of health facility planning in California provides insight into the contemporary planning process and may illuminate the path ahead.

On the passage of the Hill-Burton Act in 1946, California immediately enacted enabling legislation to participate in the program. The State Hospital Advisory Council was established to advise the Department of Public Health on the Hill-Burton program, and staff was appointed in the Department to develop the annual state plan for hospitals, later to include other facilities, and to administer the program.[30] A period of expanded hospital construction followed. The Hill-Burton program provided substantial financial assistance, $171 million from 1947 to 1968, but to only about 18 percent of all hospital facilities developed during that period.[31] Although more than 60 percent of the beds in facilities existing in 1968 had been built since 1947, the principal financing for this vast construction came from private sources. Thus, the majority of facilities built after 1946 were beyond the pale of the planning and regulatory mechanisms of the Hill-Burton program. Looking back over the history of health facility planning during this 23-year period, a distinguished committee reported to the California Legislature: "While the Hill-Burton Program implied a mechanism for planning, it had been bypassed by an enormous private investment in health facilities."[32]

Regional Planning of Facilities

In 1960 after an extensive investigation of California's health services, the Governor's Committee on Medical Aid and Health found that lack of organized planning of health facilities had led to expensive duplication of services and poor distribution of facilities.[33] The Committee proposed that

the State establish a basis through which regions of California can develop long-range programs for coordinated expansion and use of hospitals and related health facilities and services. The State Department of Public Health should be responsible for developing regional plans based on recommendations of Regional Advisory Councils composed of representatives of the public, hospitals, and physicians. State funds for administration of the program should be appropriated.[34]

In partial implementation of this recommendation, in 1961 the California Legislature authorized the State Advisory Hospital Council to establish two hospital planning regions, one for the nine counties of the San Francisco Bay Area and the other for the Southern California Region.[35] These regional planning agencies were authorized to develop standards for determining community needs for hospital beds and related facilities and services. They engaged in extensive studies of existing facilities and services, holding many public hearings. They identified key factors in effective planning: baseline information, participation of both public and private agencies, involvement of consumers, and the necessity for innovation and flexibility. In 1963, the Legislature authorized formation of a third regional hospital planning council for the South San Joaquin Valley.[36]

These regional agencies were based on the concept of voluntary planning. Freedom from "centralized governmental control" was an explicit objective of the first two regional planning agencies.[37] The invitation to participate in the South San Joaquin Valley hospital planning council referred to a resolution of the House of Delegates of the American Medical Association on November 28, 1962 in favor of formation of regional hospital planning bodies "to prevent legislation which would make the formulation and operation of these regional hospital planning boards compulsory instead of voluntary."[38]

The organization of the regional planning agencies varied, but they all shared one common feature—involvement of many professional and community groups. In the South San Joaquin Valley, the organizational form was a pyramid, consisting of seven area committees for the seven counties comprising the region and small health planning councils, with representatives of both groups forming the Regional Health Planning Council.[39] The Bay Area Health Facilities Planning Association, serving a nine-county area, was guided by a 32-member board of trustees with three technical advisory committees, one on hospitals, another on medical services, and a third on long-term care. Local planning groups in constituent counties and metropolitan areas were developed. The Bay Area Health Facilities Planning Association encouraged local planning, decentralized efforts, and coordinated work on specific projects by individual facilities and planning groups.[40] In Southern California, the Hospital Planning Association was formed in 1963 as an outgrowth of a special department of the Hospital Council of Southern California, the voluntary association of hospitals in the area.[41] In January 1968 the organization changed its name to the Health Planning Association and broadened its scope to include various kinds of facilities, health manpower, health data, and other matters.

By 1965, seven voluntary areawide hospital and health planning agencies had been developed, serving 34 counties with more than 94 percent of the state's population.[42] In that year, the Legislature established a Statewide Hospital and Related Health Facilities and Services Planning Committee, known as the "543 Committee" after the number of the bill in the Legislature that created it. Charged with promoting voluntary planning on a regional basis, the 543 Committee was directed to encourage and strengthen local voluntary hospitals and related health facilities planning groups, to correlate regional and local planning programs with statewide activities, to determine information needs for planning, and to conduct public meetings in which professional and consumer groups would participate. This impetus to voluntary planning followed the 1964 Hill-Harris amendments to the Hill-Burton Act, which strengthened and broadened the scope of planning.

The 543 Committee promoted a variety of planning activities. During its life, regional voluntary health facilities and services planning bodies came to cover 52 of California's 58 counties serving 98 percent of the people. The Committee was instrumental in developing the California Health Manpower Council, a statewide agency representing professional health organizations, the health insurance industry, educational and vocational institutions, and voluntary health planning agencies. It helped establish the California Health Data Corporation, a health data exchange for improved gathering and use of data. The 543 Committee strengthened voluntary health planning by encouraging regional groups to set priorities for facilities, by stimulating individual facilities and regional planners to link their efforts, and by helping professionals and consumers to work together.[43] Still, not a single regional plan for health facilities or health services was developed in the three years of its operation. Its legacy for future work was a recommendation that:

> Health facilities and services planning groups must now effectively relate their endeavors to planning for manpower development, personal health services, and environmental health. Under PL 89-749, in fact, planning for facilities and services now has relevance only within the context of planning to meet total health needs and by the development of comprehensive systems for delivering health services and maintaining health.[44]

More specifically, the 543 Committee recommended that the scope of health facilities and services planning be extended "beyond acute general hospitals to at least long-term care services, mental health resources, outpatient care, home care, rehabilitation, ambulance and emergency health services."[45]

Comprehensive Health Planning

By 1968, California had formally pledged itself to comprehensive health planning in place of health facility planning, although in practice the regional planning agencies exerted limited control only over planning of health facilities. Federal Comprehensive Health Planning legislation had been passed in 1966. In 1967, the State Department of Public Health was designated by the Governor as the state agency for comprehensive health planning, and the Office of Comprehensive Health Planning was established in the Department.[46] The State Health Planning Council was created to develop policy on health planning and to adopt the State Plan for Health.[47] By July 1969 the regional agencies for health facilities planning had converted to Comprehensive Health Planning agencies or, as in the case of the Bay Area Health Facilities Planning Association, were linked by contract with the Comprehensive Health Planning agency.

In 1969, too, the concept of voluntary planning underwent a notable change by linking planning and licensing of facilities. The California Legislature assigned approval of health facility construction and expansion to the Comprehensive Health Planning agencies. The legislation provided that no increase in licensed capacity, change in license category, or construction of a new facility licensed by the Departments of Public Health or Mental Hygiene could be granted until the applicant received a favorable, final decision from the voluntary area health planning group.[48] In the event of non-compliance with this requirement, 12 months would have to elapse before the facility could be licensed.[49] In 1971, the State Health Planning Council acted to integrate the Hill-Burton program for facility construction with areawide planning of health facilities, by requiring area health planning groups to abide by the state plan for health facilities until regional plans are developed and reconciled within a single state plan. A further step was taken by 1971 legislation requiring hospitals to file financial reports annually with a newly formed hospital commission. These reports will be an important component of planning, but the relationship of the new agency to the areawide comprehensive health planning agencies, if any, was not defined.

Thus, planning of health facilities in California over the last 30 years has fallen into five phases: (1) the pre-planning phase from 1941 to 1947 before enactment of the Hill-Burton program; (2) planning for construction of facilities under the Hill-Burton state plan existing side by side with unplanned construction outside of Hill-Burton from 1946 to 1960; (3) the growth of voluntary facility planning from 1960 to 1966; (4) the phase of Comprehensive Health Planning from 1966 to date; and (5) the linkage of planning to licensing and prior certification of need, without regard to specific programs.

In this sketchy review of the development of health facility planning in California, scant attention has been given to specialized facilities for the mentally ill, the mentally retarded, the disabled, the chronically ill, and for emergency care. Much activity occurred in planning for these specialized needs. For our purposes, the end result is echoed in a noted report on hospitals in New York State:

> Responsibilities for hospital affairs are now scattered among many agencies of New York State. No one agency, however, nor even the aggregate of agencies, has a comprehensive responsibility for being informed about all aspects of hospitals and related institutions and for considering institutional health care from the standpoint of the State as a whole. There is no "State" policy on hospitals and related facilities, but only a number of fragmented activities that affect these kinds of institutions. State administration in this area has, consequently, been piecemeal and inadequate.[50]

Other Regional Planning

At the regional level are two main governmental health programs, plus quasi-governmental and voluntary efforts in planning health facilities and services. The regional Comprehensive Health Planning agencies have statutory authority to review and approve new or modified health facility construction, with limited sanctions, as mentioned. Each of the areawide Regional Medical Programs plans, approves, and funds projects related to facilities, manpower, and services. Although these projects mainly concern the training of health personnel and, to some extent, the organization of specialized services, they have some influence in the planning of facilities and services.

Also at the regional level are the eight Councils of Government in California, voluntary associations of cities, counties, special districts, and planning commissions. The Southern California Association of Governments (SCAG) was established under a Joint Exercise of Powers Act to provide a forum for discussion, study, and development of recommendations on regional problems of mutual interest and concern.[51] Mainly a regional clearinghouse of information, SCAG has as its principal power the duty to review and comment on applications for federal grants. Its review of grant applications for health facilities is conducted not in terms of health needs but rather in terms of how the proposed facility fits into general regional planning, including population growth and distribution, land use, and development of transportation.

Finally, various voluntary health organizations are concerned with planning facilities and services at the regional level. One example is the Hospital Council of Southern California, which conducts surveys and planning activities and is represented on committees of the areawide Comprehensive Health Planning agencies. The geographic areas within which these regional agencies operate are all different. Throughout the state, no set of regional boundaries coincides with any other. Although some individual regions are congruent, throughout the state the boundaries of the areawide Comprehensive Health Planning agencies, the Regional Medical Programs, the Councils of Government, the Mental Retardation Services Planning Boards, and the voluntary hospital councils all differ, creating impediments to effective planning.

Local Planning

At the county and city levels of government, numerous public agencies are concerned with the planning of health facilities and services. In Los Angeles County, these include the Board of Supervisors and the Chief Administrative Officer of the County; the new unified County Department of Health Services; and non-health governmental agencies such as the County Regional Planning Commission and the Los Angeles City Department of Planning.

Each of the hundreds of voluntary health and welfare agencies in the vast metropolitan area of Los Angeles County engages in some planning of facilities and services, planning geared to its own objectives and purposes. The Welfare Planning Council, an umbrella organization representing the various health and welfare agencies, serves as coordinating link for the planning and programs of the many specialized, voluntary agencies, and its parent agency, the United Way, provides a unified fund-raising mechanism that affects planning by each agency. The areawide Comprehensive Health Planning agencies have served as a meeting ground for interchange among both voluntary and governmental health agencies.

Effective planning is impeded by multiple, noncongruent boundaries of local governmental and voluntary agencies, which may not coincide with boundaries established by state, regional, or other local public or private agencies. This multiplicity of noncongruent boundaries is a reflection of a difficult jurisdictional problem — the relationship between local planning for health facilities and services, on the one hand, and such planning at the regional, state, and federal levels, on the other hand. Required conformance to the state Hill-Burton plan has provided a unifying link for all levels of government, but this link has not stretched to include many kinds of specialized facilities nor to specialized services within general hospitals nor to a large segment of the private sector involved in construction of health facilities.

Moreover, the state plan under the Hill-Burton program was not always designed to cope equitably with local needs, as was forcefully demonstrated in 1965 when the Watts Riots occurred in south-central Los Angeles. In a wide-ranging search for the causes of the riots, the Governor's Commission on the Los Angeles Riots investigated the health resources and services in the Watts area. The Commission's Health Consultant recommended that

> a first-class voluntary or governmental hospital, with a teaching and research program, be established in the heart of the South-Southeast Districts. . . . If a new hospital is established by the Los Angeles County government, it should have the benefit of a board of directors representing the local population, and guidance on professional standards from the medical schools in Los Angeles. The geographic lines of the State Plan of Hospitals should be redrawn to take account of current human needs and social realities in this blighted area, so that necessary grant support can be properly provided.[52]

The Commission adopted this recommendation and urged "that immediate and favorable consideration should be given to a new comprehensively-equipped hospital in this area. . . ."[53] To accomplish this end, the state plan for hospitals had to be revised and new hospital planning districts delineated to show the true inadequacy of the local bed supply.[54] According to the existing state plan and districts, no new beds were needed in the hospital service area of Watts, although for the most part existing beds were in proprietary hospitals, largely inaccessible to the poor. Their only recourse was the large county hospital requiring an eight- or ten-mile automobile or ambulance trip, or a bus ride taking one hour and costing 68 cents.[55] Six years after the recommendation to redraw the hospital planning districts, a county facility, built with strong community participation, opened near Watts. Although the Hill-Burton program had enough elasticity to respond to the challenge, the state plan for hospitals had not previously and affirmatively identified the urgent need for adequate hospital services in this underserved area.

Planning of health facilities and services stands at a crossroads. Four main types of fragmentation have prevailed. First is the division between Hill-Burton planning and Comprehensive Health Planning. To some extent and in some states, the two programs merge. Second, within each is the division between planning for facilities and planning for services. In practice, the scope of planning tends to widen to include all services. Third is the separation of planning from regulation, a separation reinforced by differing philosophies, even though the two processes are related. Many professional planners would keep them sharply separate, some even rejecting governmental regulatory powers. Nevertheless, in response to consumer demand for improved and expanded services and the pressure of rising costs and prices, even stronger controls and regulation have been enacted. More than 20 states have passed so-called certificate of need legislation to require prior approval for all facility construction, not merely for construction supported by Hill-Burton funds. Fourth, the divorce of responsibility for planning from responsibility for provision of services weakens the planning process.

REGULATION OF HEALTH FACILITIES

The quality of care provided by health facilities is regulated by a variety of mechanisms.[56] These may be direct or indirect, of broad or limited impact, governmental or voluntary. Any individual facility is subject to multiple regulatory mechanisms. Licensure requires one level of inspection. Another level and different information are required for certification under Medicare. Still another approval is required for reimbursement under Medicaid, although in some places the Medicare certification suffices for Medicaid approval. Other governmental programs, such as crippled children's services, vocational rehabilitation, and workmen's compensation, specify still different standards for their beneficiaries. These multiple regulatory mechanisms may entail conflicting, contradictory, or duplicative policies, regulations, site visits, accounting procedures, and financial incentives or sanctions.

Division of authority for regulation of the quality of facilities is complicated by the many different kinds of facilities to be regulated, including general and specialized hospitals, nursing homes, residential and intermediate care facilities, public health centers, various kinds of clinics, sheltered workshops, and others. These facilities developed at different times in response to needs as they emerged. Various agencies have accordingly assumed responsibility for monitoring their quality. In California, five separate facility licensing laws are administered by three different state departments and some county departments.

Federal Programs

The Hill-Burton program was responsible initially for impelling the states to enact facility licensing laws, although no uniform minimal standards were set for these laws. It continues to exert a regulatory influence by requiring building of facilities in conformance with certain standards for construction, patient safety, and equipment. Although the Hill-Burton program has traditionally stressed the physical aspects of facilities, with little attention to staffing or organization, the current concern with the interrelationships of facilities and services may indicate a broader scope of regulation. The federal Comprehensive Health Planning program in Community Health Services of the Health Services and Mental Health Administration has no regulatory authority over facilities, but the state component in a growing number of states has power to approve new construction.

The federal government's principal mechanism for regulating facilities is certification, a process which may be undertaken by either a governmental or voluntary agency, to designate facilities that meet a prescribed standard for a special purpose, such as receipt of funds, participation in a program, or placement of patients. Under Medicare, all hospitals participating in the program must be certified. Sixteen basic Conditions of Participation for Hospitals were developed jointly by the Public Health Service and the Social Security Administration.[57] In order to participate in the Medicare program, a hospital must be certified as meeting these conditions of participation or, alternatively, must be accredited by the Joint Commission on Accreditation of Hospitals. The standards established by this national voluntary agency are thus determinative of hospital participation in Medicare. Not until late 1972, with enactment of P.L. 92-603, was there some modification of this mandatory delegation of public authority to a voluntary body.

Hospital inspection for compliance with the Conditions for Participation is not performed by the Social Security Administration but has been delegated to an agency in each state, generally the state licensing agency.[58] The application of these minimum federal standards, therefore, varies with the competence and resources of each state agency. As Worthington and Silver have pointed out,

. . . any weakness in personnel or inspection methods which exist in the state hospital licensing programs are carried over to the federal Medicare program.

Further, the application of the federal Conditions of Participation will vary, according to the varying interpretations and competencies of the state licensing authorities.[59]

To some extent, varying interpretations among the states are controlled by "validation" surveys by the Bureau of Health Insurance of the Social Security Administration or by staff in the regional offices of the Department of Health, Education, and Welfare. But hospitals accredited by the Joint Commission on Accreditation of Hospitals were automatically certified for participation in Medicare. Thus, approval of facilities for reimbursement under Medicare is fragmented among the Social Security Administration, the state licensing agency, and the voluntary Joint Commission on Accreditation of Hospitals. It should not be assumed, however, that fragmentation is solely responsible for diminishing the effectiveness of certification for Medicare. Three features of the process contribute to weak quality controls. First, failure to be certified for participation in Medicare merely prevents reimbursement by Medicare; it does not restrict the hospital from accepting patients. Second, to be certified and reimbursed, compliance with the Conditions for Participation need only be substantial. "Substantial compliance" allows deficiencies with respect to one or more Conditions of Participation, provided that the hospital is making reasonable efforts to correct the deficiencies and, despite the deficiencies, is rendering adequate care.[60] Third, hospitals that are not certified may still be reimbursed for emergency services rendered to eligible patients, and in some isolated areas hospitals that are not certified continue to be reimbursed because of lack of alternative facilities for care.

Inconsistent federal approaches to the charitable contribution of voluntary hospitals are illustrated by the differing positions taken by the Internal Revenue Service and the Department of Health, Education, and Welfare under the Hill-Burton program. Voluntary hospitals enjoy tax exemption as nonprofit, charitable enterprises. Until recently, the Internal Revenue Service interpreted "charitable" as requiring free care by hospitals in an amount between five and ten percent of gross revenues. In 1969, while the House Ways and Means Committee and the Senate Finance Committee were considering changes in the regulations, the Internal Revenue Service quietly waived the charitable requirement.

Under the Hill-Burton program, however, hospitals receiving Hill-Burton funding were obligated to provide a reasonable volume of free or below cost service to people unable to pay [61] Until challenged by lawsuits in Louisiana and other jurisdictions, hospitals were not called on to meet this requirement. In fact, what constituted "a reasonable volume of free or below cost service" had never been defined by the federal government. Settlement of the Louisiana suit in a federal circuit court provided that Hill-Burton-aided hospitals must affirmatively show provision of a reasonable amount of free or charitable services to the poor.[62] Under pressure of these and other proceedings, the Department of Health, Education, and Welfare in 1972 issued proposed and later interim regulations designed to clarify the "reasonable volume" of charitable services. These regulations require that hospitals either certify that they will not turn anyone away because of inability to pay or show that they have spent an amount at a level not less than the lesser of three percent of operating costs, minus Medicare and Medicaid reimbursement, or ten percent of all grants.[63] Implementation of this regulation will constitute a significant innovation in federal control of access to hospital care.

Some control of the quality of care provided by extended care facilities is contained in the federal mandate of Medicare for transfer agreements between hospitals and extended care facilities to assure continuity of care for patients. As in the case of hospitals, the Social Security Administration has delegated to state agencies the task of certification of extended care facilities for participation in Medicare.[64] Variability in state and local licensure requirements for nursing homes and other extended care facilities, and even greater variability in standards for inspection and enforcement, led the federal government to initiate the Health Facilities Survey Improvement Program, administered by the Community Health Service of the Health Services and Mental Health Administration, to improve the skills of state and local inspectors responsible for licensing and regulation of quality of all health facilities. Many other federal agencies also specify standards for nursing homes (see Chapter 2).

Regulation of the quality of residential care facilities is not recognized as a federal responsibility, even to the degree that certification of hospitals and extended care facilities for Medicare implies. These facilities for board and care and residential care for physically and mentally disabled children and adults, for alcoholism, and for drug rehabilitation are affected only by federal guidelines specifying standards and requirements of various categorical programs. Thus, federal standards for residential care facilities are defined in terms of the categorical objectives of programs for old age assistance, rehabilitation, services for the mentally retarded, veterans, and drug abuse and alcoholism projects, not in terms of the general quality of care these facilities provide.

Still another category of facility—the intermediate care facility— was added to the Medicaid program in 1971 for those patients who do not require hospital care or the services of a skilled nursing home but require some institutional care above the level of room and board.[65] Detailed standards and regulations of this category of facility are left to the states. In general, Medicaid turns over the control of participating facilities to the individual states with only general guidelines. It does require, however, certain minimum standards, such as licensing of facilities and compliance with recognized fire safety codes.

Other agencies within the Department of Health, Education, and Welfare specify standards for facilities for the mentally ill and the mentally retarded as a condition of grants for construction and staffing (see Chapter 5). In addition, the Departments of Commerce and of Housing and Urban Development set standards in connection with their grants for construction of facilities. Regulation of specific aspects of the quality of facilities is the responsibility of still other federal agencies: the Wage and Standards Administration of the Department of Labor, the Wage and Price Commission within the Executive Office of the President, the Bureau of Narcotics, and the Atomic Energy Commission, empowered to control use of isotopes and high-energy resources in hospitals.

Governmental regulation of facilities is supplemented by voluntary standards. Accreditation is the process by which a voluntary agency evaluates and recognizes an institution or program as meeting certain predetermined criteria or standards.[66] The principal accrediting agency for health facilities, as noted above in connection with Medicare, is the Joint Commission on Accreditation of Hospitals, a voluntary, nonprofit agency, which undertakes accreditation at the request of the facility and at its expense. After approval by a physician-surveyor or a team of surveyors, accreditation is granted for a two-year period or on a one-year provisional basis. Criticized for inadequate standards and lack of public accountability,[67] the Joint Commission has responded recently to demands for strengthened requirements and periodic upgrading of its standards.

The Joint Commission on Accreditation of Hospitals has developed and now conducts an accreditation program for nursing homes in conjunction with the American Nursing Home Association. Recently, it has begun to accredit various other long-term care facilities, rehabilitation facilities, and facilities for physical restoration, social adjustment, vocational adjustment, and sheltered employment. An accreditation program for facilities for the mentally retarded and for psychiatric facilities is under way. These efforts represent new directions at the national level to improve and expand voluntary regulation of extended care, residential, and rehabilitation facilities.

In addition to the Joint Commission on Accreditation of Hospitals, at least eight other voluntary programs, each with its own criteria, accredit or approve features of hospitals related to quality control. (1) The Council on Medical Education of the American Medical Association approves hospital internship and residency programs; (2) the American College of Surgeons approves cancer therapy programs; (3) the Liaison Committee of the American Medical Association and the Association of American Medical Colleges approve medical school affiliations of hospitals; (4) the National League for Nursing approves diploma nursing schools and practical nurse training programs; (5) the Association of American Medical Colleges approves membership in the Council of Teaching Hospitals; (6) Blue Cross and other third-party payment agencies review hospital charges and their cost-accounting basis; (7) the American Hospital Association registers hospitals of more than six beds that state that they meet certain specifications with respect to safety, staffing, medical records, nursing care, and other services;[68] and (8) various agencies provide consultative service to hospitals in the interest of promoting quality. Perhaps most important of these is the Commission on Professional and Hospital Activities (PAS), which provides periodic reports to hospitals, giving a statistical profile of their discharged patients according to various features (diagnosis, tests performed, drugs used, surgical operations, etc.) compared with national averages.[69]

State Programs

In California five departments of state government share responsibility for assuring the quality of various kinds of health facilities: the State Departments of Public Health, Health Care Services, Mental Hygiene, Social Welfare, and Rehabilitation.

In the State Department of Public Health, the Bureau of Health Facilities Licensing and Certification licenses and inspects hospitals and a wide variety of other health facilities. The Bureau is responsible for development, review, and revision of facility standards. This Bureau also inspects and licenses health facilities, certifies facilities for participation in Medicare, and approves facilities for receipt of Medicaid funds.

In addition to the Department of Public Health, two other departments license health facilities. The Department of Mental Hygiene licenses psychiatric hospitals and sets standards for other mental health facilities. The Department of Social Welfare licenses homes for the aged (for persons over 65 years of age); family, group, and institutional facilities for care of children (for those under 15 years of age); and has recently been assigned responsibility for licensing board and care facilities (for persons aged 16 to 64), formerly unlicensed except for the requirement of a business permit.[70] The division of responsibility for licensing of health facilities among three official agencies understandably resulted in problems reflecting differing purposes of different agencies. Repeated efforts have been made to consolidate the licensing function through the years.[71] Reorganization of state health programs into a single, unified department of health may assist in achieving this objective.

Other state departments are involved in the regulation of quality of facilities. The Department of Health Care Services sets standards for participation of facilities in Medicaid and determines reimbursement rates for the program. Although Medicaid is financed jointly by federal and state governments, regulation of the quality of hospital services purchased under Medicaid is a state responsibility, as mentioned. The State Department of Rehabilitation, through purchase of rehabilitation services in medical facilities, establishes standards and sets rates of reimbursement for these services. The Department of Consumer Affairs, through its 12 licensing boards for the health professions and occupations, has an important influence on quality of care provided in health facilities. A federal requirement has effectuated licensure of nursing home administrators as a condition for approval of a state plan for the Medicaid program. Other state departments and programs affect conditions for employment (Department of Industrial Relations), fee schedules for medical care (Workmen's Compensation), rates of payment for health care (Department of Human Resources Development), and certify facilities for placement of persons under their care (Department of Social Welfare, California Youth Authority, and Department of Corrections).

Two additional state mechanisms regulate costs and prices of institutional services, both directly and indirectly. The State Insurance Commissioner must approve rates of insurance companies, including all types of health insurance, thus exerting some influence on rates of remuneration for facilities. Under the California Hospital Disclosure Act of 1971, hospitals are required to file with a new commission uniform reports of hospital cost experience.[72] This requirement is designed to increase economy and efficiency in provision of hospital services and to enable public agencies that purchase hospital services to make informed decisions.

A statewide voluntary accreditation program is the Medical Staff Survey Program of the California Medical Association. Unique to California, this program is designed to supplement state licensing and voluntary accreditation of facilities by evaluating medical staff organization, policies, and procedures in each participating hospital and by recommending improvements. Similar surveys of nursing homes by the California Medical Association have also been undertaken.[73] The Bureau of Health Facilities Licensing and Certification of the State Department of Public Health has entered into contracts with the Medical Staff Survey Committee of the California Medical Association as a supplement to its licensing and certification activities. As of January 1972, a hospital is permitted to participate in the Medi-Cal program only if approved either by the Joint Commission on Accreditation of Hospitals or by the California Medical Association.

Regional Programs

Regulation of facilities at the regional level involves the same agencies as those concerned with planning: the areawide Comprehensive Health Planning agencies, the regional Councils of Governments, and the Regional Medical Programs. Each of these agencies is involved with quality of facilities in its own way. The areawide Comprehensive Health Planning agencies have authority to review grant and loan applications for Hill-Burton funding and, more broadly, to approve all new construction. The regional Councils of Governments approve all governmental grants. The Regional Medical Programs approve grants for specialized facilities and training.

Local Programs

Los Angeles County is the only county in California to which the state has delegated the function of inspecting and licensing health facilities. Under state law and with reimbursement from the state,[74] the County Health Department performs functions in hospital inspection, consultation, and enforcement with respect to approximately 750 health facilities in the county, functions that are performed in the rest of California by the State Department of Public Health. Through its Health Facilities Services Division, the County Health Department is also responsible for certification of facilities for participation in Medicare and for approval of facilities for the Medi-Cal program. The State Department of Public Health retains the functions of issuing the actual licenses, reviewing plans for new construction, examining county reports on inspection and licensing, participating in informal hearings related to noncompliance with state standards, and processing recommendations for decertification of facilities for Medicare.[75] Facilities licensed by the State Departments of Mental Hygiene and Social Welfare continue to be so licensed in Los Angeles County, including board and care homes for persons aged 16 to 64 for which licensure has only recently been required.

The county operates its own facilities—hospitals, public health centers, and mental health clinics—and thus controls the quality of these facilities directly. The county also exercises some degree of indirect control over private and voluntary facilities through contracts for emergency services, crippled children's services, rehabilitation, nursing and obstetric services, and outpatient mental health services.

County and city agencies are also involved in enforcement of local zoning ordinances, fire regulations, and other building and safety requirements. The County Engineer, Fire Department, Regional Planning Commission, and Board of Supervisors are all involved in permits, inspections, and zoning matters which affect health facilities. For the City of Los Angeles, the City Planning Commission, Board of Zoning Adjustment, Fire Department, Building and Safety Department, Public Works Department, and City Council all have some concern with sanitation, fire prevention, building inspection, and zoning.

Dispersion of responsibility to non-health agencies for technical matters, such as building safety and zoning, has been a long-standing division of authority and prerogative of local government. In some areas of the state, however, local authority over building safety and zoning is being used to thwart implementation of the state's policy, embodied in the California community mental health program, to encourage community-based treatment of the mentally ill and retarded. Under color of zoning ordinances and fire and safety regulations, some communities are excluding ex-mental patients, the retarded, the aged, and the disabled from residential areas and relegating them — 10,000 persons were living in board and care homes in Los Angeles County in 1971 — to strictly commercial zones of the county.

FACILITIES AND FRAGMENTATION

The deployment of functions related to construction, planning, and regulation of health facilities is sometimes cited as an example of the partnership of the public, voluntary, and private sectors in American health services at its best. Each level of government participates in each of the major functions related to facilities — support of construction, planning, and regulation — to varying degrees and in different ways. Voluntary and professional organizations contribute to all three functions and interrelate with government at each level.

Whether because of or in spite of this partnership, considerable progress has been made in management of this sector of health services. Minimum legal standards have been set for nearly all types of health facilities in almost all states, although the effectiveness of enforcement varies considerably. In mandating planning, the Hill-Burton program led both governmental and voluntary groups to examine aspects of facilities beyond standards for construction: the appropriate balance of different kinds of facilities, proper geographic distribution, standards of operation, and currently the relation of facilities to services. Medicare has encouraged development of national standards. While voluntary standards of the Joint Commission on Accreditation of Hospitals are still generally the ceiling for facility standards under Medicare and thus restrict the impact of federal funding on quality of care, at the same time experience under the Medicare program has contributed to demand on the part of consumers for strengthened standards. In other words, the various actors in the system of planning, building, and regulating health facilities have achieved a *modus vivendi*. Although some may disagree, probably the greatest single force contributing to this interaction of the various interests concerned with health facilities has been the far-seeing Hill-Burton program, which from the start set the pattern of integrating planning, construction, and regulation of facilities.

Recognition that the current system, with its many parts, actually works does not mean that it works optimally. Large urban public hospitals are beset with problems of providing adequate amounts and quality of care to the poor.[76] Voluntary and private hospitals have been able to shunt difficult and poor patients to public facilities.[77] Nursing homes and board and care facilities, largely the province of the private, for-profit sector, have been subjected to only minimal and belated regulation.[78] Above all, patients have been denied access to facilities, have been forced to endure inadequate or variable quality of care, and have had limited means of redress.[79]

Since 1965, various reports have analyzed the basic issues affecting the quality of facilities and the care they provide. These issues concern strengthened planning and licensing of facilities;[80] controlling escalating hospital costs;[81] assuring access to appropriate care by making available a balanced and interrelated range of health facilities;[82] using expensive resources rationally;[83] improving hospital effectiveness with respect to internal performance and external relations;[84] upgrading nursing homes and board and care facilities;[85] developing a national hospital policy, with a revitalized federal-state regulatory system and definition of gradations among hospitals;[86] and increasing the consumer voice in regulation of health facilities.[87]

Each of these issues is deeply affected by the system of categorical programs and fragmentation of functions among multiple agencies, among different levels of government, and between the public and private sectors. Although all the deficiencies of health facilities cannot be ascribed to fragmentation, nevertheless, functional and geographic fragmentation complicates the issues affecting health facilities in the following ways:

1. The multiplicity of regulatory mechanisms, both statutory and voluntary, create variable, conflicting, ambiguous, and even weak standards for quality of facilities.

2. The division of regulatory authority has left gaps in coverage. For example, certain board and care facilities were licensed in California before 1971 and still are not licensed in many states.

3. The capability of areawide Comprehensive Health Planning agencies to develop and implement area plans for facilities and services is hampered by lack of authority over health facilities, by lack of power to assure compromise of conflicting interests and compliance with a plan, by a framework for planning inappropriately conditioned by the categorical approach, and by weak linkage to financing mechanisms.

4. The dispersion of numerous categorical programs affecting facilities and services among different agencies at different levels of government creates a barrier to community participation and a muting of the consumer voice.

5. Multiple and passive financing mechanisms for construction and operation of facilities, not geared to unified purposes, necessarily fail to use the leverage of funding to improve quality and distribution of facilities.

6. Even when linkages are built among programs, such as use of approval by the Joint Commission on Accreditation of Hospitals as the equivalent of Medicare certification, the categorical approach transfers weaknesses from one program to another, rather than affirmatively strengthening the quality of facilities. The categorical approach, furthermore, provides each agency with an excuse for inaction, epitomized in the current vulgarism, "That's *his* problem."

7. In the absence of a coordinated policy governing health facilities and services, effective incentives cannot be developed for production of needed resources, for effective use of existing resources, or for improved quality of facilities and services.

NOTES

1. National Commission on Community Health Services, *Health Is A Community Affair*, pp. 103-104, Harvard University Press, Cambridge, Mass., 1966.

2. Somers, Anne R., *Hospital Regulation: The Dilemma of Public Policy*, p. ix, Industrial Relations Section, Department of Economics, Princeton University, 1969.

3. Compiled from *Health Resources Statistics, 1971*, Tables 177 and 185, U.S. Department of Health, Education, and Welfare, National Center for Health Statistics, DHEW Pub. No. (HSM) 72-1509, Feb. 1972 and from *Hospitals*, Guide Issue, Tables 1 and 2, Aug. 1, 1971.

4. Somers, supra note 2 at 76-77.

5. See Kessel, Reuben A., "The A.M.A. and the Supply of Physicians," *Law and Contemporary Problems, Health Care*, Part I, Vol. XXXV, p. 267 at 269, Spring, 1970.

6. Roemer, Milton I. and Jay W. Friedman, *Doctors in Hospitals*, pp. 35-43, Johns Hopkins Press, Baltimore, 1971.

7. Somers, supra note 2 at 104-105; Roemer and Friedman, supra note 6 at 36.

8. Ibid.

9. Fry, Hilary G., *The Operation of State Hospital Planning and Licensing Programs*, p. 25, American Hospital Association, Chicago, 1965.

10. Somers, supra note 2 at 102-103; Fry, supra note 9 at 23 ff.

11. For discussion of the provision in the Hospital Survey and Construction Act of 1946 that "if any state, prior to July 1, 1948, has not enacted legislation providing that compliance with minimum standards of maintenance and operation shall be required . . . such State shall not be entitled to further allotments," see Carlson, Rick J., "Health Manpower Licensing and Emerging Institutional Responsibility for the Quality of Care," *Law and Contemporary Problems, Health Care*, Part II, p. 849 at 872-873, note 69, Autumn 1970.

12. Roemer and Friedman, supra note 6 at 39-40.

13. Cooper, Barbara S. and Nancy L. Worthington, "National Health Expenditures, 1929-1972," *Social Security Bull.*, Vol. 36, No. 1, p. 7, Table 2, Jan. 1973.

14. See *Health Care Facilities, Existing and Needed, Hill Burton State Plan as of January 1, 1969*, p. 5, U.S. Department of Health, Education, and Welfare, Health Services and Mental Health Administration, Health Care Facilities, Services, HEW Pub. No. (HSM) 72-4004 for the statement: "Many of the facilities built under the Hill-Burton program in the early years were needed because no hospital existed within reach of critically ill patients. The original thrust of the Program was to fill this gap. Today, the priority has been shifted to the modernization of obsolete facilities to keep pace with advances in knowledge and technology and to help solve the health care crisis in urban communities."

15. Ibid.

16. *Hill-Burton Progress Report, July 1, 1947-June 30, 1969*, pp. 14-17, Department of Health, Education, and Welfare, PHS Pub. No. 930-F-3.

17. *Hospital and Health Facility Construction and Modernization*, Hearings before the Subcommittee on Public Health and Welfare of the Committee on Interstate and Foreign Commerce, H.R., 91st Cong., 1st Sess., Ser. No. 91-8, p. 100 (testimony of Dr. H. Philip Hampton, American Medical Association, based on data from the Department of Health, Education, and Welfare), 1969.

18. P.L. 84-835 (1956) (grants for construction of research facilities); P.L. 86-720 (1961) (aid for schools of public health); P.L. 88-129 (1963) (grants to professional schools); P.L. 88-581 (1964) (nursing schools); P.L. 89-751 (1966) (schools for allied health personnel).

19. *Special Analyses, Budget of the U.S. Government, Fiscal Year 1974*, pp. 158-159, Table J-26.

20. American Hospital Association, *Major Federal Aid Programs for Hospitals*, p. 13, Chicago, 1970.

21. Testimony of Dr. Vernon E. Wilson, Administrator, Health Services and Mental Health Administration, *Senate Hearings before the Committee on Appropriations, Departments of Labor and Health, Education, and Welfare and Related Agencies Appropriations, Fiscal Year 1973*. 92nd Cong., 2nd Sess., Part 2, p. 2043, 1972.

22. National Advisory Commission on Health Facilities, *A Report to the President*, p. 66, Washington, D.C., Dec. 1968.

23. *Governor's Budget, State of California, Fiscal Year 1972-1973*, passim.

24. *1972-1973 State of California Program Budget Supplement*, p. 812, Sacramento, Calif., 1972.

25. Compiled from *Hill-Burton Project Register*, July 1, 1947-June 30, 1970, pp. 43-53, U.S. Department of Health, Education, and Welfare, Washington, D.C.

26. *Monthly Report of Building Permit Activity in the Cities and Counties of California*, Research Department, Security Pacific National Bank, Los Angeles, California, 1970.

27. Fry, supra note 9 at 75.

28. See American Hospital Association, *Major Federal Aid Programs for Hospitals*, supra note 20.

29. California Government Code, sec. 34200 (West Supp. 1972).

30. *Voluntary Regional Planning: Hospitals and Related Health Facilities and Services*, Report to the California Legislature and to the State Advisory Hospital Council by the Hospitals and Related Health Facilities and Services Planning Committee, SB 543 (1965) (hereinafter referred to as the "543 Report"), p. 6, Dec. 1968.

31. Id. at 7.

32. Ibid.

33. *Health Care for California*, Report of the Governor's Committee on Medical Aid and Health, p. 37, California State Department of Public Health, Berkeley, 1960.

34. Ibid.

35. See 543 Report, supra note 30 at 8; *Regional Development of Hospitals and Related Health Facilities in California*, Report to the California Legislature and to the State Advisory Hospital Council by Southern California Regional Hospital Planning Committee and San Francisco Bay Area Regional Hospital Planning Committee, p. 10, Dec. 1962.

36. 543 Report, supra note 30 at 8.

37. Ibid.

38. See letter dated March 15, 1963 from John E. Janzen, Planning Coordinator, South San Joaquin Valley Regional Health Planning Office, Visalia, California to community groups announcing award of an initial planning grant for organization of a regional planning program.

39. See chart of organizational structure in pamphlet, "Functions of Regional Health Planning," South San Joaquin Valley Regional Health Planning, Visalia, California.

40. 543 Report, supra note 30 at 21.

41. 543 Report, supra note 30 at 24-25.

42. 543 Report, supra note 30 at 8.

43. 543 Report, supra note 30 at 2.

44. Ibid.

45. 543 Report, supra note 30 at 3.

46. *Summary of Activities, Comprehensive Health Planning in California 1969-1970*, p. 1, California State Department of Public Health.

47. Calif. Health and Safety Code, sec. 437 (West Supp. 1972).

48. Calif. Health and Safety Code, sec. 437.7(e) (West Supp. 1972).

49. Calif. Health and Safety Code, sec. 1402.1 (West Supp. 1972); Calif, Welfare and Inst. Code, sec. 7003.1 (West 1972).

50. *Report of the Governor's Committee on Hospital Costs* (Marion B. Folsom, Chairman), p. 11, New York, N.Y., 1965.

51. Southern California Association of Governments, *The Region and the Association-—1968*, p. 1.

52. Roemer, Milton I., M.D., "Health Resources and Services in the Watts Area of Los Angeles," Report of the Health Consultant to the Governor's Commission on the Los Angeles Riots, *California Health*, p. 123 at 140, Feb.-March, 1966.

53. *Violence in the City—An End or a Beginning?* A Report by the Governor's Commission on the Los Angeles Riots, p. 74, Los Angeles, 1965.

54. Kisch, Arnold I., Arthur J. Viseltear, and Milton I. Roemer, *The Watts Hospital: A Health Facility is Planned for a Metropolitan Slum Area*, Medical Care Administration Case Study No. 5, U.S. Public Health Service, Washington, D.C., Dec. 1967.

55. Roemer, supra note 52 at 126-128.

56. See Roemer, Milton I., "Controlling and Promoting Quality in Medical Care," *Law and Contemporary Problems, Health Care*, Part I, p. 284, Spring 1970.

57. 20 C.F.R. sec. 405.1001 ff. (1970). Conditions of Participation or Coverage for extended care facilities are contained in 20 C.F.R. sec. 405.1101 ff. and for home health services in 20 C.F.R. sec. 405.1201 ff.

58. See Worthington, William and Laurens H. Silver, "Regulation of Quality of Care in Hospitals: The Need for Change," *Law and Contemporary Problems, Health Care*, Part II, p. 305 at 314, Spring 1970, citing 42 U.S.C. sec. 1395aa (Supp. I, 1965).

59. Id. at 314.

60. 20 C.F.R. sec. 405.1005(c).

61. The Hospital Survey and Construction Act, 42 U.S.C. sec. 291c(e)(1968).

62. Cook et al. v. Ochsner Foundation Hospital et al., Civ. Act. No. 70-1969, E.D. La., Consent Agreement and Order of Aug. 1, 1972 (see also 319 F. Supp. 603, E.D. La. 1970).

63. 37 Fed. Reg. 14719 (Nov. 4, 1972). See Rose, Marilyn G., "The Hill-Burton Act—the Interim Regulation and Service to the Poor: A Study in Public Interest Litigation," *Clearinghouse Review*, Vol. VI, No. 6, p. 309, Oct. 1972.

64. See Worthington and Silver, supra note 58 at 314, note 40.

65. P.L. 92-223, sec. 4(a), 42 U.S.C. 1396d (1970 Edition, Supp. I).

66. See Worthington and Silver, supra note 58 at 310.

67. Id. at 319 ff. See also "The Threat to JCAH's Accreditation," *Medical World News*, May 19, 1972.

68. See Worthington and Silver, supra note 58 at 310, note 21 and at 312, note 30.

69. *High Cost of Hospitalization*, Hearings before the Subcommittee on Antitrust and Monopoly of the Committee on the Judiciary, U.S. Senate, 91st Cong., 2d Sess., Part 1, pp 449-528 (statement of Norman W. Skillman with excerpts from *PAS Reporter*), 1970.

70. Welfare and Institutions Code, secs. 16200 ff. (West 1972).

71. For efforts made to overcome the problems in division of the licensing function, see an excellent but unfortunately unpublished paper, "Licensing—Confusion or Consolidation," presented at the 1971 Conference of the California Association of Rehabilitation Facilities by

Howard A. Worley, formerly Chief, Bureau of Health Facilities Licensing and Certification, California State Department of Public Health. Excerpts from Mr. Worley's historical account follow:

In 1963 the Departments of Mental Hygiene, Public Health and Social Welfare at the request of the Health and Welfare Agency Administrator agreed to establish a "Joint Licensing Service" in the Department of Public Health. The plan was to become effective in July 1964, but as questions were raised as to the legality of the agreement, the plan was abandoned. . . .

In 1965 a "Committee on the Consolidation of Licensing" was established in the Health and Welfare Agency. The report of this Committee in December 1966 recommended the establishment of a permanent "Licensing Coordinating Committee," the modification and revision of classifications, regulations, standards and procedures, and the transfer of licensing responsibilities where necessary to bring facilities under the most appropriate health, substitute home or other grouping. This has only been partially accomplished.

The Senate Subcommittee on Social Welfare reported in 1967 the same conditions and problems emphasizing the inconsistencies between related programs and noticeable gaps mentioned earlier. The report cited the operational problems of dual licenses being required in certain instances and the difficulties of attempting to classify facilities into distinct bins which deter the development of comprehensive programs.

The Subcommittee's recommendations included the establishment of a new Department of Facility Licensing, the expansion of coverage to include halfway homes, and out-of-home care for persons between the ages of 16 and 65, and the establishment of a licensing advisory board. The Subcommittee's recommendations were embodied in a legislative bill the following year. The proposal was referred for interim study with a legislative resolution requesting the Health and Welfare Agency "to simplify and consolidate licensing functions" and to submit a report to the Legislature in 1969.

The 1969 report reemphasized the many existing problems particularly duplication and inconsistency. An additional report by the Agency submitted in 1970 suggested legislation to consolidate health facility licensing in the Department of Public Health and residential care facility licensing in the Department of Social Welfare with identical language for similar functions in each program. A legislative bill was not, however, submitted for consideration.

Also during 1968 and 1969 an Agency Task Force was studying duplicative and overlapping responsibilities in the health field especially for programs for the mentally retarded, alcoholism, research and facility licensing. The culmination of the Task Force reports and that of a subsequent task force was the recommendation to the Governor for the reorganization of health and related programs into a single Department of Health.

72. Calif. Health and Safety Code, secs. 440 ff. (West Supp. 1972).

73. California Medical Association, *CMA News*, 17 Feb. 1971.

74. *Future Directions for Health Services, County of Los Angeles/1970*, Review of the Program of the Los Angeles County Health Department, undertaken at the request of the Los Angeles County Board of Supervisors (Malcolm H. Merrill, M.D., Director of study). p. 155, Los Angeles, 1970.

75. Ibid.

76. See Worthington and Silver, supra note 58 at 305-306 for failure of Boston City Hospital and St. Louis City Hospital to meet accreditation standards of the Joint Commission on Accreditation of Hospitals; for statement of the house staff of the D.C. General Hospital in the District of Columbia that that hospital was rendering inadequate and inferior patient care; for account of suit filed by residents at Los Angeles County-University of Southern California Medical Center seeking to enjoin overcrowding at that hospital which resulted in patient beds

being placed in corridors. See also *The Contemporary Status of Large Urban Public Hospitals—Ambulatory Services,* Summary Report, Large Urban Public Hospitals, Ambulatory Services Project (James P. Cooney, Jr., Ph.D., Principal Investigator, Milton I. Roemer, M.D., Co-Principal Investigator, and Martin B. Ross, Project Director), School of Public Health, University of California, Los Angeles, Nov. 1971 and Piore, Nora, Deborah Lewis, and Jeannie Seeliger, *A Statistical Profile of Hospital Outpatient Services in the United States: Present Scope and Potential Role,* Association for the Aid of Crippled Children, New York, Aug. 1971.

77. Roemer, Milton I., M.D., "Patient Dumping and Other Contributions of Voluntary Agencies to Public Agency Problems," *Medical Care,* Vol. 11, No. 1, p. 30, Jan.-Feb. 1973.

78. See *Trends in Long-Term Care,* Hearings before the Subcommittee on Long-Term Care of the Special Committee on Aging, U.S. Senate, 91st and 92nd Congs., July 1969-Oct. 1971.

79. Ibid.

80. Fry, Hilary G., *The Operation of State Hospital Planning and Licensing Programs,* American Hospital Association, Chicago, 1965.

81. *Report of the Governor's Committee on Hospital Costs* (Marion B. Folsom, Chairman), New York, 1965.

82. National Commission on Community Health Services, *Health Care Facilities, The Community Bridge to Effective Health Services,* Report of the Task Force on Health Care Facilities, Public Affairs Press, Washington, D.C., 1967.

83. National Advisory Commission on Health Facilities, *A Report to the President,* Washington, D.C., 1968.

84. Secretary's Advisory Committee on Hospital Effectiveness, *Report,* U.S. Department of Health, Education, and Welfare, 1968.

85. *Nursing Homes for the Aged: The Agony of One Million Americans,* Task Force Report on Nursing Homes (Kate Blackwell, Ed.), Preliminary Draft, Center for the Study of Responsive Law, Washington, D.C., 1970.

86. Somers, Anne R., *Hospital Regulation: The Dilemma of Public Policy,* Industrial Relations Section, Department of Economics, Princeton University, Princeton, N.J., 1969.

87. See *Report of the Task Force on Medicaid and Related Programs,* p. 71, U.S. Department of Health, Education, and Welfare, June 27, 1970.

CHAPTER 8

Problems of Fragmented
Health Services

*Escalating costs; uneven geographic distribution of health care
personnel and facilities; increased specialization among health
professionals, side by side with a scarcity of primary care practitioners; too much devotion to exotic, seldom-used facilities
combined with too little concentration on the prevention of
illness; overworked physicians and under-utilized assistants—
all of these are part of a litany.* . . .[1]

—Elliot L. Richardson
Secretary, U.S. Department of
Health, Education, and Welfare,
1972

The many-faceted system of health care, grown both incrementally and by
leaps, has unusual merits. Action by devoted groups and individuals has
expanded care and furthered innovations. Research has pushed into new
frontiers. Training has been made possible for more professional and allied
health workers. Hospital beds have been provided where none had existed
before. Preventive health services have been strengthened. A sizeable amount
of care has been insured for the working population. Services have been
extended to the poor and the aged. The quality of care, drugs, and medical
technology has been noticeably improved. Many disparate groups, with their
differing and sometimes competitive inputs, have contributed to better
health services, reducing mortality, lessening morbidity, and lengthening the
life-span.

Despite these many advances over the past half-century, deep and
persistent problems in the health service system affect the provision of care
for the total population. Contributing heavily to each of the problems listed
by Secretary Richardson above, and to other problems as well, is the frag-

mented structure of the health service system, both public and private. While there is justifiable concern over the rising costs of health care, these high costs are symptoms of deep structural deficiencies of the systems of financing and delivering health services. Fragmented programs, divergent funding policies, and splintered organization of services are crucial elements that make the system something less than economical, efficient, and responsive.

The effects of fragmentation are pervasive, restricting the quantity and quality of services for consumers and limiting the capability of providers to furnish them. Fragmentation contributes to unequal access to care, gaps and inequities in services, a dearth of preventive care, discontinuous and sometimes inappropriate care, and considerable lag in responding to changing needs. Fragmentation also impedes economical use of scarce resources, effective planning and evaluating of programs of care, and controlling their costs and quality. All these problems bear on all sections of the population but most grievously on the disadvantaged.

POOR ACCESS TO CARE

Of the many factors affecting access to health care, two principal factors are ability to pay for service and availability of providers.[2] The increase in expendable income and the greater share of health care underwritten by private insurance and public funding have expanded access to medical care for a large portion of the population. But for far too many, access to care is impeded by the maldistribution of services and compounded by fragmentation. Fewer physicians serve the one-fourth of the population living in rural areas and those poor and nonpoor who live in central cities of metropolitan complexes.[3] Physicians are generally not available nights and weekends, and the specialist is financially inaccessible to many. Unavailability of physicians, in turn, restricts access to community hospitals and compels reliance on overcrowded public hospitals, adding the further impediments of longer travel time and waiting for care. Fragmented efforts have not redressed this inequity.

Introduction of new forms of ambulatory care under various auspices has improved access only for a limited number of people. The 500 publicly financed health centers, most in urban settings, have provided access for a relatively small proportion of the population in need.[4] Some health centers, it is true, have served as models of new forms of care, but the multiplicity of public and private agencies has not provided multiple points of entry into the system as a whole.

Eligibility requirements of various agencies and programs present successively higher barriers to access. A community hospital may require proof of ability to pay before admittance, a physician assurance of source of income. The neighborhood health centers funded by the U.S. Office of Economic Opportunity restrict services to those below the poverty level. Medicaid imposes numerous and variable eligibility barriers, depending upon the state or the county of residence.[5] Means tests require repeated determinations of eligibility, without regard to the individual's need for medical care. At one income level, a person may be eligible; if he earns a dollar more, he may lose eligibility no matter what his medical condition. When increases in Social Security benefits raised incomes above levels set by the state, the medically needy aged were ousted from medical benefits. Judicial action was necessary to enforce a federal mandate to the contrary.[6] In 20 states the medically needy are not eligible for services under Medicaid; and in those states that provide benefits, access is increasingly limited by requirements for prior authorization before services can be provided. Ever tightening eligibility requirements in welfare or cash assistance programs also restrict access of the welfare poor to medical care, regardless of health needs.[7]

In some instances, eligibility is further fragmented by diagnostic category. The kind of care that the handicapped child in California receives is determined by 25 diagnostic categories, imposed in addition to 14 different age hurdles and 14 different financial tests.[8] The multiple diagnoses of many handicapped children make the eligibility requirement of diagnostic categories "no longer a service . . . it is a barrier to service."[9] Access to mental care is similarly entangled, fragmented not only by age but by type of hospital in which care is provided and by source of financing. The net effect of such division and complicated eligibility requirements is that, despite growing welfare rolls, half of the poor are barred from access to medical services except through public hospitals.[10]

Both private insurance and public programs limit access to certain services and introduce income barriers through coinsurance and deductibles.[11] Medicare, the largest public program, interposes a three-day hospital stay, which may be medically questionable, before allowing reimbursable admission to a nursing home and then limits length of stay. Such limitations work hardships on all, not only on the poor, as in the case of the widow of a Supreme Court Justice, with a $5,000 a year pension as well as Medicare benefits, who was unable to afford a prolonged, medically prescribed stay in a nursing home.[12] Occasionally publicized examples of such hardship reveal only the tip of the iceberg.

Lack of access is a geographic, as well as an economic, problem. It is also not confined to the poor but seriously affects the entire population, particularly the work force. For example, some 14,000 persons are killed annually in industrial accidents, and two million are disabled. Many of these victims of industrial accidents work in places where facilities for emergency care are not readily available.[13] Moreover, the numerous, different, and overlapping geographic areas for provision of services by various agencies create what has been called a "thicket of district boundaries."[14] The 30 different sets of administrative districts for health and social services in Los Angeles County present a challenge to the most talented social worker and a confusing maze to the citizen whom these districts are designed to serve.[15]

Multiple agencies and fragmented services place not only economic and geographic roadblocks in the way of obtaining care but more subtle socio-cultural barriers that make health services inaccessible and unacceptable in many instances. Categorical prerequisites for care are associated with an inflexibility that inhibits development of services sensitive to varying cultural attitudes.

GAPS AND INEQUITIES

Increased spending within a fragmented system does not reach all who need care. Categorical programs and episodic care are designed to cover specified persons, specified diseases, specified services, or specified geographic areas — and not others. Gaps and inequities are built into the system, both the public and private sectors. As Secretary Richardson of the U.S. Department of Health, Education, and Welfare pointed out with respect to the public sector,

> [T]he problem of fragmentation is not unique to the grants-in-aid programs of the Federal Government. It does have its counterparts in the diffusion of services and lack of communications at the local level. . . . with respect to many kinds of services, we are reaching only a fraction of those who, in principle, are eligible.[16]

Private insurance has notable gaps in coverage of the poor, the low paid, the chronically ill, the unemployed, and the aged, in the extent of benefits provided, and in limited coverage for mental illness, dental services, drugs, and rehabilitation. In California in 1968, 20 percent of the population was not covered by hospital insurance, 27 percent had no surgical coverage, and 35 percent had no physician's coverage.[17] Even for those covered, waiting periods, deductibles, coinsurance, and extremely limited psychiatric and dental benefits create gaps. Medicare pays for less than half the medical costs of the aged.[18] Medicaid in 1969 reached approximately half of those on welfare and less than a third of the poor.[19] By 1972, possibly half the poor were reached. These gaps led the national Task Force on Medicaid and Related Programs to conclude:

> A new look at public and private financing of programs is needed. If Medicaid, Medicare and Maternal and Child Health programs have provided less coverage and

benefits than desirable, so too, have private carriers. Uncovered population represents a failure of both the public and private sectors.[20]

In California, some 500,000 children live in families too poor to pay for medical care but not eligible for care under the Medicaid program.[21] In the fragmented system, two of every three poor children do not receive care either under Title V of the Social Security Act, which provides basic support for maternal and child health services, or under the Medicaid program. Moreover, as the Task Force on Medicaid noted, "there is some question of the extent of need which is met even where they are reached."[22]

In addition to such documented gaps in health services, two significant types of inequity in the delivery of services have their roots in fragmentation. One type is the persistent geographic inequity in implementing almost every national program that is subject to state and local control. The other is the fundamental inequity in the quantity and quality of services received by the poor in contrast to that received by the general population.

The geographic inequity is pronounced in the Medicaid program, with its state variability in eligibility and benefits. Twenty-five years after federal legislation established services for crippled children, major inequities in the kind of care provided by the states, not wholly related to differing state income levels, persist in this ostensibly nationwide program.[23] In the rubella immunization program conducted throughout the United States, more than a fifth of the target population was not reached because of the wide variations in state efforts, both public and private.

Despite continual addition of programs to correct inequities in care of the poor, fewer low-income persons, nonwhites, and central city residents had regular sources of medical care and were less likely to see a physician than the rest of the population.[24] This inequity is made more serious by the higher rates of illness and disability among the poor than in the population as a whole.[25]

Public programs that reach only a portion of their eligibles reveal only some of the unmet need. The entire population is affected by gaps in service. Some needs are unknown or unmeasurable; some surface only episodically. Even when need is known, or can be projected with some accuracy, the gap between need and available care may be serious. A nationwide survey concludes that

[B]y our best available estimates, only 10 percent of those in need can be served by our present professional mental health services and personnel. Further, many of our present care arrangements are little more than custodial institutions which offer little in the way of habilitation or rehabilitation.[26]

DEFICIENT PREVENTION

A paradox of health care is that preventive health services, although largely
responsible for decreased morbidity and mortality, receive the least in funds
in the fragmented system. Less than five percent of the federal budget for
health goes for preventive activities.[27] Public financing of medical care
generally fails to pay for preventive measures. The same neglect of prevention
pervades the entire system of health care. Private insurance covers little for
prevention; hospitals provide limited preventive services; private physicians
provide only minimal preventive care.

Paucity of preventive efforts in the field of industrial accidents and
diseases affects the great majority of the working population: the millions of
workers in factories, construction, mines, transport, agriculture, and governmental blue collar employment. Not only are there wide state disparities in
such preventive activities, but the total effort is limited. Nationally, 1600
state and 100 federal inspectors can provide only limited surveillance over the
four million work places for occupational accidents and disease.[28] The efforts
of industry and government have failed, except in some branches of manufacturing, to stem the rising rate of both accidents and industrial disease.

Health education, nutrition, family planning, and procedures for early
detection of disease have become separate measures, rather than being built
into the structure of the system of health care. As long as they remain fragmented and detached, they do not reach their target populations, let alone
the submerged majority who cannot be reached by current health agencies.
Thus, by 1972, approximately half the five million low-income women
targeted in the special message on population of 1969 were served by categorical programs for family planning;[29] and Medicaid, the major program of
health care for the poor, spent less than one-half of one percent on family
planning services in 1971.[30]

Understandably, sound preventive measures are inhibited by categorical
and fragmented programs. The separation of health education, nutritional
services, immunizations, diagnostic screening, and family planning services
in public programs from curative services tends to assign a low priority to
prevention. Many of these services could be provided effectively in the course
of providing regular medical care, perhaps more effectively. Currently,
financial incentives are lacking for individual providers in a segmented
system to keep patients well. Moreover, prevention of disease and disability
involves programs outside the system of personal health services: programs
for proper food, sanitary housing, clean neighborhoods, recreational areas,
better education, and employment. Fragmentation within the health service
system is hardly conducive to creating effective links with nonhealth but
related programs.

DISCONTINUOUS AND INAPPROPRIATE CARE

Fragmentation contributes to lack of continuous, comprehensive, and appropriate care for both rich and poor. Plural funding sources, multiple agencies, and numerous programs intended to supplement each other may, in fact, lead to discontinuity or support inappropriate levels of care. The consumer has neither knowledge nor power, the insurer neither incentive nor organization, the isolated providers not the means, and the fragmented public system but few mechanisms to remedy this condition that pervades the system. Thus, school health examinations are separated from follow-up medical care, preventive public health clinics from curative treatment, ambulatory care generally from hospital care, hospitals from nursing homes and home care despite prescriptions to link them, and home care is divided between paid-for nursing services and unpaid additional services that are needed.

The level of care provided is often medically inappropriate. Private insurance and public funding promote hospitalization, although a fourth or more of hospital stays, perhaps a larger proportion of surgery, may not be appropriate.[31] According to the Comptroller General of the United States,

[T]he health care system is oriented primarily toward treatment of the acute phase of illness and does not offer a complete spectrum of health care by providing available alternatives to acute care, financing for the alternatives, and educating physicians and patients in accepting alternatives.[32]

Neither insurance nor public programs pay adequately for nursing home care or for home care.[33] No program pays for custodial care. As the Task Force on Medicaid noted, no program has provided the appropriate long-term care required by the aged.[34] The same comment applies to other groups.

Various programs, such as the OEO neighborhood health centers, the family health centers, and the Model Cities projects, have attempted to assure continuity of care. Blue Cross has moved toward broader insurance coverage, community hospitals in the direction of increased outpatient care. Health maintenance organizations are designed to assure access to a full spectrum of services for a defined population. But variable payment mechanisms, eligibility requirements, and scope of services covered block achievement of continuous care. The sheer number of agencies that must be brought under one umbrella, the diversity of federal and state regulations, the even more diverse insurance programs and financing mechanisms constitute formidable obstacles. Medicaid builds in discontinuity with its division between five required and ten optional services and its welfare and nonwelfare categories. Medicare prescribes discontinuity by its division between hospital and physician's care.

With the exception of Veterans and military hospitals and some group practices, the capacity to organize continuous and appropriate care is impeded by fragmentation. Rarely does a single patient record follow the patient through different stages of care. More importantly, responsibility for assuring a full range of services for each patient's needs is seldom defined. Decisions on care are basically a function of physicians. The consumer has little opportunity and less knowledge to influence the quality of care he receives. He generally cannot distinguish necessary from unnecessary surgery or good from poor surgery. He must accept drugs as prescribed. He may not substitute a lower priced, generic drug for a higher-priced brand name product. He is, moreover, bombarded with misleading claims for non-prescribed remedies for countless ailments. Depending on the physician's hospital staff affiliations, the patient may receive care, on the one hand, in a university-based, leading hospital or even in a crowded public hospital, or, on the other hand, in an unaccredited voluntary hospital or a small, proprietary hospital. In each of these institutions there may be a range of quality, although the likelihood of good care is greater in the former than in the latter. In both private and public sectors episodic, discontinuous care is the product of numerous individual providers and segmented programs.

POOR RESPONSIVENESS TO CONSUMER NEEDS

The irony of fragmented and categorical programs is that although each program has been enacted in response to a specific need, the fragmented and categorical system as a whole proves too cumbersome to respond readily to unmet and changing health needs. Each agency or program is accountable for a specific function, but none, singly or in combination, has the responsibility or authority to coordinate or reorient the elements of the system as needed.

Delayed responsiveness may be seen in the lag in providing care for the poor, the aged, and the disabled. Their needs have been persuasively set forth and almost endlessly elaborated for two generations in reports, special investigations, Congressional hearings, and national conferences. It has taken more than a generation of critical needs to enact Medicare and Medicaid and almost another generation to assure medical care to the disabled. National health insurance that would cover the total population is still in the future, despite both the need and expressed desire of the majority of the people, not only the poor.

Lagging responsiveness to consumer needs is, in part, related to inadequate involvement of consumers in the decisions of agencies and providers.[35] This lack of consumer involvement is notable at every stage, from the preparation of health legislation, through all aspects of the delivery of services to surveillance of their quality. It contributes significantly to the slowness of change. Despite requirements of many public programs that advisory councils contain consumer representatives, participation of consumers tends to be formal rather than active. Comprehensive Health Planning agencies are required to have a majority of consumer representatives, but they are often selected haphazardly or even by the providers.[36] Consumer representation on hospital boards is infrequent. Consumers have little voice in the operation of group practice plans. Union officials, with expertise in bargaining and a large stake in the way that health and welfare trust funds are used, exert few pressures on the health care delivery system. Nor do public agencies utilize their leverage sufficiently on behalf of the public to this end.

Only the neighborhood health centers, funded by the U.S. Office of Economic Opportunity, have encouraged significant consumer involvement. Despite some abrasive experiences, the result has been increased knowledge and activity on the part of consumers with respect to their health services. A recent experiment extending consumer representation on advisory boards of 22 voluntary hospitals, with the participation of a *"funding* and *regulatory* agency [emphasis in original], accelerated the promulgation of long overdue reforms in voluntary hospital ambulatory care."[37]

In the drive to make health services more responsive to people's needs, public agencies have undertaken to decentralize delivery of care to communities and even to neighborhoods. Decentralization has the merit of placing the administration of programs close to the people served by them, but it has not succeeded in overcoming the divergent directions of multiple programs established for categorical purposes. Decentralization affects the locale and perhaps the acceptability of services, but it cannot per se enhance the capacity of the system to respond to health needs in the absence of effective allocation of resources and planning of services — functions that require authority at a level of government higher than that of the community or the neighborhood.

INEFFICIENT USE OF SCARCE RESOURCES

Fragmentation in the organization of health services contributes to misuse of scarce resources — personnel, facilities, and financing. In both the private and public sectors, divided authority and responsibility present serious hindrances to optimal use of resources. Although public funding pays one-third of the cost of hospital care and one-fourth of the cost of physicians' care and all other health services, fragmented governmental policy has blocked use of this single largest source of funds for organizational change. Private insurance, even more intricately divided, also serves as a passive conduit of funds. Although these two largest funding sources have marked impact in other ways on the system of health care, their segmented structure is at variance with efforts to make the system more economical and efficient. As a leading economist has noted,

[T]he real function of the cost increases of the past decade and those in process should be to compel vast structural changes in the organization of medical care. Nothing could be worse in our society today than to say we need another three to five billion for medical care, and then simply duplicate or multiply the arrangements that we now have. This would get us nowhere. It is the fundamental transformation in a variety of our arrangements that I think is signalled by these cost changes . . . brought about by structural changes in the practice and organization of medicine.[38]

The private sector presents a broad spectrum of organizational forms in response to increasing specialization and a wide market. Each hospital is, of course, an organization of diverse capabilities. In many instances, costly facilities and specialized equipment are duplicated for the same population and geographic area, even though they may not be fully utilized. In recognition of the extravagance that such duplication may entail, hospitals are undertaking a variety of cooperative efforts that range from shared administrative and housekeeping services to mergers.[39] For example, with declining birth rates, stand-by beds for maternity care are being maintained by hospitals jointly. Moreover, joint provision of highly specialized services by two or more hospitals is being impelled by expert opinion that a certain number of cases is necessary to maintain medical and surgical skills for superspecialty care.[40] Corporate entry into the hospital and nursing home field, including hospital supplies, indicates that larger-scale, more economical operation is emerging, but the most efficient operation of expensive facilities does not address the problem of the use of costly hospital services in place of preventive, ambulatory, and extended care.

The slowly expanding proportion of physicians engaged in some form of organized practice is a trend toward more effective use of the scarce and expensive resource of physicians' skills.[41] This increasing organization of physicians into a variety of patterns constitutes recognition, to some extent, of the need to deliver services economically and efficiently. Group practice permits far greater division of labor than does solo practice and expanded use of allied and auxiliary personnel. It also permits effective use of capital investment in technological advances, such as the large computer and the automated clinical laboratory.[42] One element in the movement to provide comprehensive care through health maintenance organizations, or prepaid group practice, is exercise of increased control over the use of facilities. Thus, health maintenance organizations are, in part, a response to the inability of the present fragmented system to substitute adequate, less costly alternatives for expensive hospital care.

Fragmentation has also been a barrier to improved use of resources by public agencies, despite numerous cooperative and managerial techniques. One federal mechanism to spur improved use of resources and integrated delivery of services is joint funding of a single project by several agencies. The unifying advantages of joint funding, however, tend to be dissipated by diverse state requirements and divergent federal policies and funding formulas.[43] Revenue sharing, promoted as a means of eliminating categorical strictures and of returning decision-making authority to the states, has not been proposed, however, for health services primarily because the major federal funding programs fall outside the grants-in-aid structure.

Another and recurring response to the need for improved use of resources and integrated services has been administrative reorganization of agencies. Reorganizations improve executive controls but do not automatically result in integrated services at the place where they are provided.[44] Successive reorganizations at federal, state, and local levels must still contend with the differing mandates of their categorical programs. Nevertheless, reorganization can improve the capacity to use resources economically and to provide services on an integrated basis. Current efforts to merge departments of hospitals, public health, and mental health at the state, county, and metropolitan levels across the country can contribute to unified, comprehensive services in public medical care, if not in the private sector. If this result is achieved, it will be because reorganizations are undertaken not merely as a means of reordering administrative units but as a means of implementing explicit plans for unified public services in the communities where these services are provided.

INEFFECTIVE PLANNING AND EVALUATION

Planning and evaluation of health services, despite many advances, are seriously hampered by the numbers of discrete agencies and programs with differing requirements. The extreme variability in medical records of unrelated providers and programs severely limits meaningful and multiple uses of data for evaluation and planning. Although single programs or individual facilities may be well evaluated at some level in terms of their specific goals, the sheer numbers of different programs with innumerable variables defy evaluation in terms of adequacy and effectiveness of health services.

Evaluation—the basis of planning—is made more difficult by multiple, categorical programs. Measuring either the process or outcome of health services does not reach the critical question of just how much each of the many programs contributes to the better health of its recipients. It yields more valuable insights to measure the outcome of a comprehensive health program than to measure the differential contributions of many single programs.

Fragmented programs also entail gaps as well as overlaps in data collection. Reporting of venereal disease or adverse drug reactions by private practitioners is deficient.[45] Blue Cross, Blue Shield, and private insurance companies have excellent, modern data systems intended primarily for processing claims. Their adaptation for utilization review and for examination of provider or patient profiles has barely been explored, in part because of the separation of responsibility between public agencies and fiscal intermediaries. Uniform data based on patient and provider records are emerging slowly in both public and private systems. The Commission on Professional and Hospital Activities, which began in 1953, enlists fewer than half of the voluntary hospitals in its Professional Activity Study (PAS) and fewer than a fourth of the hospitals in its Medical Audit Program (MAP).[46] Data on nursing home services and costs on a national basis are a serious lack.

Even within the public sector, fragmented programs yield an inadequate data base for effective planning. Three years after Medicare and Medicaid were in operation, the two agencies responsible for their administration within the Department of Health, Education, and Welfare exchanged little information on the same providers; nor, in fact, did they use the same fiscal intermediaries in certain states to simplify processing of claims and data. Medicaid records, invaluable for planning and evaluation, differ by state, sometimes by county, and also by administrative agency, giving rise to controversial estimates for budgeting. Nationally, Medicaid has not been able to determine with any accuracy the number of persons eligible for services in each category of the cash assistance group, let alone the numbers eligible in the medically needy group.[47]

Many federal programs require a state plan in the particular field to be approved by the Secretary of the Department of Health, Education, and Welfare as a condition of receipt of federal funds. Many of these plans have been indicted as "not actually planning" but "meaningless statistics and geographical descriptions."[48] Nevertheless, a joint federal-state-local statistical system, which would facilitate effective state plans and is well within the capabilities of modern computers, has not been established. Divisions between state and local jurisdictions with multiple agencies at each level stand as a barrier. The frustrations of Comprehensive Health Planning agencies, in attempting to plan for a full range of services, can be attributed in part to the numbers of programs and agencies, with differing boundaries, jurisdictions, and accountability, that are beyond the scope of authority of the planners.

Each agency operates on the basis of its own definitions of goals, target populations, and services. Each governmental agency tailors its data to its own administrative needs. Each voluntary agency uses a data base or region that suits its administrative and fund-raising potential. California has more than 100 different geographic regions for various planning efforts by public agencies. In one county, with a single governing body, each major health agency has a different data base; some agencies have two or three for different administrative purposes. If to these county agencies are added the regions for community mental health centers, the areas served by regional mental retardation centers, the areas for hospital construction of the state Hill-Burton plans, the various administrative regions of state agencies concerned with health services, and the many and differing districts of voluntary agencies, these many regional boundaries impede effective planning and evaluation. To provide comparable data from the latest Census, with vital statistics, patterns of morbidity, patient origins, income and welfare status, and meaningful socioeconomic data from each agency for any group in the population entails expensive and intricate computer preparation and processing. Moreover, even when the data are processed and rearranged for various uses, no single agency in the county has the authority to use the data for planning the totality of services but only for partial planning.

ESCALATING COSTS

Separated agencies, diverse financing, and fragmented programs contribute to inability to restrain rising costs of health care. Both public and private funding, accounting for almost two-thirds of total expenditures, favor high-cost hospitalization at the expense of lower cost alternatives, provide no incentive for cost reductions, and use cost-raising formulas, such as "reasonable" costs and "customary" and "prevailing" fees, as bases for payment. Incorporation of these cost-plus formulas in Medicare and Medicaid resulted in the escalation of costs out of proportion to the increased service provided. Where responsibility is joined and not divided, however, effective controls are possible not only over costs but over quality of care. Such unified control was incorporated in the Medicaid program in New York City, where the health department also acted as fiscal agent, with excellent results.[49]

The Medicare and Medicaid experience has exposed the folly of attempting to control costs of health services without changing the organization of services.[50] Both Medicare and Medicaid have attempted to constrain the rise of prevailing fees, made limited use of drug formularies, entered into a certain number of prepayment contracts, and worked with fiscal intermediaries to detect overcharging. General price controls were also in effect for a time. These measures were insufficient, however, to prevent increased costs of these programs. In the absence of a changed pattern of organizing services, the recourse was to decrease services and to shift an increased proportion of the cost of the programs to the beneficiaries.

The financial costs of fragmentation are revealed through the examination of potential economies achievable from a universal payments system and from an articulated system of delivering comprehensive care. Some of the savings to be realized might include the following:

1. Many million hospital days per year (some estimate 80,000,000) could be replaced by suitable alternatives to hospital care at a saving, in 1970 figures, of $3 billion. Another billion dollars could be saved by reducing the average hospital stay by one day without impairing the quality of care. Under the current fragmented system, these alternatives are not readily available.

2. Greater use of ambulatory services, costing less than half of hospital care, would relieve hospitals of an additional 10 to 20 percent of their inpatient utilization. But only three in ten hospitals have organized outpatient departments.

3. Extension of prepaid group medical practice, with its demonstrated economies, would reduce materially costs of both inpatient and ambulatory care. Surgical and hospitalization rates of prepaid group practices are substantially less than those under Blue Cross or private insurance; their physician ratios are two-thirds the national average, feasible with a team approach and greater use of allied health manpower.

4. Increased sharing of services, particularly expensive specialized ones, by hospitals and other facilities would permit further cost reductions but require improved organization and linkages. The costs of duplicated and underutilized specialized services are substantial.

5. Important savings could be achieved by expanding use of preventive and rehabilitative services.

6. The potential savings in administrative costs under a comprehensive system would eliminate (a) the cost of eligibility determinations under means test programs, which are currently four to eight times more expensive than administrative costs under Social Security; (b) duplications and overlaps both in private insurance and in major public programs, which result in multiple billings and claims procedures, estimated to waste $1.5 billion; (c) numerous administrative mechanisms attempting to coordinate fragmented programs; and (d) the present duplication of patient records and information systems.

Effective solutions to mounting costs are thus inhibited by a fragmented system drawn in different directions. Although regulation of hospital charges or rates and prospective budgeting for this most expensive component of health care have been demonstrated to be feasible and effective financial controls, they have been applied only spottily in the United States. As the National Conference on Medical Costs pointed out in 1967, "no single controllable factor escalates medical costs more than poor organization for the delivery of health services."[51] Five years later, the office of the Comptroller General, examining the costs of hospital construction, was led to enlarge the scope of its inquiry to include the entire organization of services, of which hospital costs are only a part, and in the end prescribed a "massive overhaul" of the nation's system of health services in order to reduce costs.[52]

INADEQUATE QUALITY CONTROLS

Multiplicity characterizes all aspects of controlling quality of health services. Although quality has been improved significantly in recent years, multiple mechanisms and agencies involved in safeguarding the quality of health services block further advances. Almost one-third of hospitals and more than two-thirds of extended care facilities certified for participation in Medicare in 1970 were not in full compliance with all requirements.[53] In many instances, standards are not sufficiently rigorous or uniformly enforced among the states. Responsibility is divided, gaps occur, and varying standards have been established. Superimposed on these basic faults in surveillance are the limited purposes and segmented authority of the various regulatory mechanisms and agencies. Not all the deficiencies in quality control, however, can be ascribed to fragmentation. For example, personnel assigned to surveillance are generally too few and may be inadequately qualified to do the job.[54]

A number of fragmenting features of the regulatory system impede effective quality controls. First, multiple kinds of regulatory mechanisms govern the health system. Some, like licensure, certification, and accreditation, constitute a form of prior approval, which must or may be met prior to operation. These same mechanisms or others, such as tissue committees of hospitals or accreditation committees for educational institutions or programs, may operate on an on-going or periodic basis to oversee performance. Still others, such as disciplinary action by personnel licensing boards or malpractice suits, intervene after the fact.

This variety in form of social control has the advantage of extending surveillance at different times to the sequence of providing health services. Nevertheless, the multiplicity of mechanisms invoked in specific ways, for specific purposes, and with differing effects results in erratic surveillance. Some individuals and institutions are held by licensure to a prescribed standard; others may meet less rigorous criteria. Some institutions may insist on close scrutiny of performance by hospital staff committees; in others the functioning of the committees may be *pro forma*. Worse than the variability is the fact that the multiplicity of mechanisms with specialized impact allows some individuals, some institutions, and some parts of the system to escape regulation that could be applied through one or another mechanism.

Second, the same aspect of the health system is regulated by multiple and different mechanisms. Credentialing of personnel, the unifying word given currency by a recent federal report,[55] actually consists of licensure by licensing boards of state government, certification by professional organizations, and accreditation of educational programs or institutions by professional organizations or accrediting agencies. Health facilities are subject to state facility licensing laws that set minimum standards that must be met as a prerequisite to their operating. In addition, they may meet standards set by the voluntary Joint Commission on Accreditation of Hospitals, the requirements of the Medicare legislation for certification as a provider, and the requirements of the state Medicaid program.[56] Also, hospitals may be subject to supervision of their nursing education or other training programs, and all facilities must meet requirements of federal narcotics controls, state labor legislation, local public health or sanitary regulation, and requirements of fire prevention codes.[57] As Anne Somers points out,

[H]ardly any aspect of hospital operations—from the organization and responsibilities of the medical staff, to the method of cost finding and accounting, to the overtime pay and union rights of the lowliest orderly—escapes the scrutiny of some public official.

Most of this regulation has grown like Topsy, without any deliberate cultivation and without any relation to an overall hospital policy. . . .[58]

One might think that such all-embracing surveillance, even if provided "without any relation to an overall hospital policy," would result in an effective regulatory system, but Mrs. Somers concludes:

. . . piecemeal regulation is almost inevitably incomplete as well as contradictory. Some regional variation is necessary in a nation as large as ours. But the present extent of variation, even contradiction, in current state licensing laws, tax laws, labor laws, and in judicial interpretation of hospital negligence and medical staff privileges, etc., borders on anarchy.

Whatever balancing advantages we have derived from the present conglomeration of laws and regulatory bodies—and there have been some—and whatever the extenuating circumstances for our failure to approach the problem of hospital regulation more positively and constructively in the past, the time has clearly come for a systematic overhaul of the entire apparatus.[59]

Regulation of drug safety and efficacy is also characterized by fragmented responsibility of multiple federal, state, and local programs and of numerous scientific, professional, and industrial organizations. Associated with this fragmentation are serious gaps. No single repository for information on the results of drug research has been established, not even a single repository for reports on side-effects from physicians, hospitals, and other institutions.[60] Coordination among scientists in the Food and Drug Administration, the National Institutes of Health, the Veterans Administration, and the Department of Defense on experimental and clinical trials of drugs has been conspicuously lacking.[61] Division of responsibility for quality of biological serums and vaccines between the Food and Drug Administration and the Division of Biological Standards of the National Institutes of Health resulted in transfer in 1972 of the Division of Biological Standards to the Food and Drug Administration.

Perhaps the most serious result of fragmentation in regulation of drugs, mentioned in Chapter 2, is the dichotomy between regulation of the safety and efficacy of drugs by public and voluntary agencies, on the one hand, and the prescribing practices of physicians and organized programs of health care, on the other. The enormous duplication of drug preparations under different trade names results in variable practices by hospitals and physicians. Each hospital has its own pharmacy committee, which operates independently of any national formulary. Each physician has his own prescribing habits, which may respond slowly to the "Dear Doctor" letters from the Food and Drug Administration warning against the deficiencies of certain preparations. This segmentation of the regulatory system for drugs from the medical care system that utilizes them affects both the cost and the quality of care.

Third, regulatory bodies may be governmental or voluntary, with differing sanctions. Official regulatory agencies exist at all levels of government. Voluntary agencies are generally professional associations or organizations of providers. Only recently, with increased powers for Comprehensive Health Planning agencies, have consumers become involved in regulation to a limited degree. This mixture of public and private regulation opens the door to differing standards and interpretations of measures of quality control. With enactment of P.L. 92-603, a new opportunity for voluntary monitoring of the quality of care is presented by requirements that Professional Standards Review Organizations (PSROs) be established to monitor and evaluate care provided to beneficiaries of Medicare and Medicaid. Experience with PSROs should reveal whether peer review, mandated by the federal government but operated voluntarily by the medical profession, can provide effective surveillance of the quality of care.

Fourth, it is not surprising that, with the multiplicity of programs and agencies regulating the quality of care, varying standards have been set and then enforced in varying ways. Social controls vary among the states. For example, three states have enacted comprehensive health facility licensure laws,[62] and this study is replete with examples of differing state provisions under the federal Medicaid program. Even within states, interpretations and enforcement of similar standards may result in critical differences in quality.

Fifth, the many measures of quality control, applied with great variability, are addressed to a fragmented health service system. At best, each measure can reach only a portion of the system. At worst, the regulatory system results in such complexity and confusion that bad actors may escape, good actors may be harrassed, and protection of the public is inadequate. Fortunately, the increasing provision of health services in organized frameworks tends to enhance the quality of care.[63] Just as highly organized hospitals are capable of providing specialized and sophisticated care, so organization of preventive services, emergency medical systems, and ambulatory care tends to improve the quality of these services. Thus, the trend towards organization gives promise of new, and perhaps innate, mechanisms of quality control.

FRAGMENTED POLICY

In the continuing national debate on health policy, it has become clear that lack of a unified health policy is at the root of fragmented services and underlies each of the problems discussed above. Policy is an ordering of priorities to achieve agreed-upon goals. At the federal level of government, however, no single arena or mechanism exists, either in the executive or the legislative branch, for central consideration of national health policy. This void is filled by bargaining by competing interests with divergent goals and unequal strength, which eventuates in an accumulation of disparate health programs, rather than a rational ordering of priorities.

The effects of limited purposes and contending objectives of categorical programs are particularly plain in the public sector, where legislation, regulations, and the activities of civil servants are open to public scrutiny. The President's own Panel Report on the Scientific and Educational Basis for Improving Health criticized the lack of national goals and priorities in the health system thus:

At present, no individual or group of individuals within the Executive Branch of the Federal Government has responsibility for monitoring the heterogeneous federal activities in the health field or for establishing national goals and priorities in relation to which the various programs can be evaluated, coordinated, or directed. Central control and evaluation consist largely of a retrospective tabulation of the sum of the many budgetary decisions to foster or to limit growth of individual programs.[64]

Similar fragmentation in the Legislative Branch is reflected by the 31 committees of the Congress concerned with different segments of health policy.

Perhaps the more obdurate effects of fragmented policy are to be found not in the relatively visible public sector but in the private sector, where government has long attempted to fill the gaps in the private delivery of health care and the private payment system. Fundamental to consideration of this fusing of the fragmented system is the changing relation of the private and public sectors. In funding, the public function has expanded from a minor to a major one, possibly the dominant one. But in providing services, the private sector dominates. Chiefly responsible for delivery and organization, it is also responsible in large measure for the gaps and inequities.

The public obligation has widened in increments. It has sought to fill the gaps in financing left by the private sector. It has attempted to fill the gaps in the delivery of services, particularly for the poor, the aged, and the chronically ill. It is just beginning to face the broader responsibility, inevitably assumed with costly spending, to reshape the system of care. Regulatory devices, like administrative controls, coordinating mechanisms, and even policy analysis, are further fragmented efforts in meeting this responsibility to restructure the system in the absence of a comprehensive program of financing and a deliberate effort to develop a sound, coherent national health policy.

NOTES

1. Address by the Honorable Elliot L. Richardson, Secretary of Health, Education, and Welfare before the Institute of Medicine, Washington, D.C., May 10, 1972.

2. See Cantor, Norman L., "The Law and Poor People's Access to Health Care," *Law and Contemporary Problems, Health Care*, Part II, Vol. XXXV, No. 4, p. 901, Autumn, 1970 for a summary of voluminous studies of income and health. For detailed personal narratives, see *Health Care Crisis in America, 1971*, Hearings before the Subcommittee on Health of the Committee on Labor and Public Welfare. U.S. Senate. 92nd Cong.. 1st Sess.. Parts 1-13. 1971; see also *Delivery of Health Services for the Poor*, Program Analysis 1967-72, U.S. Department of Health, Education, and Welfare, Office of the Assistant Secretary for Program Coordination, Dec. 1967.

3, See *Health Care Delivery in Rural Areas, Selected Models*, prepared by the Council on Rural Health, Division of Health Services, American Medical Association, Chicago, September 1970 for statement that rural populations have half as many health professionals and facilities available to them as the rest of the nation. See also Lesser, Arthur J., "A Look at Maternal and Child Health: 1970," *MCH Exchange*, Vol. 1, No. 1, p. 2, July 1970.

4. Merten. W. and S. Nothman. "Implications of the Neighborhood Health Center Experience for Future Investment of Federal Funds in the Delivery of Health Services," paper presented at the Annual Meeting of the American Public Health Association, Atlantic City, N.J., Nov. 15, 1972 showing that 408 selected ambulatory care programs, including neighborhood health centers, Maternity and Infant Care projects, Children and Youth projects, and free clinics. with a total target population of 9.4 million. enrolled or registered only 2 million.

5. McNerney, Walter J., "The Bronfman Lecture to the American Public Health Association," *Am. J. Public Health*, Vol. 61, No. 2, p. 223, Feb. 1971:

> Whereas Medicaid legislation promised access to health care for the poor and near poor, the promise had, in fact, "vanished into the obscurity of State determinations of eligibility and the limitations of State resources and priorities." How completely this had happened is seen in the fact that in 1971, it is estimated that Medicaid will cover only 13 million of the 30 to 40 million poor and near poor, and currently one of three children in the poor or near poor families is under Maternal and Child Health or Medicaid programs.

See also English, Joseph T., M.D., *Health Care Crisis in America, 1971*, supra note 2 at Part 3, pp. 471–472 for the point of view of the Administrator of the New York Municipal Hospital Corporation:

> Most disturbing of all, however, is the snarl of eligibility determination procedures which must be mastered before hospitals can complete the massive paperwork needed for reimbursement. . . . Frightened, disoriented, occasionally accompanied by distraught families, our patients often cannot prove their eligibility for coverage through the maze of paperwork and questions that confront them.

6. "State Told to Reinstate Medi–Cal to 10,000," *Los Angeles Times*, Part 3, p. 6, Dec. 19, 1972 in which Superior Court Judge Robert A. Wenke said that the State Department of Health Care Services is obligated to restore categorical aid under P.L. 92-603, which requires states to restore Medicaid benefits to those ruled ineligible because the Social Security increase put their incomes over welfare department computed need. See Dils v. Geduldig, Los Angeles County Superior Court, No. C-44371, Dec. 27, 1972.

7. For example, the requirement of Notice to Law Enforcement Officials (NOLEO) imposes on welfare recipients the obligation to identify and give information about a father who has deserted or abandoned a family; some states require that the mother also file a legal claim against the father, although the only requirements under Medicaid are proof of need and dependency. See Silver, Laurens H. and Mary Ann Efroymson, "Suggested Attacks on the NOLEO Requirement," *Clearinghouse Review*, Vol. 4, No. 1, p. 12 and No. 2, p. 55, May and June, 1970.

8. *A Report to the Assembly Select Committee on Mentally Ill and Handicapped Children*, pp. 42, 7, Arthur Bolton Associates, Sacramento, 1970.

9. Id. at 42.

10. See Cantor, supra note 2 at 902; McNerney, Walter J., supra note 5 at 223; English, supra note 5 at 469-470; Cooney, James P., Milton I. Roemer, and Martin B. Ross, *The Contemporary Status of Large Urban Public Hospitals— Ambulatory Services*, pp. vi-xi, xxvii-li, School of Public Health, University of California, Los Angeles, 1971; and Roemer, Milton I. and Jorge A. Mera, "Patient-Dumping and Other Voluntary Agency Contributions to Public Agency Problems," *Medical Care*, Vol. 11, No. 1, p. 30, Jan.-Feb. 1973.

11. McNerney, Walter J., "Today's Problems in Voluntary Financing Mechanisms," *Closing the Gaps in the Availability and Accessibility of Health Services*, 1965 Health Conference, *Bull. N.Y. Acad. Med.*, Vol. 41, No. 12, p. 1301, 1967, noting that limited payments, deductibles, co-payments, and similar devices thrust the burden on the patient and are "often too burdensome to be desirable medically. . . . It is becoming increasingly evident that for several reasons, expenses should be paid comprehensively and controls should be worked out between carrier and provider rather than allowing the burden to fall on the relatively ill-equipped individual." Testifying six years later, Dr. English, supra note 5 at 479, noted: "In relation to co-insurance, our experience in New York would indicate that it presents a barrier to care and an administrative nightmare."

12. "Frankfurter Widow Ailing, Near Charity on $5,000 U.S. Pension," *Los Angeles Times,* p. 1, May 27, 1972:

> Living for years at a Washington nursing home, Mrs. Frankfurter has all but exhausted a modest income from her husband's estate (and) is bedridden, running out of money needed for her care and in danger of becoming a charity case.

13. McKiever, Margaret F., *National Health Survey Findings of Occupational Health Interest,* PHS Pub. No. 1418, p. 1, U.S. Department of Health, Education, and Welfare, 1966.

14. Los Angeles County Health Services Planning Committee, Task Force on District Boundaries and Coordination, "Progress Report," May 27, 1968.

15. Frink, Jeanne Ewy, M.P.H. and Ruth Roemer, J.D., "Multipurpose Districts for Health and Social Services: A Proposal for Metropolitan Areas," *Public Affairs Report,* Bulletin of the Institute of Governmental Studies, Vol. 13, No. 1, Feb. 1972.

16. Departments of Labor and Health, Education, and Welfare Appropriations for 1973, Hearings before a Subcommittee of the Committee on Appropriations. H.R., 92nd Cong., 2d Sess., Part 1, p. 172.

17. California Medical Association, Bureau of Research and Planning, Socio-Economic Report, Vol. IX, No. 3, Table 5, San Francisco, March 1969.

18. *Report of the Task Force on Medicaid and Related Programs,* p. 41, U.S. Department of Health, Education, and Welfare, June 29, 1970.

19. Ibid.

20. Id. at 9.

21. California Legislature, Assembly Committee on Health and Welfare, *Malnutrition: One Key to the Poverty Cycle,* p. 13, Jan. 12, 1970.

22. *Report of the Task Force on Medicaid and Related Programs,* supra note 18 at 11.

23. See *Children Who Received Physicians' Services under the Crippled Children's Program,* Fiscal Year 1969, p. 4, PHS Pub. No. 2163, MCHS Statistical Series, No. 1, U.S. Department of Health, Education, and Welfare for the statement: "Interstate variation in percent of children reported to have multiple conditions . . . probably reflects differences in the scope of services provided and record keeping rather than differences in children." The percent of children with multiple conditions reported by the states varied from 1 percent in Rhode Island to 55.6 percent in Minnesota, against a national average of 19.8 percent.

24. Andersen, Ronald, Rachel McL. Greeley, Joanna Kravits, and Odin W. Anderson, *Health Service Use, National Trends and Variations,* DHEW Pub. No. (HSM) 73-3004, pp. 33-34, Health Services and Mental Health Administration, U.S. Department of Health, Education, and Welfare, Oct. 1972.

25. Id. at 34. See also Roemer, Milton I. and Arnold I. Kisch, "Health, Poverty, and the Medical Mainstream," *Power, Poverty and Urban Policy* (Bloomberg, Warner, Jr. and Henry J. Schmandt, Eds.), p. 181, Vol. 2, Urban Affairs Annual Reviews, Sage Publications, Inc., Beverly Hills, Ca., 1968.

26. Bobbitt, Joseph K., "Preview of the Findings and Recommendations of the Joint Commission on Mental Health of Children," *Interdepartmental Committee on Children and Youth, the 21st Year of Work,* pp. 63-64, Children's Bureau, Social and Rehabilitation Service, U.S. Department of Health, Education, and Welfare, 1969.

27. *Special Analyses of the Budget of the U.S. Government, Fiscal Year 1974,* pp. 158-159, Table J-26.

28. See *Occupational Safety and Health Act, 1970,* Hearings before the Subcommittee on Labor of the Committee on Labor and Public Welfare, U.S. Senate, 91st Cong., 1st and 2d Sess., Part 1, p. 85, Sept. 30, 1969; Page, Joseph A. and Mary-Win O'Brien, *Bitter Wages: Ralph Nader's Study Group Report on Disease and Injury on the Job,* Grossman, New York, N.Y., 1972.

29. *Special Analyses, Budget of the U.S. Government, Fiscal Year 1971*, p. 166.

30. Ibid.

31. Comptroller General of the United States, *Study of Health Facilities Construction Costs,* Report to the Congress of the United States, 92nd Cong., 2d Sess., Joint Committee Print, p. 769, Dec. 1972.

32. Ibid.

33. Van Dyke, Frank and Virginia Brown, "Organized Home Care: An Alternative to Institutions." *Inquiry*, Vol. IX, No. 2, p. 4, June 1972.

34. *Report of the Task Force on Medicaid and Related Programs*, supra note 18 at 83.

35. McNerney, Walter J., in *Health Care Crisis in America, 1971*, supra note 2 at 915:

> Government and private programs need consumer input. Both tend to become obsessed with internal needs rather than effective services if all decisions are made by "professionals." To assure that care is rendered at a time and place and in a way satisfactory to the consumer, the consumer must participate in decisions and be taught what his rights are and how to purchase care. None of this will come about without concerted programs involving organizational change and health education.

See also *Heal Yourself, Report of the Citizens Board of Inquiry into Health Services for Americans*, Lester Breslow, School of Public Health, University of California, Los Angeles and C. Arden Miller, University of North Carolina, Chapel Hill, 1972.

36. Mott, Basil, "Consumer Participation in Comprehensive Health Planning," *Quarterly Bulletin on Health Politics*, Vol. 2, No. 4, p. 3, Feb. 1972.

37. Bellin, L. E., Florence Kavaler, and Al Schwarz, "Phase One of Consumer Participation in Policies of 22 Voluntary Hospitals in New York City," *Am. J. Public Health*, Vol. 62, No. 10, p. 1370, Oct. 1972.

38. Dunlop, John T., "The Capacity of the U.S. to Provide and Finance Expanding Health Services," *Closing the Gaps in Availability and Accessibility of Health Services, Bull. N.Y. Acad. Med.*, pp. 1326-1327, 1965.

39. Starkweather, David B., "Health Facility Merger and Integration: A Typology and Some Hypotheses," paper presented to Conference on Interorganizational Relations, The Johns Hopkins University, 1970; Starkweather, David B. (Ed.), *Analysis of Hospital Mergers, Conference Proceedings*, Pub. HSRD 71-28, PB 203-458, National Center for Health Services Research and Development, U.S. Department of Health, Education, and Welfare, Oct. 1971.

40. See, for example, *Guidelines for Cancer Care*, prepared by Committee on Guidelines for Cancer Care, Commission on Cancer-American College of Surgeons, Chicago.

41. Greenberg, Ira G. and Michael L. Rodburg, "The Role of Prepaid Group Practice in Relieving the Medical Care Crisis," Note, *Harvard Law Review*, Vol. 84, No. 4, p. 889, February 1971.

42. Ibid.

43. See Flashner, Bruce A., Gene Garguilo, Shirley Reed, and Philip R. Fine, "Prepaid Health Care for the Indigent: The Problem of State Government," paper presented at the Annual Meeting of the American Public Health Association, Nov. 15, 1972 on the difficulties of agreements between states and providers posed by the "multitude of counterproductive and divisive Federal requirements."

44. See Williams, Spencer, "Final Report—Organizing for Health Services," California Human Relations Agency, Sacramento, May 1969.

45. See Cornely, Paul B., in *High Costs of Hospitalization*, Hearings before the Subcommittee on Antitrust and Monopoly of the Committee on Judiciary, U.S. Senate, 91st Cong., 2d Sess., Part 1, pp. 427-428 stating that, according to the March 16, 1970 issue of the Journal of the American Medical Association, private physicians report only one of every nine cases of venereal disease to public health officials.

46. *High Cost of Hospitalization*, supra note 45 at 591.

47. Medical Assistance Advisory Council, Committee on Evaluation of Title XIX Programs, pp. 256-272, March 15, 1969.

48. See statement on the Federal Assistance Streamlining Task Force submitted by Secretary Finch, *Hearings on Appropriations of the Departments of Labor and Health, Education, and Welfare for 1971* before a Subcommittee of the U.S. House of Representatives, Committee on Appropriations, 91st Cong., 2d Sess., Part 1, p. 108, 1970.

49. Bellin, L. E. and Florence Kavaler, "Policing Publicly Funded Health Care for Poor Quality, Overutilization, and Fraud—the New York City Medicaid Experience," *Am. J. Public Health*, Vol. 10, No. 5, p. 811, May 1970.

50. Greenfield, Margaret, *Meeting the Costs of Health Care: The Bay Area Experience and the National Issues*, pp. 124 ff., Institute of Governmental Studies, University of California, Berkeley, 1972.

51. *Report of the National Conference on Medical Costs*, Summary of Panel on Hospital Costs, p. 88, Washington, D.C., June 1967.

52. See *Study of Health Facilities Construction Costs*, supra note 31 at 114-116. "Massive overhaul" is from the *Los Angeles Times* story on the report, p. 1, Nov. 23, 1972.

53. See *Social Security Amendments of 1970*, Hearings before the U.S. Senate Committee on Finance, 91st Cong., 2d Sess., Part 1, p. 149 and Part 2, p. 894, June 1970.

54. Roemer, Milton I., "Controlling and Promoting Quality in Medical Care," *Law and Contemporary Problems, Health Care, Part I*, Vol. XXXV, No. 2, p. 284 at 290, Spring 1970; Somers, Anne R., *Hospital Regulation: The Dilemma of Public Policy*, p. 109, Industrial Relations Section, Princeton University, Princeton, N.J., 1969.

55. *Report on Licensure and Related Health Personnel Credentialing*, DHEW Pub. No. (HSM) 72-11, Office of Assistant Secretary for Health and Scientific Affairs, U.S. Department of Health, Education, and Welfare, 1971.

56. See Worthington, William and Laurens H. Silver, "Regulation of Quality of Care in Hospitals: The Need for Change," *Law and Contemporary Problems*, Vol. XXXV, No. 2, p. 305 at 308-317, Spring 1970.

57. Roemer, supra note 54 at 291.

58. Somers, supra note 54 at 192.

59. Id. at 196-197.

60. See *Interagency Coordination in Drug Research and Regulation*, Hearings before the Subcommittee on Reorganization and International Organizations of the Committee on Government Operations, U.S. Senate, 87th Cong., 2d Sess., Agency Coordination Study, p. 33, Aug. 1, 1962: "There is no formal mechanism existing either inside or outside of the government for the central collection of information on adverse reactions to medications either old or new." Successive committees since then have repeated this observation (see Chapter 2).

61. Id. at 147.

62. N.Y. Hospital Code, 10 N.Y.C.R.R., Sec. 700.1 et seq. (1969); Mich., Comp. Laws Ann., Sec. 331.411 et seq. (Supp. 1970). For discussion of these laws, see Worthington and Silver, supra note 56 at 317 ff. and Somers, supra note 54 at 110 ff. Also, Calif. Health and Safety Code, Secs. 1250-1318 (West Supp. 1974).

63. Roemer, supra note 54 at 292-294.

64. *President's Panel Report on Scientific and Educational Basis for Improving Health*, p. 7, Washington, D.C., 1972.

CHAPTER 9

More Rational Systems of Health Care

The search for a way out of the jungle of fragmented and uncoordinated health services and its problems, described in the preceding chapters, leads to consideration of more rational systems of health care. Proposed in various forms for the United States and contained in the experience of other countries, more rational systems have one feature in common. They avoid categorical prescriptions of disease, person, kind of service, and method of payment. They are based, rather, on the concept of total care for all the people within a specific geographic area.

From this research emerges the view that more rational systems of health services share, to a greater or lesser degree, two basic components: (1) a social system of financing care that assures universal access to services and (2) a hierarchical system of organizing the provision of services within a defined geographic region.

While a system of universal health insurance may not be able per se to restructure the delivery system, it is basic to that restructuring.[1] It can be shaped toward the following ends: to remove financial barriers to care; to embrace all health risks, not just selected ones; to achieve a more equitable sharing of the financial burden of illness; and to encourage more effective and economical patterns of providing care. Alternative methods of financing health services have been a matter of national debate since the 1930s, a debate sharpened in recent years by rising expenditures and escalating public and private costs. The financing mechanisms proposed, no matter how diversely conceived, are all in the direction of removing financial barriers to services. Since enactment of some system of national health insurance seems to be a question of time (hopefully less rather than more time), that issue is put aside in this consideration of more rational delivery systems. Emphasis is placed here not on the system of financing services but on more rational systems of organizing services.

The essence of all more rational delivery systems is regionalization, which has been defined as "the organization and coordination of all health resources and services within a defined area."[2] A regional system consists of an integrated network of services within a defined geographic area, based on the health needs of the population to be served and on the technical capacity to provide needed services. Health needs vary in frequency of occurrence and in complexity of medical condition involved. Resources for health care are finite. A regional system allocates and organizes available and appropriate health resources so as to meet the total health needs of a given population. Shorn of political constraints and historical antecedents, a regional system is governed by three factors: (1) health needs, both pathological and behavioral; (2) geographic location of services; and (3) technical requirements for different kinds of care.

Thus the key feature of a regionalized system consists in organization of services within a defined geographic area by levels of care. Primary care, using basic and relatively simple resources, is provided on a neighborhood basis, close to the homes of the people to be served. Secondary and tertiary care, using increasingly sophisticated resources for less frequently occurring and more complex conditions, is provided to serve larger geographic areas. The size of the population required for effective provision of different levels of care tends, with a few exceptions, to increase with the complexity of the medical condition involved.

In the United States, the principle of regionalization has been applied with increasing frequency to specific kinds of services. Regional hospital services were first demonstrated with the initiation of the Bingham Associates Fund in New England in 1931, and the Rochester Regional Hospital Council was formed in 1946 with the assistance of the Commonwealth Fund.[2] The Hill-Burton program for hospital planning and construction was one of the first national programs to be developed on a regional basis.[4] The original intent of the Regional Medical Programs legislation was to encourage regionalization of services and resources for treatment of the three leading causes of death — heart disease, cancer, and stroke.[5] As described in earlier chapters, federally funded Community Mental Health Centers, mental retardation centers, and programs for control of alcoholism and drug dependence have been organized on a regional basis to some extent.

But all these regional efforts have been specialized and limited. The Bingham Associates program linked only a few hospitals and not other resources for health care in its regional network. The Hill-Burton program was able to affect only the 25 percent of hospitals receiving Hill-Burton grants. Perhaps because of political constraints, the Regional Medical Programs as implemented turned away from regionalization to other activities concerned with improving the quality of care. Regionalization of federally funded Community Mental Health Centers excludes the community mental health resources supported by state, local, and private funding. Similarly, other programs attempting a regional approach, such as those concerned with alcoholism and drug dependence, have been organized separately and apart from related services. Although the Comprehensive Health Planning program was designed to encompass planning for health services generally, in actuality its emphasis thus far has been on planning of facilities. The manifest limitations of all such regionalization led Dr. Kerr L. White to comment sarcastically, ". . . if the United States succeeds in regionalizing its services along the lines of categorical diseases, it will be the first country in history to do so."[6]

In contrast to what may be called "categorical regionalization," then, attention is directed here to comprehensive regionalization. First, models proposed for the United States are mentioned. Then the experience of other countries with regional systems is reviewed briefly.

REGIONAL MODELS PROPOSED FOR THE UNITED STATES

Nearly 30 years ago, the far-seeing public health leader, Dr. Joseph W. Mountin, and his associates, Elliott Pennell and Vane Hoge, projected a plan for an integrated scheme of hospitals and related facilities for the nation.[7] Mapping the United States into an integrated, regionalized system, these pioneers envisaged a hierarchical system consisting of health centers for diagnosis and treatment of ambulatory patients, rural hospitals serving ordinary demands for health services, large, well-equipped district hospitals providing general and specialty services, and base hospitals providing super-specialty care. Under this system, weights would be assigned to different types and degrees of need, hospitals would be designated in accordance with their capacity to provide services, and health unit boundaries would be determined on the basis of the minimum population necessary to support the services, the size of the area that could be administered effectively, appropriate travel time, and other factors.

Thus, the flow for health services would be a natural one, going from the simple to the complex, the routine to the specialized, from the small local hospital to the sizable and integrated medical center.[8]

The past is prologue, and contemporary problems in health services cry out for reexamination of the Mountin approach.

Numerous graphic models of regional health organization have been proposed over the years. All of them embody the same basic principle of peripheral, intermediate, and central facilities paralleling a rising degree of complexity of service. One of the most noted recent models is perhaps the proposal of the American Hospital Association. Its Ameriplan would establish 400 health care corporations responsible for health maintenance, primary care, specialty care, restorative care, and health-related custodial care within defined geographic areas.[9]

Despite differences among the various regional models proposed, all are based on the principle of what Anne Somers calls "rationalization of health facilities and services — in the interest both of cost controls and better patient care."[10] All involve implementation of the concept of levels of care. Let us suppose that no health services existed in a geographic region for a defined population. What services would be provided? Where would they be provided? And how would they be provided to assure accessibility of the total population to a full range of services and efficient use of resources? The outlines of such a system have been described as follows.[11]

Primary Care

In such a system, the primary level of care consists of general ambulatory services — both preventive and curative. It is at this level that immunizations, well-baby care, prenatal check-ups, family planning, health education, nutrition counseling, general physical examinations, screening, and treatment for simple illnesses and minor injuries take place. Emergency services for minor conditions are available at this level. Routine dental care and some mental health care, at least screening and counseling, are also provided.

The patient's first contact with the health team occurs at the primary level. It is to these resources that the person comes while he is still well or when he becomes sick with "symptoms, complaints, and problems, not with specific diseases."[12] Providing medical care for the large volume of complaints that do not require sophisticated technical capacity is one function of the primary level of care.

An equally important function of the primary level is referral of patients for further diagnostic procedures, for treatment that cannot be provided on an ambulatory basis in the relatively simple facilities of the primary level of care, and for other community services. While patients will be evaluated and referred to other sources of care, at the same time the primary providers will retain responsibility for their patients on a continuing basis.

Resources at the primary level may be neighborhood health centers, staffed by primary practitioners, including specialists in family practice and nurse practitioners working in teams with other health personnel as the dominant form of primary care. Such neighborhood health centers might be sponsored by community health groups, by unions, by consumer councils, or other organizations. Primary care may also be provided by outpatient departments of hospitals, by group practices, and transitionally by solo physicians' offices until they evolve into sounder patterns of health services. Specialized clinics, such as those for family planning, veneral disease control, or treatment of drug dependence, may be retained to handle heavy case loads in an efficient manner or to provide visibility in the community.

The optimum demographic size of the level of primary care may vary from 10,000 to 30,000 people, depending on the age distribution of the population, its socioeconomic status, and its health needs. A large factor in determining the appropriate geographic size of this level will be travel time from patients' homes to the nearest source of continuously available care.

The important feature of the primary level of care is that each person served will have a specified physician or group of physicians, with an associated team of allied health personnel, for providing care and assuring care from other resources. In this way, a mechanism will exist for strengthening the weakest link in the current system of health services — access to a primary provider. As Dr. Vicente Navarro points out, concern will be extended from the individual who seeks care to all patients for whom the physician or group of physicians is responsible.[13]

Secondary Care

The next echelon of care required by a population consists of specialists' services and inpatient care in a hospital. Most patients will be referred to this level of care by their primary physicians. Diagnostic and consultant services will be provided on an outpatient basis by specialists in their offices and at the hospital. These services will also be provided, when needed, on an inpatient basis, and hospitalization for moderately complex conditions will be provided in community hospitals at this level of care. Maternity cases, second trimester abortion cases, trauma, abdominal surgery of lesser complexity, certain psychoneuroses, most cardiovascular cases, and severe respiratory infections will be treated at the community hospital.

It has been suggested that the second echelon of care might serve a population four or five times the size of the primary level, so as to encompass this many units of primary care.[14] Thus, if the population of the primary level is 10,000, then the secondary level will serve 40,000 to 50,000 people.

The community hospital might be a facility of 200 to 300 beds, depending on the size of the population served, with a full range of specialists' services. It should contain beds for short-term care of the mentally ill, a detoxification unit for drug dependence, and more sophisticated emergency services than are provided at the primary level. Links between the primary and secondary levels of care will be furnished by the referral system, a unified record system, and policies relating to case conferences, professional education, and exchange of personnel among facilities.

In the same geographic area served by the hospital will be located extended care facilities of various kinds, nursing homes, halfway houses, intermediate care facilities, and board and care homes. The community hospital will maintain horizontal links with these facilities for the aged, the chronically ill, and the handicapped, just as it will maintain vertical links with the primary level of care and with the more specialized and sophisticated tertiary level of care. Similarly, the ambulatory care resources will relate directly to the extended care facilities for patients who could be referred directly to these resources.

Home care services will also be provided at the secondary level of care. Both the staff of the community hospital and that of the ambulatory care network will contribute to home care services of the aged and chronically ill. In this effort, use of nurse practitioners and specialized rehabilitation personnel will be of paramount importance.

Although the trend in a regionalized system may be to provide all hospital services within a community hospital,[15] some specialized hospitals for mental illness or chronic disease will still be required at the secondary level. These hospitals will probably serve a larger population and geographic area than the community hospital, which will refer patients to these specialized resources and maintain close administrative and professional liaison with them.

Tertiary Care

This level of care will be centered in two kinds of facilities: (1) regional hospitals of about 500 beds (one bed per 1,000 people) serving a population of 500,000 or the service areas of ten community hospitals and (2) university medical centers serving a population of three to five regional hospitals, or from 1,500,000 to 2,500,000 people.

At this level of care are treated conditions occurring less frequently in the population but requiring a high degree of specialization, expertise, and sophisticated technical resources. Patients needing complex diagnostic work-ups, chest surgery, complicated abdominal surgery, cancer radiation therapy, kidney dialysis, or other sophisticated or expensive procedures would be referred either to the regional hospital or the university medical center. In order to make expensive services geographically accessible, some flexibility in their location may be desirable. For example, cancer radiation therapy might be authorized in certain community hospitals, provided links are maintained with the radiology service in a regional hospital. Also, it has been suggested that the university medical center should accept both the most complex cases and other patients usually treated at the primary level, in order to provide a proper perspective of medical practice for medical students, to yield appropriate diagnostic categories for research, and to serve the needs of the surrounding community.[16]

In addition to provision of direct services, personnel and facilities at the tertiary level of care will have an important role in influencing the quality of health care throughout the region. Certainly, these resources will provide continuing education training programs for personnel from the entire region. In addition, exchanges of personnel might be developed on a regular basis, to permit regional personnel to work at the primary and secondary levels and personnel from community hospitals to work in regional hospitals. In this way, administrative and clinical links would be strengthened among all the levels of care.

In short, a regionalized system of health care in the United States would ideally consist of a pyramidal hierarchy of facilities from primary to secondary to tertiary levels, serving increasingly greater populations with increasingly more complex resources. The essence of a noncategorical system of health services has been well summarized thus:

> The subdivisions of disease categories, population classes and agency jurisdictions are terribly complex, but the basic requirements of delivering health service to the people in communities are conceptually simple. For the ambulatory services, health centers are needed, with a spectrum of personnel for medical, dental, psychiatric and related services both curative and preventive. For the institutional services networks of hospitals and related facilities are necessary. The financial support must be on some social basis—by insurance or taxation—if everyone is to get the care he needs. The quality promotion must be systematized through some form of teamwork with smooth communication and discipline, if uniform standards are to be maintained.[17]

REGIONALIZATION IN THE HEALTH SERVICE SYSTEMS OF OTHER COUNTRIES

The foregoing theoretical construct of a more rational system has the virtues of clarity and simplicity. For more realistic delineation of regional systems, with all their variations, one must turn to actual systems in operation in different countries. Brief comments are presented here on regionalization as it has been developed in the health services of Czechoslovakia, the United Kingdom, and Sweden, and as it has been proposed recently for the Province of Quebec.

Czechoslovakia

Following World War II, Czechoslovakia undertook to transform its "heterogeneous, spontaneously developed conglomeration of dispersed hospital and outpatient facilities, lacking any system" into an integrated system of health institutions.[18] A hierarchy of services is provided, ranging from basic services to the most sophisticated. Although many kinds of facilities and services are part of the system, its feature of regionalization is best described in terms of the kind of hospital at each level of care.

The Type 1 hospital in Czechoslovakia is the basic unit providing ambulatory and inpatient care to a population of 50,000. It has 240 to 300 beds and provides at least four basic inpatient services—medicine, pediatrics, surgical gynecology, and obstetrics. Outpatient services provided in the polyclinics include the same four basic departments and additional ones: ear, nose, and throat, ophthalmology, dermatovenereology, tuberculosis, dentistry, and neurology. Integration of hospital and outpatient care is assured by a single team in every branch of health service, using uniform methods in hospital and outpatient care.

The Type 2 hospital serves a population of 50,000 to 70,000 people and has 700 to 800 beds. It encompasses the areas of ten Type 1 hospitals. It provides specialist services that cannot be obtained in Type 1 hospitals for its own population of approximately 70,000 and consultant services to a secondary population of 130,000 to 200,000. Hospitals of Type 2 are associated with specialized hospitals and sanatoria providing long-term treatment. Training and monitoring functions are also provided for the entire district. All the facilities in the district are linked into a functional unit, and the district institute of national health, in which all district facilities participate, ensures the unity of preventive and therapeutic care.

The Type 3 hospital, serving one to one and a half million, is usually a teaching hospital, with 17 to 23 departments and extensive complementary facilities. All the sophisticated medical specialties, including cardiology, endocrinology, thoracic surgery, and neurosurgery, are provided at this level. The regional institute of national health performs important functions in health statistics, postgraduate training, scientific control of health services, teaching, and research. Institutes of national health exist at both the district and regional levels as functional and organizational units "for rapidly and promptly transmitting the results of research into practice and for the smooth link of science and training with practice."[19] On a national level, several postgraduate institutes for medical and paramedical training exist and also 30 research institutes of the Ministry of Health.

In developing the regional structure of its health services, Czechoslovakia took into account the following factors: the size and demographic structure of the population, its health status, living and working conditions, economic and cultural level of the population, number and qualifications of health workers, density of health resources, and rate at which scientific advances are incorporated into practice.[20] A combination of two methods is used to estimate the need for medical care: the experimental method, which assesses demand for health services on the basis of actual utilization in an area with defined favorable conditions anticipated to prevail generally in the future, and the analytical method, which analyzes the morbidity of a population by diagnosis on the basis of previous experience, medical examinations, and estimates of probable future changes in disease and utilization.

A distinguished American observer, the late Dr. E. Richard Weinerman, summarized the organization of health services in Czechoslovakia and other Eastern European countries in this succinct way:

> The design is characterized by central policy definition, regional organization and local delivery of personal services. Primary emphasis is on direct provision of medical care through organized staffs in publicly-owned facilities, with priority of attention directed to maternal and child welfare and industrial hygiene.[21]

Dr. Weinerman's assessment of this regional system pinpointed both strengths and weaknesses.[22] On the positive side he found (1) extension of general medical care to the total population through a free, publicly operated, and functionally coordinated program; (2) allocation of functions among various echelons of administration; (3) unity of preventive, therapeutic, and educational services within the department of health; (4) emphasis on health protection of workers, mothers, and children; and (5) use of the neighborhood health unit for provision of basic medical care. The difficulties related more to particular economic and professional conditions than to defects in the regional model: (1) obsolescent facilities and shortages in equipment and supplies; (2) administrative rigidity; (3) over-reliance on medical specialization, and (4) the relative weakness of the primary level of care. Significant for the United States is Dr. Weinerman's conclusion: "In the potential to be realized from a *combination* of rational structure and excellent resources lies the challenge to our own country."[23]

The United Kingdom

Under the British National Health Service, the tripartite pattern of organization that evolved included 14 Regional Hospital Boards in England and six in Scotland responsible for hospitals and specialist services; 119 Executive Councils responsible for general practitioner services; and 158 local health authorities responsible for maternal and child health services, home nursing, social work, and related services.[24] Outside the National Health Service is the school health service provided by local education authorities. This fragmented responsibility was found to create serious problems: lack of public accountability, divided health services, and health care separated from essential related services.[25] Reorganization of the National Health Service, and of local government, is designed to integrate this tripartite system of health services in the United Kingdom.[26]

Under the current reorganization, set forth in the National Health Service Reorganization Bill of 1973, health services will be administered in a unified system; the distinction between hospital and specialist services, previously the responsibility of the Regional Hospital Boards, and preventive health services, previously the function of local health authorities, is to be removed.[27] All services, including school health services, previously the responsibility of local education authorities, will be administered in a unified system, with ultimate responsibility lodged in the national Ministry of Health. The administration of this unified system below the national level will consist of two echelons: (1) 15 Regional Health Authorities, each serving a population of two to three million, and replacing the former Regional Hospital Authorities; and (2) approximately 90 Area Health Authorities or Area Health Authorities (Teaching), with facilities for undergraduate and postgraduate clinical teaching, serving smaller populations and subdivided into districts, with catchment areas substantially those of district general hospitals.

This major reorganization of the British National Health Service is designed to strengthen central controls over the money spent and to ensure that maximum value is obtained for it and, at the same time, to decentralize administration to local and regional agencies, operating with strong local and professional participation consistently with national plans and priorities.[28] This bold but deliberate step to unify the three separate parts of the British health system, undertaken "to facilitate the flexible development of the service to meet changing needs,"[29] will provide invaluable experience on the functioning of a nationwide system of integrated, regionalized care.

Regionalization has two basic aspects. One concerns the organization of services into echelons of care. The other concerns the interrelationships among the various actors within each region: providers, consumers, and government. Definition of optimum demographic and geographic sizes for different levels of care presents a technical question, which can be solved. Rearrangement of existing facilities to fit a regionalized scheme involves political constraints that can be overcome. Perhaps the most difficult problems concern integrating different kinds and levels of service, assuring public accountability and consumer participation, and defining the roles of different governmental units in the provision of care. The current reorganization of the British National Health Service addresses these issues.

Sweden

Development of the Swedish regional system of health services began in 1960 with the Parliamentary recommendation that county councils cooperate to provide hospital care in seven hospital regions, each serving a population of from 70,000 to 1,500,000. The system consists of four levels of care, as follows:[30]

1. Health centers serving a population of 10,000 to 20,000, providing both preventive and curative services, linked to district hospitals.
2. Local district hospitals of 300 beds serving 60,000 to 90,000 people, with small hospitals either closed or converted into nursing homes, health centers, or a combination of the two.
3. County central hospitals of 800 to 1,000 beds serving a population of 250,000 to 300,000, with large outpatient departments providing specialist care, rehabilitation, and welfare services.
4. Regional hospitals serving a population of a million or more and providing tertiary or superspecialty services. Voluntary arrangements may be made among several county councils for provision of tertiary services.

The methodology used for developing this regionalized system was based on demographic analysis of hospital utilization.[31] The optimum demographic size of a region was determined "by ascertaining the minimum number of persons needed to supply a clientele large enough for teaching, research, and services activities for the minimum size of the superspecialized department (neurosurgery, plastic surgery, thoracic surgery, child surgery, special cardiology) at the regional hospital center."[32] Definition of optimum geographic size of a region was based on the principle of maximum accessibility to regional hospitals for the largest number of people living in the region. No person in the region should have to travel more than four hours, round trip, by car to reach the regional center.[33]

The Swedish system has been justified not only on the ground of rational use of resources and rational organization of services but on the ground of economy in use of personnel and funds.[34] The architect of the Swedish regional system, Dr. Arthur Engel, pointed out that

[T]he main goal is to provide qualified medical treatment for the population of every area of the country. . . . If we had not launched the regional hospital system we would have witnessed the growth of small specialist services in many places. They would not have had the capacity to develop the highest quality of care and to keep abreast of scientific progress. They would have meant a bad investment of capital and medical personnel.[35]

In describing Sweden's hierarchical system of health services and the planning carried out at the regional level by planning councils working in close cooperation with the directors of clinical services, Dr. Leonard Rosenfeld concluded:

In Sweden, there has been a relatively smooth adaptation of organization to medical, social and economic change. This may be attributed in large degree to historic factors, and to geographic, social and economic characteristics of the country. The population is relatively homogeneous. The country is relatively small, with most of its 8,000,000 inhabitants residing in the southern half of the country. Approximately 75% of costs of health services are borne by governmental agencies.

The two tier system, with a tradition of effective cooperative relations between the National and county levels of government, lends itself to orderly public policy formulation. The absence of powerful private organizations and agencies with vested interests in the system facilitates accommodation to change.[36]

The guiding principle of the Swedish planners is that care should be provided at the lowest acceptable organizational level of care.[37] In the United States, this principle has been widely recognized with respect to use of personnel, that is, that tasks should be performed by the person with the requisite but minimum skills necessary to do the job adequately.[38] Regionalization extends this principle to the total health care system.

The Province of Quebec

An exhaustive investigation of the health services of the Province of Quebec led in 1970 to recommendations of the Quebec Commission of Inquiry on Health and Social Medicine for a regionalized health plan for the entire province.[39] Finding serious organizational defects in the health system, the Castonguay-Nepveu Commission set out to remedy "the absence of systematic organization in care distribution,"[40] with its attendant gaps and inadequacies in services, separateness of elements of the distribution care network, parallel systems, duplicate record systems, and lack of focused responsibility for first-line care. These problems in the system emerged, in the opinion of the Commission, because

. . . the organization of the health system did not evolve at the same pace as medical progress. There was fragmentation, dispersal, with overlapping, redundancy, serious lucunae, high costs and wasted effort, instead of a coordinated plan. . . .

We believe the shortcomings of the Quebec health system are due to the absence of a true system of care distribution. Partial systems have developed, favoring one category of the sick, certain institutions, particular aspects in one case or the other, leaving the physician free to practice according to his tastes and habits, often aloof from any structured system.[41]

The health plan recommended by the Commission is composed of three levels of care.

1. General care includes prevention, advice, health education, diagnosis, treatment, and rehabilitation for emotional, mental, and physical problems. It is designed to meet the health needs of people without resorting to specialized facilities and care. Moreover, the general level of care assumes responsibility for distribution of care and for making it accessible at all times for all needs. An estimated 80 to 90 percent of patients can be fully cared for by health teams at this general care level.[42]

2. Specialized care, including diagnosis, treatment, and rehabilitation, will be provided at the secondary level for the approximately ten percent of patients in a population of 100,000 to 150,000 requiring this type of service. The number and duration of episodes of illness for these patients are not indicated, though many will require care several times during a single year.[43] A full range of specialties will be available to treat patients in accordance with the needs of their conditions.

3. Highly specialized care for the rarer and most costly health problems requires concentration of hospital strength and equipment. This tertiary level of care generally will involve a population of one to one and a half million, but in certain cases the population base may be as great as six to seven million.[44] The Commission points out that the demarcation between specialized and highly specialized care follows the evolution of scientific knowledge and frequency of illness; certain types of care, now considered highly specialized, will be treated at the specialized level as care is improved.[45]

Common Elements of Regionalized Systems

These four systems illustrate the principle of regional organization of echelons of care that characterizes many health service systems in the world. Although these systems have developed at different times and in different ways, certain common elements stand out—elements also contained in the model of primary, secondary, and tertiary care sketched at the beginning of this chapter. These common elements of a regionalized system may be described as (1) structuring of services into levels of care, according to health needs and degree of professional skill required; (2) horizontal and vertical linkages among segments of the system at all levels of care; (3) provision of total services to a total population, without distinction as to kind of service or kind of recipient; (4) combining central authority for standard and quality of services with decentralized delivery of services; and (5) use of available resources with maximum effectiveness and equity.

Organization of resources so as to provide a full spectrum of continuous and coordinated health care for a defined population requires rejection of the categorical approach. As Dr. Kerr L. White has pointed out,

[E]mphasis on building standards and on the "number of beds," which preoccupies the Hill-Burton programs, or on the search for "doctors" in the central city or the rural village, which preoccupies community leaders, needs to give way to concern for the provision of adequate balanced health services systems.[46]

In a sense, the regional system embodies for a geographic area what has already occurred within the walls of hospitals. Implementation of the principle of progressive patient care has resulted in organization of hospitals into intensive care units, intermediate care sections, and long-term care wings and special facilities rather than by diagnostic categories. The social application of progressive patient care to a defined population requires similar organization by levels of care needed. Under this organization, the patient will be able to move from ambulatory care to general hospital care, to specialized services, to extended care, to home care, and back among these components, as his health needs dictate. The regionalized system is not monolithic. Just as many hospitals exist today, so under a regionalized system numerous subsystems will serve defined populations.

CONSTRAINTS ON IMPLEMENTATION

Implementation of more rational systems of health service faces a number of constraints. Political, professional, and economic forces tend to resist change and support the status quo.

Political Constraints

The main political impediment to implementation of a rational system of health services lies in the established preserves of the various levels of government. The legal functions and traditional roles of the federal, state, and local governments require revision if a regional system is to be organized in new geographic areas and with new powers.

Particularly at the local level of government, transformation into a regional system will encounter obstacles in legislatively established responsibilities of local government. Compounding the statutory mandate of local government are multiple geographic boundaries of cities and counties, domains of special districts, and overlapping administrative areas of governmental agencies. A regional system would undoubtedly change, and perhaps diminish, the authority of local government in health services. It would certainly alter the geographic districts and the interrelationships of many agencies, both public and private.

Resistance of local government to yielding some of its authority to a larger regional agency is not the only political constraint. All levels of government will need to revise their functions, for a regional system cannot be developed voluntarily. It can be developed only if government has the mandate and powers to establish new organization, to encourage new relationships, and to resolve conflicting interests.

Professional Constraints

The main professional impediment to implementation of a more rational system of health services lies in the vested interests of various professional groups. Organized private medicine has for years (until quite recently) opposed group practice, salaried physicians, and national health insurance. Hospitals and other health facilities have only recently accepted the necessity for regulation of their location, services, and prices. A rational system means more — not less — organization of services, and free enterprise in medicine and health care will need to be replaced by socially organized services.

Voluntary organizations also have vested interests. Accustomed to autonomous functioning, they may operate as a constraint on development of a regionalized, integrated system unless they fit their resources into the totality of the system and recognize the potential for achieving their goals within such a framework.

Within the public sector, too, professional constraints exist. Public employees have long ingrained ways of working, and the civil service system tends to reinforce the status quo. Governmental agencies and their personnel have acquired vested interests in particular programs. Development of a regionalized system will require imaginative leadership from public servants, unfettered by the requirements of job classifications designed in former times for different settings.

Economic Constraints

Financing of health services from multiple sources, each with its own prescription, tends to bar development of an integrated, unified system of care. While it is not impossible to design a rational system financed from many pockets, it is much more difficult to do so than if all funding came through a universal payments system. Enactment of a system of national health insurance will remove one of the greatest constraints on development of a more rational system by assuring universal access to care.

Moreover, enactment of national health insurance will provide the basis for resolving other economic problems: the existing and perhaps inappropriate location of facilities and, more importantly, the relation of the large private sector of health care to a regionalized system. Control over the financial resources for support of health services will permit facilities to be used or transformed in accordance with the needs of a regional system. Similarly, a universal payments mechanism will allow incentives to be developed for integrating different kinds of professionals and facilities of different capacities within the private sector into a unified, regionalized system of care.

It would be unrealistic to overlook the enormous social price of the profits and high incomes that accrue to corporations and individuals in the present fragmented system. These range from the exceptionally high profits of the pharmaceutical companies (the highest rate among all categories of U.S. industry)[47] and appliance manufacturers to the generous profits of proprietary hospitals and nursing homes (many in corporate chains),[48] and the very high earnings of many private medical and dental practitioners. At the same time, it should be recognized that a regional system, based on a program of national health insurance, does not eliminate private profits, although it might better control them.

Necessity for Compromise

The complexity of the present categorical system of health services and the significant constraints on change necessitate some compromise of goals. Perhaps the better part of valor is to aim not for an ideally rational system but rather for a realistic system of improved health services.

No *tabula rasa* exists on which a brave new world can be built. Rather, we must start where we are and build on the base of existing services and institutions, attempting to improve them and realign them in the direction of comprehensive health services for the total population. Fortunately, emerging patterns of health service embodied in comprehensive programs of maternal and child health, neighborhood health centers, health maintenance organizations, community networks of service, and expanded health insurance point the way. Let us turn, therefore, to the features of a realistic system of health services that may incorporate, to some extent, the principles of more rational systems.

NOTES

1. See Roemer, Milton I., M.D., "Social Insurance as Leverage for Changing Health Care Systems: International Experience," *Bull. N. Y. Acad. Med.*, Vol. 48. No. 1, p.93, Jan. 1972.

2. President's Commission on the Health Needs of the Nation, *Building America's Health*, Vol. 2, p. 246, U.S. Government Printing Office, 1952, cited in Bodenheimer, Thomas S., M.D., "Regional Medical Programs: No Road to Regionalization," *Medical Care Review*, Vol. 26, No. 11, p. 1125 at 1127, Dec. 1969.

3. Rosenfeld, Leonard S. and Henry B. Makover, *The Rochester Regional Hospital Council*, pp. 5, 9, The Commonwealth Fund, Harvard University Press, Cambridge, Massachusetts, 1956.

4. See Abbe, Leslie Morgan and Anna Mae Baney, *The Nation's Health Facilities, Ten Years of the Hill-Burton Hospital and Medical Facilities Program, 1946-1956*, p. 33, PHS Pub. No. 616, U.S. Department of Health, Education, and Welfare, Division of Hospital and Medical Facilities, Program Evaluation and Reports Branch, Washington, D.C., 1958.

5. See The President's Commission on Heart Disease, Cancer and Stroke, *A National Program to Conquer Heart Disease, Cancer and Stroke*, Vols. I and II, U.S. Government Printing Office, Washington, D.C., 1964 and 1965.

6. White, Kerr L., "Organization and Delivery of Personal Health Services, Public Policy Issues," *Milbank Mem. Fund Q.*, Vol. XLVI, No. 1, Pt. 2, p. 225 at 235, Jan. 1968.

7. Mountin, Joseph W., Elliott H. Pennell, Vane M. Hoge, *Health Service Areas, Requirements for General Hospitals and Health Centers*, Pub. H. Bull. No. 292, U.S. Government Printing Office, 1945. See also Mountin, Joseph W. and Clifford H. Greve, *Public Health Areas and Hospital Facilities*, PHS Pub. No. 42, Federal Security Agency, Public Health Service, Washington, D.C., 1950.

8. Mountin, Pennell, and Hoge, supra note 7 at 5.

9. *Ameriplan—A Proposal for the Delivery and Financing of Health Services in the United States*, Report of a Special Committee on the Provision of Health Services (Earl Perloff, Chairman), American Hospital Association, Chicago, 1970.

10. Somers, Anne R., "The Rationalization of Health Services: A Universal Priority," *Inquiry*, Vol. VIII, No. 1, p. 48, Jan. 1971.

11. The description of proposed levels of care is drawn from Roemer, Milton I., M.D., "An Ideal Health Care System for America," *Where Medicine Fails* (Strauss, Anselm L., Ed.), p. 77, Transaction Books, New Brunswick, N.J., 1973.

12. White, Kerr L., M.D., "Primary Medical Care for Families—Organization and Evaluation," *New Engl. J. Med.*, Vol. 277, p. 847 at 850, Oct. 19, 1967.

13. Navarro, Vicente, M.D., "The City and the Region—A Critical Relationship in the Distribution of Health Resources," paper presented at the seminar, "World Cities of the Future," American Association for the Advancement of Science, p. 16, Chicago, Dec. 27, 1970 (processed).

14. Roemer, supra note 11.

15. Navarro, supra note 13 at 17-18.

16. Roemer, supra note 11 and White, Kerr L., M.D., Franklin Williams, M.D., and Bernard G. Greenberg, Ph.D., "The Ecology of Medical Care," *New Eng. J. Med.*, Vol. 265, p. 885 at 892, Nov. 2, 1961.

17. Roemer, Milton I., M.D., "Planning Health Services: Substance Versus Form," *Can. J. Public Health*, Vol. 59, p. 431 at 435, Nov. 1968.

18. Palec, Rudolf, "The Regional System and Postgraduate Medical Training in Czechoslovakia," *Milbank Mem. Fund Q.*, Vol. XLIV, No. 4, Pt. 1, p. 414, Oct. 1966.

19. Id. at 421.

20. For discussion of methods of planning in Czechoslovakia, see the excellent paper by Vacek, Milos and Emilie Skrbkova, "Methods of Planning Health Services in Czechoslovakia," *Milbank Mem. Fund Q.*, Vol. XLIV, No. 3, Pt. 1, pp. 307-317, July 1966.

21. Weinerman, E. Richard, M.D., "The Organization of Health Services in Eastern Europe, Report of a Study in Czechoslovakia, Hungary, and Poland, Spring, 1967," *Med. Care*, Vol. 6, p. 267, July-Aug. 1968, reprinted in *Yale J. Biol. Med.*, E. Richard Weinerman Issue, Vol. 44, No. 1, p. 81 at 84, Aug. 1971.

22. Id. at 89-92. For fuller discussion, see Weinerman, E. Richard, M.D., with the assistance of Shirley B. Weinerman, *Social Medicine in Eastern Europe*, Harvard University Press, Cambridge, Mass., 1969.

23. Weinerman, supra note 21 at 92.

24. United Kingdom, Department of Health and Social Security, *National Health Service, The Futue Structure of the National Health Service*. p. 4, Her Majesty's Stationery Office, London, 1970. See Brotherston, John H. F., M.D., "Trends in the British National Health Service," *Bull. N.Y. Acad. Med.*, Vol. 48, No. 1, p. 58 at 61 ff., Jan. 1972.

25. Galloway, James, "The State of the Union," *Lancet*, p. 88, July 1970.

26. See White Papers, *National Health Service Reorganization: England* (Cmnd. 5055) and *National Health Service Reorganization: Wales* (Cmnd. 5057), Aug. 1972.

27. Explanatory and Financial Memorandum, National Health Service Reorganization Bill (House of Lords), as amended in Committee, 1973.

28. *The Future Structure of the National Health Service*, supra note 24 at 2-3.

29. Explanatory and Financial Memorandum, supra note 27 at ii:

30. Navarro, Vicente, M.D., "Methodology on Regional Planning of Personal Health Services: A Case Study: Sweden," *Med. Care*, Vol. 8, No. 5, p. 386 at 388 ff., Sept.-Oct. 1970; Engel, Arthur W., "Planning and Spontaneity in the Development of the Swedish Health System," The 1968 Michael M. Davis Lecture, Center for Health Administration Studies, Graduate School of Business, University of Chicago.

31. Navarro, Vicente, M.D., "Planning for the Distribution of Personal Health Services," *Public Health Reports*, Vol. 84, No. 7, p. 573 at 576-578, July 1969.

32. Navarro, supra note 30 at 389.

33. Id. at 390.

34. *Regional Hospital Planning, Current Trends in Health Services, In Honor of Arthur Engel*, The National Board of Health, Sweden, 1967.

35. Somers, Anne R., "The Rationalization of Health Services: A Universal Priority," *Inquiry*, Vol. VIII, No. 1, p. 48 at 53-54, Jan. 1971.

36. Rosenfeld, Leonard S., M.D., "Regional Organization of Health Services in the United States: An International Perspective," paper presented at the Third International Conference on Social Science and Medicine, Elsinore, Denmark, Aug. 14-18, 1972.

37. Somers, supra note 35 at 53.

38. *Health Manpower, Action to Meet Community Needs*, Report of the Task Force on Health Manpower (Chairman, L. S. Goerke, M.D.), National Commission on Community Health Services, p. 65, Public Affairs Press, Washington, D.C., 1967.

39. *Report of the Commission of Inquiry on Health and Social Welfare*, Government of Quebec, 1970.

40. *Report of the Commission of Inquiry on Health and Social Welfare*, Vol. IV, Tome I, p. 88, Government of Quebec, 1970.

41. Ibid.

42. *Report of the Commission of Inquiry on Health and Social Welfare*, Vol. IV, Tome II, pp. 28, 32, Government of Quebec, 1970.

43. Id. at 33.

44. Id. at 36.

45. Ibid.

46. White, Kerr L., M.D. "Organization and Delivery of Personal Health Services: Public Policy Issues," *Milbank Mem. Fund Q.*, Vol. XLVI, No. 1, Part 2, p. 225 at 243, 1968.

47. See Harris, Richard, *The Real Voice*, The Macmillan Company, New York, 1964.

48. "Annual Check-Up, Proprietary Hospital Chains Continue to Thrive," *Barron's*, July 31, 1972.

CHAPTER 10

A Realistic System: Health Maintenance Organizations in a Regionalized Framework

With the numerous constraints operating against achievement of an ideal or thoroughly rational health care system in the United States, what is a realistic approach toward improvement, in the sociopolitical setting of the 1970s? In spite of systems actually instituted in Europe, what can be reasonably planned for in America?

A BALANCED APPROACH

The most sensible and effective social strategy on the spectrum of choices between idealism and practicality can be endlessly debated. It is sometimes implied that an effort to achieve rationality in the pluralistic American setting is a kind of naive utopianism.[1] A planned, equitable, and efficient health care system, it is argued, cannot be expected in this country, but only a conglomerate of diversified and uncoordinated local actions in both public and private sectors. Another related view, bordering on cynicism, is that health service is not so important after all; our energies should go instead to improving the larger social environment: employment, housing, education, and so on.[2] Obviously medical care is only one of many influences on health, but struggling for its improvement does not imply a denial of the probably greater importance of an effective economic and social system as a whole. Those of us concerned with personal health services cannot simply await the social millennium in larger spheres; until full employment, good standards of living, and social justice are achieved, there is much to be done here and now for bettering the health care system.

This chapter was contributed by Milton I. Roemer, M.D.

To determine the appropriate point of compromise between idealism and pragmatism requires, first of all, a clear picture of the ideal goal, such as has been drawn in the previous chapter. The decision depends, of course, on the political and economic forces at each time and place. A propos of time, witness the great steps forward taken through the Social Security Act of 1935, at the depth of the Depression, and through the Medicare and Medicaid Amendments in 1965 soon after the landslide victory of Lyndon Johnson. The relevance of "place" is well illustrated by the action in 1947 of one Canadian province, Saskatchewan, to launch the first social insurance program covering a whole population for health care in North America.[3] The movement started under the impetus of a local semi-Socialist party; within a decade all of Canada had enacted a governmental hospital insurance program covering virtually everyone; and by 1968, physician's care insurance had also become nationwide in that country. By the same token, judgment in 1973 must be tempered by recognizing the generally conservative political climate in the United States.

Despite the fragmentation and inefficiencies documented in earlier chapters, the health improvements of the past cannot be denied. Associated with the organization of countless subsectors of health service, personal and environmental, under both private and public auspices, improvements have been notable. Age-specific mortality rates have declined and life expectancy has lengthened.[4] In spite of the persistent deficiencies, more people are getting more health services, both preventive and curative, than ever before. This is true not only in absolute numbers, but in terms of proportions of the total population, including the poor as well as the affluent.

Yet, it is not a cliché to recognize the rising expectations of the American population for health care, as for other elements of life. The escalating costs, rising more rapidly than over-all costs of living, cause personal anger and public concern. Relative inaccessibility of doctor's service at many times and places has highlighted the inadequacies of manpower resources, and their maldistribution, in relation to the mounting demands. Expectations rise continually regarding the quality of services, reflected by spiraling malpractice actions and national clamor for more "peer review," consumer participation or other forms of social control. The multiplicity of programs and agencies, their incoordination and confusion, give a steadily hollower sound to apologetics for the "pluralism" of the American way in health care.

And so the pressures mount, despite the generally cautious and conservative temper of the 1970s, for an improved system of health service delivery. The new cliché has become "more than money is needed." Medicare for the aged has had its predictable double effect of (1) leading to demands for equivalent social insurance protection for the other age groups, yet (2) highlighting the need to "change the system" instead of simply pouring more money into the old system. Almost every legislative proposal for "national health insurance," as we will see below, incorporates various incentives toward changing the patterns of health care delivery. Along with the appreciation that more health money alone is not enough, the power of fiscal legislation as leverage to change delivery patterns is also widely recognized.

What then is the reasonable point of compromise along the spectrum of possible decisions on changing the health care system? One formulation of this spectrum defines its two poles as: (1) the bureaucratic, rational, and hierarchical approach—that seen in the Socialist countries or even the European "welfare states"; and (2) the open market approach with major emphasis on local initiative and free competition—that seen as more appropriately American. It has been under the spirit of the latter approach that the promotion of "health maintenance organizations" has been prominently put forward.[5]

In our view, the appropriate strategy to achieve a realistic health care system in America must embody *both* of these approaches. It must contain certain features of centralized planning, along with a great deal of local free enterprise. Incentives must be provided for changing the delivery patterns toward greater teamwork, while not mandating these mechanisms overnight for everyone. Economic support must be forthcoming to achieve greater equity between the rich and the poor, the well and the sick, but the degree of egalitarianism is subject to a range of options. Social controls over costs and quality are necessary, but they need not all emanate from a central governmental authority.

Accordingly, we can draw the outlines of a realistic health service system along four dimensions:

1. Planning
2. Delivery patterns
3. Financing
4. Controls

Taken together, actions proposed along each of these paths could yield a system of personal health services that would be attainable in America within the coming decade and would mobilize our resources for human welfare far more effectively than we do today.

PLANNING

By its very nature, planning must be mainly a centralized process, although one may argue about *how* centralized, and what degree of input should be expected from peripheral bodies. In the realistic system we propose, the ultimate planning authority should be exercised at the national level. At the same time, the planning decisions should be made only after consideration of information, ideas, and demands flowing from the states and localities.

Planning of the realistic system, as discussed here, has two principal tasks: (a) delineation of sound health *regions* to blanket the nation; and (b) policy decisions on the production and distribution of *resources*, especially health manpower and facilities.

Lest this national locale for planning be considered revolutionary or unrealistic, we may take note of how extensively and successfully this approach has been used in the past. The Flexner Report on medical education, for example, was a national planning action, even though a large private foundation rather than the central government provided the leadership. No more sweeping modification of the entire system of training physicians in a nation could have come from governmental edict. Within the orbit of the medical profession itself, the specialty boards to improve standards in clinical medicine and surgery constituted national, albeit non-governmental, actions, in contrast to ordinary licensure which was and is operative at the state governmental level. When the problem of massive entry of foreign medical graduates became prominent after World War II, the ECFMG (Examining Council for Foreign Medical Graduates) program was another professional planning action involving health manpower taken at a national level. The Joint Commission on Accreditation of Hospitals established national quality standards in 1951, following from still another national but nongovernmental precedent in the program of the American College of Surgeons, started in 1917.

National planning emanating from the central government itself has come, of course, in a variety of sectors of health service. The Sheppard-Towner Act in 1924 gave national tax support to the establishment of infant health clinics everywhere. With the Social Security Act of 1935, while a fully centralized system was applied only to old-age pensions (later extended to several other benefits), Titles V and VI were the beginnings of a long series of federal grants to the states for various health purposes. These grants typically called for "state plans" on the use of the several categorical funds; the schemes for 'alloting grants under formulas considering state population, per capita income levels, measures of health need, and so on clearly constituted *national* planning strategies. The Hill-Burton Act of 1946 was a national planning program to improve the supply and distribution of hospital resources, implemented through grants to the states. Mandatory state "master plans" established scaled priorities of local bed need within each state, in relation to a national recommended bed-population ratio. Medicare and Medicaid in 1965, of course, constituted further national planning with respect to financing of medical care for the aged and the poor; while Medicare delegates administrative operations to private "fiscal intermediaries" and Medicaid to state governments, the standards and the funds conditional on meeting them emanate from the national government.[6]

While each of these national health planning precedents is categorical, rather than comprehensive, the principle is similar. Indeed, the Comprehensive Health Planning Act of 1966 once again used federal grant incentives, in effect, to induce each state to undertake its own generalized planning at the state and "areawide" (regional) levels. Our proposal for further extension of health planning at the national level, then, has plenty of antecedents.

Delineation of Health Regions

In a vast nation of over 200,000,000 population, effective delivery of personal health services requires first of all the delineation of manageable health regions. A region may be defined as a geographic area containing a population for which a full range of needed health services may reasonably be provided within the borders. The definition of "full range," as composed of primary, secondary, and tertiary levels, will be discussed below. With rare exceptions, however, the concept of a health region is similar to that of a "trade area," in which, with acceptable amounts of transportation and time, all needed services can be obtained by all the residents.[7]

In a sense, the 50 states of the union provide a "first cut" into the delineation of regions, except for a number of special circumstances. Some of the states, such as South Dakota or Nevada, are too sparsely settled to yield all the resources of a proper health region within their borders; combinations with adjacent states would be necessary. In other locales, there are metropolitan centers on the edge of a state—like Memphis, Tennessee or Kansas City, Missouri—which logically should serve as the technical centers of regions encompassing two or more states. In still other states, like New York or California, the populations are so large and the subcenters of population so important as to require the establishment of several health regions. For all these reasons, delineation of sound health regions should be a federal task.

Such mapping of the nation into reasonable health regions should not, of course, be done autocratically or unilaterally, but only following consultation with knowledgeable representatives from the states and localities. There is adequate precedent for this process in the experience of the Regional Medical Programs (RMP), enacted in 1965. By the same token, the experience of the Comprehensive Health Planning (CHP) program and its difficulties in defining manageable borders of "area-wide" jurisdictions suggests the wisdom of having the final mapping decisions made at a higher level, after consideration of all the facts.[8]

Considering the constraints of distance and travel time, and the technical requirements of modern comprehensive personal health service, we propose that health regions contain populations of between about 500,000 to 3,000,000 population. Estimating a rough average of about 2,000,000 people, there would be about 100 health regions in the nation. (It may be noted that there is approximately one medical school for each 2,000,000 population in the United States today.) Taking account of political realities, many of these regions would be whole states, even if an occasional county at the borders might logistically fit better into a neighboring region. Mindful of current realities also, the regional boundaries should ordinarily encompass whole counties and not cut across county lines — with the exception of the super-metropolitan counties (like New York City or Los Angeles) where subdivisions of the metropolis might serve as the technical centers of two or more regions. In general, however, congruence with state and county lines should determine the boundaries of regions, in the interests of realistic governance, communications, statistical analysis, etc., even at some small sacrifice of logistical convenience.

The delineation of health regions should be one of many tasks of a National Department of Health. In our view, the responsibilities of an effective health service for the United States are large, complex, and varied enough to warrant cabinet and departmental status in the federal government. In spite of the relationships between health and welfare or education, calling for coordination, the enormity of the current U.S. Department of Health, Education, and Welfare is too great for effective management. The conglomeration of functions in the Department of HEW reflects essentially an earlier period, when no one of these major fields was important enough at the federal level to warrant cabinet status by itself. This is no longer true today, and the United States now stands as one of the few nations of the world lacking a discrete Ministry of Health. The steady rise of the public sector in health services, the need for greater planning, and the generally higher priority that health care has achieved in American values all emphasize the need for a Department of Health at the national level.

This is not the place to discuss the overall structure or full range of functions of a national Department of Health. Its responsibilities would obviously include all health functions now under the HEW Health Services and Mental Health Administration*. We would also assign to it the health functions of the Social Security Administration (Medicare) and the Social and Rehabilitation Service (Medicaid), since the essential decisions in these programs should be shaped by medical more than fiscal expertise. Beyond the national planning task of delineating health regions of the nation, discussed above, a larger and more complex planning responsibility concerns the production and distribution of health resources.

Health Resources—Production and Distribution

The entire delivery of personal health services depends on the number and types of health manpower and facilities in the nation, and their distribution.

*Subsequent reorganization of this Administration (HSMHA) does not alter the need for a National Department of Health.

The production of these resources has long been recognized to require national action, as well as action at the state and local levels. The Hill-Burton Act on facilities and the numerous health manpower training acts from the 1950s to the 1970s reflect a growing national consensus that health needs in the 50 states and 3,100 counties, of great diversity in socioeconomic strength, cannot be equitably met without the redistributional powers of the national government.[9]

Current national programs on resource production and distribution, however, require great extension if an effective though realistic health care system is to be achieved. The National Commission on Health Manpower in 1967 considered and made recommendations on many though not all the relevant issues. Progress has been real with respect to an increased output of physicians and many types of allied health personnel; it need not be reviewed here.[10] Some of the deficiencies in resource planning, however, require serious attention.

If all the health regions are to be staffed with necessary manpower, the impediments of state-by-state professional licensure laws should be lifted. Mobility of health workers is not only a fact of American life, it is a necessary policy if needs are to be met. The National Board of Medical Examiners, the FLEX (Federation of Licensure Examining Boards) examinations, and the State Board Test Pool Examinations in Nursing are well-established steps in the direction of national licensure, but the concept should be applied to regulation of all the health professions and occupations. A moratorium on the accretion of new state licensure requirements for additional categories of personnel and the achievement of greater flexibility through institutional (mainly hospital) legal responsibility for personnel have been discussed elsewhere, and we see such moves as necessary steps forward.[11]

The new Area Health Education Centers (AHEC) are a recognition of the continuing needs for expanded training of allied health workers and for continuing lifetime education of all health personnel. Regardless of where they are trained, however, health workers should be free to move to locations where they are needed and, indeed, to which they may be attracted by various incentives.

Where incentives, financial or otherwise, fail to achieve reasonable distribution of human resources, other methods should be used. The Emergency Health Personnel Act of 1971 was recognition of this principle — one long accepted in the field of national defense. Although its quantitative impact has so far been small, this program established the important policy that the powers of the national government should be utilized to send physicians and others to rural or urban localities in grave need of them.[12] This principle should be implemented, if necessary, on a much larger scale. Many nations require all new medical and dental graduates to serve in areas of need as a condition of licensure; as public support of professional education becomes more predominant, such a policy is always more socially acceptable.

National planning and influence must also play a much greater role with respect to another form of resource distribution: the distribution among the several specialties of medicine and dentistry, perhaps of other fields as well. The enormous swing of the medical pendulum toward specialization, particularly in the surgical specialties, is widely recognized, and the last decade has shown a rising realization of the need for a better balance. The Coggeshall and Millis Reports and the establishment of a Specialty Board in Family Practice were major moves in the direction of increasing the relative proportions of generalists and primary care doctors so badly needed.[13]

But more direct and comprehensive action is necessary. The output of specialists in some 40 specialty or subspecialty fields in America is now largely determined by the hundreds of residency training programs in teaching hospitals. Decisions on the qualifications in each of these programs are made by a national nongovernmental body, the American Medical Association, but there is no national policy on the numbers of residencies to be authorized in each field. If the people's health needs, rather than academic or professional interests and ambitions, are to be reasonably satisfied, a national policy is needed on the proportional outputs of the several types of specialists. The proposed national Department of Health should formulate and implement such a policy, with advice of course from the numerous specialty groups. Implementation will naturally require national review of and constraints on the programs of all teaching hospitals and professional schools.

Similar national planning influence would be needed to achieve proper supplies of other health service resources in each health region of the nation. Regarding hospital construction, for example, the Hill-Burton Act yielded improved urban-rural distribution of beds over its first 25 years of operation, but the greater problems have now shifted to the bed supply in the large cities.[14] Since New York State's legislation on "certification of bed need" in 1962, about 20 other states have enacted similar laws requiring official approval of all new hospital construction, irrespective of the receipt of Hill-Burton subsidy.[15] These are all somewhat negative influences on hospital planning, however, and more affirmative measures are needed to assure that facilities are, in fact, constructed where they are needed. Such facilities should include health centers for ambulatory care, as well as bed units. National channelization of funds for such purposes (as will be discussed below) should be a function of the federal Department of Health, as well as the establishment of resource standards.

There are other resources demanding national planning that may only be mentioned, although the policy questions involved are large and complex. The whole field of production and distribution of drugs is important.[16] Deeply imbedded in the entire capitalist economy, the pharmaceutical industry has been subject to only limited public controls (although increasing ones) and its output has been mainly determined by the operations of the free market. Yet cost and quality problems in drug utilization are enormous, tackled only here and there by policies of certain hospitals or health care programs requiring "drug formularies" or the use of "generic" products. Much more extensive national planning is required in this field, through regulation of a large private industry so involved in the public interest. The same applies to the manufacture and distribution of eyeglasses, hearing aids, and other medical appliances.

Another resource demanding greater national planning is medical knowledge, produced through scientific research. Through enlarging federal subsidy programs since World War II, the nation's research efforts have increasingly been influenced by the U.S. National Institutes of Health, which in turn reflect the priority decisions of Congress. The strategy of this whole effort has long attempted to strike ·a balance between the local scientist's individual freedom to do what he likes and considerations of social need.[17] Recent thinking, with respect to such top problems as cancer or heart disease, has been swinging toward greater emphasis to the side of social need; this is implementable more by a policy of specific research "contracts" than by the open-ended research "grant" mechanism. In our view, the trend of this changing research policy is sound and should be pursued further.

Beyond these two major planning functions of a national Department of Health, on health regions and health resources, there are other responsibilities to be met in connection with planning at the national, state, and regional levels. Basically these involve establishment of technical *standards* in the numerous components of health service. Below we will discuss health service delivery patterns, financing, and social controls; with respect to all these functions, standards are necessary if nationwide equity is to be achieved. Reasonable minimum levels of all forms of health resources and also health services must be stipulated and updated periodically. Such standards are necessary if there are to be objective criteria for evaluation of how the whole health service system is operating. The formulation of standards must, of course, take account of the competing demands of society in nonhealth sectors, in relation to the nation's economic capacity. Priorities are obviously influenced by political dynamics. Within these constraints, the formulation of technical standards will be a duty permeating the entire operation of a national Department of Health.

HEALTH SERVICE DELIVERY

Within the framework of health regions, described above, we propose that a realistic system would put major emphasis on the promotion and development of "health maintenance organizations" (HMO) throughout the nation. Such a strategy, enunciated by President Nixon in his health message to Congress of February 1971, would recognize the imperatives of American pluralism and local initiative, while still constituting planned social change to achieve health improvements.

The mounting discussion of HMOs over the last few years cannot all be summarized here. Like many health slogans, the meaning of HMO is subject to a wide range of interpretations. In its simplest terms, as Dr. Paul Ellwood has stated it, "An HMO is a health care organization that is capable of providing a full range of medical services to a defined, or enrolled, population in return for a fixed annual fee paid in advance."[18] The very flexibility of the idea, it has been argued, is one of its great assets in the American setting, for it would permit many different delivery patterns — ranging from individualistic to collectivized — although our recommendation will hope to sharpen the more desirable alternatives.

Since the President's advocacy of HMOs, a special unit of the Department of HEW has been established to promote them. The HMO Service, as it is called, has been encouraging establishment of new HMOs through developmental grants.[19] Beyond the HMOs or HMO-like entities that already exist, about 110 new ones are in developmental or operational stages throughout the nation by reason of these grants, and an indeterminate additional number (probably several hundred) are being organized on their own. Numerous conferences have been held on the HMO concept, and countless articles have been written. Group practice clinics, medical societies, consumer groups, hospitals, insurance companies, and other bodies are exploring possibilities of joining the movement. Several bills have been introduced in the U.S. Congress on promotion of HMOs, to be backed up with larger federal funding, and extensive hearings on them have been held in both the Senate and House of Representatives.* In late 1972, furthermore, P.L. 92-603 (formerly H.R. 1) was enacted, providing for extensive amendments to the Medicare and Medicaid laws, including specific provision for furnishing statutory benefits to aged Medicare beneficiaries through the HMO mechanism.[20]

Thus, the HMO idea is by no means a speculative goal in a brave new world, but an enlarging part of current health service realities. As an alternative to individualistic fee-for-service health care delivery, it is of course not a new idea, but a newly respectable phrase for an old one — an old idea that was formerly marginal and contending with much opposition, especially from the private medical profession.[21] Prototypes, like the Kaiser-Permanente Health Plan or the Health Insurance Plan of Greater New York, have been operating, in spite of professional opposition, for 30 years. Other approaches, embodied in the "medical foundations" of San Joaquin County,

---

*In December 1973, after the above was written, Congress passed legislation authorizing expenditure of $375,000,000 for promotion of health maintenance organizations.

California, and elsewhere, have also offered a wide range of medical and hospital services through the mainstream of private doctors and existing facilities for a prepaid annual premium. The task in designing a future realistic system is to define more clearly the scope of health services that would be provided by HMOs, the way they would operate, their place in the Health Regions previously outlined, and the large problem of planning services for populations not enrolled in HMOs.

The Range of Health Services in a Region

Before considering a reasonable scope of health services and other features to be expected in HMOs, the total range of services to be offered in a Health Region should be reviewed. As outlined in the previous chapter, an ideal system — or indeed any health care system — can be construed to offer services of three degrees of complexity. In the context of a realistic system, these would be as follows.

Primary care constitutes both curative and preventive service on a regular basis to the ambulatory person. For illness, it constitutes the attention of first contact by a general practitioner or one of the new specialists in family practice, or alternatively by an internist or pediatrician. Under the direction of these physicians, the actual initial encounter might be with a physician's assistant, nurse practitioner, or another such allied health worker. These primary care personnel would deal with the conditions of high frequency in the population and relatively low technical complexity.

For prevention, primary care must include immunizations, personal health education, case-finding procedures (including multiphasic screening tests), and other health maintenance measures applied routinely. Emergency service (including ambulance transportation) on a 24-hour basis must also be part of primary care, although it might sometimes require prompt referral to secondary care (see below). Primary care should also include relatively simple laboratory, X-ray, or other diagnostic procedures not demanding highly specialized skills. Pharmacy services must also accompany primary care for filling the prescriptions of the primary doctor. Likewise dental care, restorative and preventive, for simple conditions is part of primary care. Obviously all these primary services should be close at hand to where people live — 30-minute travel time ought to be the usual maximum. Since primary health care, despite its basic importance, has come to be relatively neglected in the current era of specialized medicine, it deserves high priority emphasis in the Health Regions of the future.

Secondary care consists only of curative services; these are ordinarily obtained on referral from the primary care level. Secondary care includes the services of specialists (beyond the primary-type internist or pediatrician), whether the patient is ambulatory or hospitalized. All inpatient hospital services constitute part of secondary care if they are of sufficient frequency to be provided in a peripheral or district general hospital (as distinguished from a regional medical center, as described below). Thus the commoner forms of surgery or management of uncomplicated medical conditions are at this level. Likewise, long-term care of chronic illness in a nursing home or ECF (extended care facility) is part of secondary care, since such cases are nowadays of relatively high frequency and require a moderately skilled but not highly complicated level of technique. By the same token, organized home health services, under the aegis of a general hospital or other community agency, are part of secondary care. Physical, occupational, or speech therapy for relatively frequent disorders (such as stroke or post-trauma cases) is a component of secondary care, as are special services for visual refraction (optometry) or foot conditions (podiatry).

Tertiary care includes the services of the "super-specialists" for rare disorders or the care of serious long-term conditions of relatively low frequency. This level of care in a Health Region would include the treatment of cases requiring brain or cardiac surgery, kidney dialysis, cobalt radiation therapy, or other modalities that can economically be offered only at a regional medical center. Such centers would often be parts of medical schools. Tertiary care would also include elaborate programs of rehabilitation (such as for paraplegics) and mental hospital care of long-term serious psychotics, which could not be handled in the average general hospital or nursing home. The designation of these several types of patient as requiring "tertiary" level care is in the interests of both economy and quality — economy, because the expensive modalities required for their care (such as heart-lung machines) must be used at high capacity to avoid extravagant waste of resources; quality, because proper skills in the staff can be maintained only if a relatively high volume of cases is seen. The surgeon and hospital performing open-heart surgery only once a month or so, for example, constitute both a high-cost and a high-risk enterprise.

Physical and professional linkages among primary, secondary, and tertiary services in a health region have been described in many accounts of regionalization. Primary care services might be ideally rendered by a health team in a local community health center, but realistically for some time to come many will be furnished at the premises of private medical and allied practitioners. Secondary or "back-up" specialist and hospital services would come largely from community general hospitals, as well as from nursing homes and other units. Professionally, the primary health workers should be affiliated with the general hospitals for educational and consultative purposes. The general hospitals, in turn, should operate as professional satellites to the regional medical centers, where tertiary care services are concentrated. Education and consultation should emanate from the regional centers throughout the region, in response to specific problems as well as on a systematic quality-promotion basis.

This, then, is a brief accounting of the three levels of health service to be offered within each Health Region. It is doubtless an oversimplified description that would require adjustment or modification in each local circumstance. Within each Health Region, the regional authority would be immediately responsible for assuring that services at all three levels were available, and that any special deficiencies perceived would summon priority attention. A particularly high incidence of alcoholism, for example, or of accidents or infantile diarrhea or lung cancer would presumably justify special efforts to cope with these problems preventively and therapeutically.

Scope of Health Maintenance Organizations

Recognizing this three-tier composite of services to be offered in each health region, what would be the scope of the Health Maintenance Organization in the delivery process? In our view, a realistic system would expect the HMO to offer many but not all these services.[22] Federal legislation will probably mandate a minimum scope of services to be offered by HMOs (which would be subsidized with public funds), or this may be left to future regulation.* A feasible expectation of services from HMOs, in our view, would be as follows:

"Basic services" to be mandated in all HMOs should include most, but not all, services at the primary and secondary levels described above. The preventive service and emergency service constituents (including ambulances) of primary care would be essential, as well as day-to-day primary care of physicians (or allied health workers) for common illness. Simple laboratory and other diagnostic tests at the primary care level should be offered. At the secondary care level, most specialist service, both ambulatory and inpatient, should be offered, as well as hospitalization in local general hospitals. This range of "basic services" should be required as a financial and legal responsibility of all HMOs.

"Extended services," in our view, should be mandated under the HMO model only if a sufficiently large membership group (perhaps 5,000 persons) requests them and is willing to pay for them. These should include certain primary care services, such as prescribed drugs or simple dental care (preventive and curative), and various secondary care services, such as nursing home care, vision (optometric) care, or podiatry. Ambulatory psychiatric services at this stage of American medicine are sufficiently expensive and infrequent to be included among the "extended" rather than the "basic" services required of HMOs.

"Arranged services" of HMOs, finally, should not be a mandated

*In the HMO Act of 1973 (P.L. 93-222), the requirements for "basic" and "supplemental" services are not very different from those proposed here (before the law was enacted).

financial responsibility of the organization, but only subject to arrangement by appropriate referral. These would include certain services at the secondary care technical level, such as specialized dental care (prosthodontics, orthodontia, etc.). Beyond this the "arranged services" should include the superspecialities and the long-term psychiatric and rehabilitation modalities, at the tertiary care level. As stated earlier, these services should indeed be available within each region, but should not be expected to fall within the financial or legal responsibility of the HMO.

A schema of these three possible types of HMO service, in relation to the three technical levels of care in each Health Region, is shown in Table 1.

This schedule of basic, extended, and arranged services is recommended as a reasonable legal scope for HMOs, in the interest of promoting maximum nationwide development of the HMO idea. If legislation should demand of all HMOs more than the services suggested as "basic," the model would be idealistic but rarely applied; if less than this scope, the improvement over current patterns would be slight. The objective of an HMO strategy, in our view, should be to strike a realistic compromise between the ideal and the feasible, toward the objective of rationalizing the health care delivery system.

Regarding the _tertiary care services_ necessary in each Health Region, yet not expected to be offered as either "basic" or "extended" HMO benefits, special commentary is required. Many of these services, such as psychiatric hospital care, long-term rehabilitation of severely disabled patients, and recently kidney dialysis (for Medicare beneficiaries under P.L. 92-603) are typically financed by governmental programs. We propose that general revenue or social insurance financing be used to support all these high-cost, though relatively infrequently used, services in all Health Regions. In some regions, this might be done through direct operation by a regional medical center of the necessary facilities, with engagement of all personnel on salaries. In other regions, the Regional Health Authority (see below) might purchase the services for its residents from independent providers on a traditional fee basis. Still another device might be through arrangement for these services by consortiums of several HMOs, with appropriate public subsidy. Under whatever mechanism is used, however, the resources needed (neurosurgeons, kidney dialysis equipment, cobalt therapy units, etc.) to serve the needs of each regional population should be subject to allocation geographically by the national health planning authority, discussed in the previous section, and financed by public funds. Only in this way could there be assurance that total health needs would be properly met in each region.

Organizing HMOs

The above definition of scope of services within HMOs still leaves many questions to be answered about these mechanisms for moving toward a better

Table 1. Types of Health Service Recommended under "Health Maintenance Organizations" (HMOs), by Technical Level in a Health Region

HMO Services	Technical Level in a Health Region		
	Primary	Secondary	Tertiary
"Basic"	Prevention — Immunization — Health education — Screening tests — Family planning Emergency services First contact doctor's care Simple diagnostic tests	Most ambulatory specialist care Elaborate diagnostic procedures In patient specialist care: surgical and medical Hospitalization in general facilities	—
"Extended"	Prescribed drugs Simple dental care	Home care Rehab. therapies: — Physical — Occupational — Speech Optometry Podiatry Ambulatory psychiatry Nursing homes (ECF)	—
"Arranged"	—	Specialized dental care	Long-term psychiatric care Super-specialties — Renal dialysis — Cardiac surgery, etc. Complex rehabilitation

delivery system. The most important of these are: HMO sponsorship, enrollment methods, the precise patterns of delivery, and monitoring of HMO hazards.

Regarding *sponsorship,* the American health system would allow many possibilities. An American Public Health Association policy statement on HMOs listed these possible sponsoring entities:

—— consumer associations (including labor unions)
—— employer-employee groups (including health and welfare trust funds)
—— industrial corporations
—— medical societies
—— medical group clinics
—— neighborhood health centers
——community hospitals
—— teaching hospitals and/or medical schools
—— local government agencies (such as Health Departments)
—— nonprofit health insurance plans (such as Blue Cross or Blue Shield)
—— commercial insurance companies
—— other private medical enterprises.

Other types of organization could doubtless be named. In our view a wide range of HMO sponsorships should, indeed, be allowed, but we believe there are certain considerations making some forms preferable to others.

A basic consideration is the profit motive. In a theoretical sense, there might be no objection to profit-making bodies sponsoring HMOs, so long as there is adequate surveillance against abuse. Some even argue forcefully that the profit motive can promote efficiencies not found in lax nonprofit organizations. The problem is, however, that to be effective against the abuses of commercialization in our society, the surveillance must be continuous and rigorous—so much so that it is costly and onerous; as a practical matter, governmental surveillance in the health care industry, for these very reasons, is seldom effective.[23] Witness the sordid history of the pharmaceutical industry, with the saga of commercial drug control legislation enacted since 1906 to limit the harms emanating from the profit motive.[24] Witness the American nursing home situation, a sector of health care largely in proprietary hands and replete with problems of poor quality and commercialized practices.[25]

One hears the rejoinder that ordinary medical or dental practice is profit-making, and that such practice would be included under many nonprofit HMO sponsorships. The individual physician, whether in solo or group practice, however, is subject to the constraints of medical ethics and professional peer review, not to mention the incentives to economy and quality of the HMO mechanism itself. An HMO sponsoring body, on the other hand, is a third party, once-removed from the doctor and the patient. Constraints at this level are more distant from the point of service. They are accordingly less likely to be operative, and discipline would be solely dependent on the weak hand of governmental surveillance. Lest these be considered only idle speculations, one may point to the recent rise, in the California Medicaid program, of a number of profit-oriented HMO programs of highly dubious quality and integrity.[26]

A safer social policy therefore, in our view, is to limit HMO sponsorship to nonprofit bodies. Granted, there may be legal subterfuges by which the "nonprofit" cloak can be worn by a commercialized HMO operation, but insofar as possible the nonprofit tradition in the organized health services — seen most venerably in the hospital field — should be upheld.

Hospitals, indeed, are potentially important sponsors of HMOs, with many advantages that have been recognized. The Ullman Bill for national health insurance, introduced in the House of Representatives in 1972, embodies concepts put forward by the American Hospital Association, under which "health care corporations," very much like HMOs, would presumably be set up by hospitals. A sophisticated observer of the health scene like Anne Somers has spoken forcefully of the wisdom of hospital sponsorship of HMO-like programs of comprehensive care.[27] Hospitals certainly have a strong technical base for HMO sponsorship, both in their facilities and their medical staffs, not to mention all their employed nursing and technical personnel. Their governing boards, furthermore, are intended to represent the community population, although the range of this representation may be somewhat narrowly confined to the upper-middle-class business world.

Organized ambulatory service units, like the "neighborhood health centers" initiated by the U.S. Office of Economic Opportunity, are other obvious nuclei for development of HMOs. The new centers offering comprehensive ambulatory services for maternal and infant care (MIC) or for children and youth (C and Y), which could expand their scope to reach total populations, are further possibilities. Outside of government, large private group medical clinics — whether or not affiliated with particular hospitals — are probably the most numerous type of antecedent structure from which HMOs could be developed. Labor unions, labor-management trust funds, and other consumer organizations, with or without ties to existing health care facilities, are logical sponsors. In general, the Regional Health Authority should promote organization of HMOs under public and voluntary nonprofit sponsorships to cover the largest possible proportion of its population.

Whatever diverse sponsorships of HMOs evolve in a health region, we advocate a strong, if not dominant, voice for consumers. Although some of the most important pioneers of the HMO idea, through "prepaid group practice health plans," were consumer associations, the new wave of HMOs has unfortunately contained relatively few such sponsors. Perhaps a practical solution is to encourage sponsorship of HMOs by groups representing a mixture of health care providers and consumers in varying proportions.

Enrollment policies and practices are another important aspect of the

HMO strategy. Health insurance plans in America have typically grown most rapidly by enrollment of organic membership groups, rather than of isolated individuals or families; this approach helps to assure, of course, a diversified spread of "insurance risks." The same would apply to enrollment in HMOs which are, after all, a type of risk-spreading organization.

The population to be included in an HMO, however, should be subject to certain regulations, if equitable services are to be assured. Geographic boundaries are important; since services should be geographically accessible to the members, limits of distance and travel time would have to be set. The numbers of enrollees to be permitted in any HMO, of course, must be related to the health personnel and other resources available, according to minimum resource standards (such as ratios of pediatricians per 10,000 children), if quality of service is to be maintained.

The minimum number of persons necessary to insure actuarial stability in an HMO has been subject to much discussion. A common estimate has been 20,000 to 30,000, if high-cost events of relatively low frequency, such as hospitalizations, are to be safely financed.[28] Yet, with the group provider model, enrollments of as few as 5,000 persons have proved viable; "losses" that may be incurred in one year can be compensated for the next. Perhaps a maximum enrollment might also be stipulated for an HMO in a health region, to avoid the impersonalities of large bureaucratic structures. Much depends, of course, on the use of sub-centers in an HMO, to achieve geographic convenience for members. Once more than 100 physicians or more than 100,000 consumers are involved, logistical difficulties are created, even though economies of scale may be enjoyed.

The "marketing" techniques for attracting subscribers into HMOs present special problems. The great majority of the American population is accustomed to an open-market free-choice pattern of obtaining medical care, so that the innovative HMO design requires educational persuasion. The behavioral changes, implicit in the use of a group practice delivery pattern (see below), doubtless require greater educational efforts than the individual practice setting of the "medical foundation" pattern, but even the latter would demand "salesmanship" since not all local doctors would ordinarily participate. To carry out the actual marketing and enrollment process, an HMO might subcontract with experienced health insurance organizations, such as the current Blue Cross or Blue Shield plans or even insurance companies (this was done, for example, by the Harvard Community Health Plan). The methods used will ultimately have to depend on the availability of "start up" administrative funds for the organization of new HMOs, such as are to be, indeed, available under the provisions of the Health Maintenance Organization Act of 1973.

The precise mechanisms or *patterns for providing the scope of health services,* outlined above for HMOs, would be subject to numerous variations. Broadly speaking, one may refer to the "individual provider model" and the "group provider model." In a realistic system both of these models must be expected to develop.

Under the individual provider model, identified commonly with the "medical society foundations," HMO members would have free choice of all participating physicians, who would mainly be engaged in solo practice (although some private group practices would also doubtless participate). The elements of primary and secondary care required would be offered by these providers, including the preventive as well as therapeutic services. Hospital care would typically be furnished in the existing local facilities. If prescribed drugs were among the benefits, they would be obtained in regular pharmacies, and corresponding open-market arrangements would be applied to laboratory or X-ray examinations, optometry, physiotherapy, and so on. Since a fixed annual premium would be payable for all these services, financial incentives would theoretically induce the physician to use hospitals or other doctor-prescribed services prudently. Remuneration of the physicians on a fee-for-service basis, however, would have to be subject to possible proration of fees, if the annual fund was not adequate to pay all bills at 100 percent. On the other hand, an unexpended balance in premium income could yield "bonuses" to the providers, refunds to the subscribers, reserve funds for future expansion of benefits, or other uses—depending on legislative requirements and the particular HMO's policies.

The "group provider model" of HMO in its pure form would deliver primary and secondary services through various forms of health center or clinic. Teams of doctors, technicians, nurses, social workers, and other personnel at one or several facilities would work together for provision of curative and preventive services. If prescribed drugs were a benefit, they would be furnished from an in-house pharmacy. Similar direct provision would be made for diagnostic tests, rehabilitation therapy, vision care, and so on. Hospitalization would be provided in facilities directly controlled by the HMO, as in the prototype illustrated by the Kaiser–Permanente Health Plan, or in local institutions as under the Health Insurance Plan of Greater New York. The latter arrangement entails a much lower capital investment for the HMO and has other advantages, but creates various problems in the way of conflicts between HMO physicians and other members of the hospital's medical staff. Under the "group provider model," the physicians, along with all other health personnel, are ordinarily paid by salary, but the disposition of earnings or losses, in relation to premium income, could also follow several options, as discussed above.

These are over-simplified descriptions of the two basic HMO delivery patterns, and within each type numerous variations would be possible. The individual provider model, for example, might be associated with one or more directly controlled pharmacies or laboratories; the group provider model, on the other hand, might allow free choice of local pharmacy or optometrist for prescribed drugs or eyeglasses. Great flexibility is one of the assets of the HMO concept in the pluralistic American setting, so long as certain minimum standards are met with respect to the scope of services, resources, costs, and other features of care.

There is much evidence that the group provider HMO model can probably achieve economies, quality standards, and a preventive orientation more effectively than the individual provider model.[29] The organizational and administrative mechanisms for reaching people routinely to perform case-detection tests or immunizations, to carry out epidemiological follow-up on communicable diseases (tuberculosis, venereal disease, or acute infections), to offer health education, and so forth, can hardly be applied in numerous individual medical offices as efficiently as in clinic setups.

Yet in a realistic system, both types of delivery pattern must be expected and, indeed, encouraged. Competition, it is presumed, will operate to promote the best possible performance under both types of model and under multiple demonstrations of the same model. The effective operation of competition, of course, depends on consumers being properly informed, and this must be an obligation of the governmental authority in each health region.

Monitoring of HMOs in each health region is the final aspect of their operation that must be considered. Beyond the inducements of free competition, a system of governmental surveillance must be set in motion to assure application of minimum technical standards and to inform consumers of the operational effects or health outcomes of HMOs, which the average patient could not be expected to assess. While maximum promotion of HMOs, as noted earlier, should be carried out in each region as a general rule, in certain thinly settled areas this might be unwise; where competition for enrollment of a small population leads to duplication and waste, official franchising of one or another HMO may be in the best public interest. This whole question of social controls over HMOs, as well as over the entire health care system, will be discussed more fully below.

Insofar as HMOs are developed to provide a wide range of services to defined populations, it is obvious that for their members a great deal — perhaps nearly all — of the fragmented, categorical health programs, which this study has analyzed, would disappear. More cogently, the services of the previous categorical programs would become absorbed into and integrated within the overall program of the HMO. Thus, the well-baby conference or the venereal disease clinic of the Health Department would, for these HMO members, have no further purposes. The OEO neighborhood health center, the crippled children's service, the voluntary cancer detection facility, the mental health clinic, the hospital emergency room, the V.A. facility, the migrant family clinic, these and many specialized units will gradually lose their markets as more people become enrolled in HMOs providing these services. In effect, the countless categorical programs that compose the

American health care system have been a response to the deficiencies of the private medical market; if those deficiencies are corrected in the entitlements of HMO enrollees, the rationale for much of our complicated pluralism disappears.

Such benefits of integration would apply, of course, only to those persons who join HMOs, and only to the extent that these HMOs provide adequately comprehensive services. In a realistic world, we cannot be too sanguine about either the extent of population coverage or the range of benefits, unless governmental policy is dedicated and forceful. If it is, however, we may look to the time within 10 or 20 years when the people not enrolled in HMOs would constitute a minority—a sort of "social remainder" outside the mainstream of the prevailing health care system. The resources and services within this side-stream would still have to be subject to planning and social controls, as discussed below, but the strategy of national planning would be to reduce the volume of non-HMO activity to the smallest possible proportions.

Certain types of health service, even under a realistic but integrated system, should remain separately administered. First-aid and health educational activities in schools and workplaces should continue under. the auspices of educational or industrial bodies. This would be merely for the sake of physical convenience to children or adults while they are at school or at work. Overall responsibility for the diagnosis and treatment of these people, however, can be best assumed and integrated through the HMO to which they belong.

Could one envision the time in America when membership in an approved HMO would be made mandatory for everyone? So long as such a requirement were linked to financial support for services, it would not be so outlandish. In Great Britain, everyone is expected to choose a general practitioner (to become a member on his panel) if he is to enjoy the financial protection of the National Health Service for primary ambulatory care; if he does not wish to make such a choice, then he must pay the practitioner personally. Under the National Health Insurance Standards Act submitted in the 92nd Congress and supported by President Nixon (see below), enrollment of workers by their employers in some approved health insurance plan would be mandated—a requirement not very far from mandatory enrollment in an HMO. Perhaps when 60 to 80 percent of the population becomes enrolled in HMOs, the political dynamics would point toward mandatory enrollment of the remainder, in the interest of economy and social welfare.

Such a question, and indeed the whole proposal of health maintenance organizations, is intimately related to the basic issue of financial support. The entire prospect of HMO growth and encouragement depends directly on the availability of stable financing. A realistic system must, therefore, next consider the economic framework of the whole structure of health services.

FINANCING

The national planning and improved organization for delivery of health services discussed so far must rest on a firm economic foundation. Otherwise, accessibility and equity of health services remain a hollow rhetoric. An improved but realistic system must have a sound framework of financing which provides support for all needed services to the entire population.

The multiplicity of financing mechanisms and their sustenance of fragmented delivery patterns have been reviewed in Chapter 3. In a very theoretical sense, multiple origins of moneys should not matter, so long as all contingencies are covered and the spending is channelized through an organized system of delivery. In practice, however, such organization of a sound delivery system must remain very difficult without systematization of most, if not all, of the flow of economic support. Vested interests tied to the origins of funds are too strong and obstructive of integration.

The numerous existing sources of health care financing—private payment, voluntary insurance, social insurance (Medicare and Workmen's Compensation), philanthropy, government revenues at several levels and of several types—are each encrusted with all sorts of pride and sovereignties. The many collectivized methods, now paying for more than 60 percent of personal health services in the nation, have undoubtedly increased the accessibility and utilization of services, but they have also accentuated the fragmentation of the delivery process. The challenge remains, therefore, to develop a system of health service financing that not only fills the many gaps but also provides a power base for rationalizing the health care delivery system. Indeed, the political realities in the United States suggest that the strongest leverage for improving the delivery system is probably the enactment of national legislation to strengthen and streamline the social financing of health services.

The usual description of such legislative strategy is the approach of national health insurance (NHI). Since enactment of Medicare for the aged in 1965, the demand for similar social insurance protection of the rest of the population has predictably been rekindled. In the 92nd Congress, at least a dozen bills were introduced that, in one degree or another, would expand the financial access of the American population to medical services. When so many proposals appear, from all points on the political spectrum, one may conclude that some action will be taken in the near future.

The contents and mechanisms of the several proposals for NHI have been reviewed in many other places, and here we need only take note of their underlying concepts.[30] Considering the proposals along a range from minimum to maximum impact on existing processes of health care financing, one can identify four main approaches: First, there are the bills that would rest on a perpetuation of the current voluntary health insurance plans, but strengthen them through financial inducements to enrollment of more people, subsidy for enrollment of low-income families, and encouragement of wider scopes of benefits. This approach is illustrated by the "Medicredit" bill backed by the American Medical Association and the "National Health Care Act" backed by the commercial insurance industry. Secondly, there are the bills which would mandate enrollment of all employed persons—the great majority of the population, counting their dependents—in voluntary insurance plans meeting certain standards. This approach is illustrated by the "National Health Insurance and Health Improvements Act," introduced by Senator Javits, and the "National Health Insurance Partnership Act," introduced by Senator Bennett pursuant to President Nixon's "Health Strategy" message of February 1971. Another bill of this general philosophy is the "National Health Care Services Reorganization and Financing Act," introduced by Representative Ullman and backed by the American Hospital Association. All these bills entail various limitations in benefits (deductibles and co-payments, for instance), but they also include incentives toward modifying delivery patterns, especially by way of encouraging HMOs.

Thirdly and in contrast to the two previous types of bill, which would build upon existing voluntary health plans, another type would establish a new national health insurance fund, protecting virtually the entire population, but for limited benefits. This is illustrated by the "Catastrophic Health Insurance Program" bill introduced by Senator Long. The strategy behind this approach may well be like that of Canada, where the first national health insurance legislation was mandatory but covered only hospitalization; it was soon followed, however, by amendments to cover physicians' services—with further benefits now under discussion. The fourth NHI approach would apply the social insurance principle of covering the entire national population and offer virtually comprehensive health services. This is illustrated by the "Health Security Act" introduced by Senator Edward Kennedy and backed by the AFL-CIO labor movement. Beyond its wide financial scope, this bill would introduce substantial incentives for modifying patterns of health care delivery and for monitoring the quality of all services.*

The promotion of HMO or HMO-like organizations under bills of the second and fourth types would be through the operation of incentives for both providers and consumers. For providers, there would be the opportunity for enhanced earnings, if superfluous or unnecessary services were curtailed; for consumers, there would be the entitlement to a wider scope of benefits. These incentives, it is hoped, would overcome the natural inertia of people to depart from traditional open market health-care patterns.

*In the 93rd Congress (1973-74) modifications of almost all these bills were introduced, along with some new ones.

It is hardly likely that any of these NHI bills will be enacted in precisely the form in which it was originally written. Congressional and general public debate is bound to produce compromises of many sorts; after enactment, furthermore, numerous amendments may be expected, as lessons of experience are learned and problems become visible. Any of the bills, nevertheless, even the most modest, would have the effect of strengthening the social financing of most health services. This would include support for HMOs. The degree of strengthening would obviously vary among the bills, especially insofar as inequities were to be corrected among different regions of the nation and different socioeconomic groups. The strongest leverage for correcting geographic inequities in the location and use of resources (especially health manpower) would be offered by the social insurance strategy of the "Health Security Act." Under this bill, nationwide funds would all flow to a central point, from which they could be redistributed in some reasonable proportion to local health needs.

In any event, NHI legislation of some type to improve financing must be part of a realistic system of personal health care. We would advocate its coverage of at least the scope of services discussed earlier as coming under primary and secondary care. If so, it would also automatically cover all services likely to be mandated under any probable definition of an HMO. Regarding tertiary care, there are compelling arguments for its support from national general revenues. Many of such services (mental hospitals and high-cost rehabilitation services, for example) are now provided through public revenues and are typically excluded from voluntary insurance plans. More important, the deployment of resources for such services—especially the super-specialties of surgery and medicine—in relation to regional needs requires decisions from a central level. If the scarce resources for tertiary care are to be equitably distributed throughout the nation, government should have the power to use funds flexibly. Such mechanisms are permitted, in fact, in the "Health Security" NHI proposal, but we suggest that under any NHI bill that is enacted, the tertiary care services be supported from general revenues.

Just as HMOs would reduce fragmentation in delivery of health care, national health insurance would doubtless reduce the segmentation of care for certain population groups, particularly the indigent. It is noteworthy that nearly all the NHI proposals in Congress would have the effect of enrolling recipients of public assistance into a mainstream of medical care, whether through local insurance plans or a national social insurance fund. Government revenues would be used for paying "insurance premiums" on behalf of the poor. Thus, a truly single system of health care for all could be achieved. Moreover, most of the bills would use only federal revenues for this purpose, rather than shared federal-state revenues as at present under Medicaid.

Whatever NHI legislation is enacted, it would doubtless not finance all health services initially—for example, all dental services, noncritically necessary drugs, or nursing home care. Under several bills, moreover, cost-sharing or maximum benefits would be imposed. Much would remain, therefore, for private insurance financing. Moreover, even after benefits are extended with time (as has occurred in all other industrialized nations after NHI has been started), some non-essential services, such as private rooms in hospitals or certain types of prosthetic dentistry, would doubtless be left to private financing. Furthermore, even for the insured benefits, wealthy persons may still wish to use the services of a handful of doctors or other resources that remain outside the general system, as one sees for a tiny fraction of services in Great Britain today. Such private sector services can act as a "safety valve" for pressures that can arise in any large system. As long as these services are not of large proportions, they will not create serious inequities, and should be regarded as an appropriate aspect of a realistic system.

This combination of NHI financing for the great bulk of primary and secondary care, public revenue financing for most tertiary care, and private financing for non-essential or "luxury" services would foster the expansion of HMOs and also improve the access to personal health services for those remaining outside HMOs. Depending on the details of NHI legislation enacted, the economic mechanisms proposed would lay the foundation for massive changes in the American health care system to better meet population needs.

SOCIAL CONTROLS

No system of health services in a complex, continually changing society will operate effectively over the years without constant surveillance and controls. The operation of numerous controls in our current pluralistic system reviewed in previous chapters—licensure laws, food and drug control legislation, accreditation programs, "comprehensive health planning" constraints on hospital construction, etc.—indicate the many measures evolving even in a largely free enterprise setting. In a realistic system that aims to assure services of good quality at reasonable cost to everyone, the need for controls would be somewhat greater.

The requirements of centralized national planning for resource production, delineation of health regions, and establishment of quality standards have been discussed. Implementation of those standards, along with many other duties concerning HMOs, and the surveillance of services outside HMOs, would devolve in a realistic system largely upon regional health authorities. Between the regional and the national levels, however, many functions of state governments would still remain.

At the state government level, established functions of professional surveillance would continue. The states would also be the logical intermediary channels through which funds from a national health insurance program or from federal general revenues would be allocated to the health regions. Many of the states, indeed being less than 2,000,000 population, would serve essentially in the role of health regions, as described earlier; the larger states containing two or more health regions would give technical advice to the health regions within their borders. The Comprehensive Health Planning (CHP) bodies set up at the state level under the 1966 legislation provide a precedent vis-à-vis the area-wide (regional) CHP agencies.

In our view, the responsible agency for social controls at the state level should be the Department of Health. Under this agency should be placed the licensure functions now often lodged in separate boards, dominated by the very professional groups that are to be controlled. State Health Departments, in theory, are intended to represent the will of the total population, rather than one or another class of health care provider; where their governing boards do not reflect this philosophy, they should be appropriately modified in their composition to do so. The realities of all the accumulated federal grant-in-aid legislation for health services, along with the recent federal-state revenue-sharing laws, require that any realistic health care system must recognize the role of state governments.[31]

Regional Health Authorities

The major responsibilities for social controls in the system we advocate would nevertheless be vested in the regional authorities, governing an average of 2,000,000 population, as defined at the outset of this chapter. These regional health authorities should be designed and built from the resources of our present network of state and local public health agencies. The tradition of public trust, the orientation to prevention, the community viewpoint, the technical competencies associated with Health Departments, these offer the combination of characteristics needed.[32] Where these established agencies are weak, we are confident that they can and will be strengthened by assignment of the responsibilities here proposed.

Regional Health Authorities (RHA) should be governed by boards representing both technical expertise and the interests of consumers as a whole. Various approaches to this concept are possible. We favor appointment of technical experts by the State Director of Health, on the basis of established criteria; such persons ought to constitute 40 to 45 percent of the RHA Board composition. The balance of Board members ought to be elected, in the same sense that Boards of Education are often elective. In this way, the interests of consumers can be represented through the usual mechanisms of the political process. Conceivably the strategy of "proportional representation" on a district basis could be implemented, so that various ethnic groups with special health needs could be virtually assured of representation. Citizen advisory boards on special problems would also be in order. Under the RHA Board, of course, would be a purely technical staff to carry out the on-going work.

The Regional Health Authority, unlike the state or local Health Department of the past, should not be engaged in the direct provision of personal health services through various clinics; under the realistic system all these services would be furnished by HMOs or non-HMO providers. Environmental health services, on the other hand, would be the function of the Regional Environmental Quality Control Boards, mentioned elsewhere in this volume. The functions of the RHA should instead consist of planning, controlling, consulting on, and evaluating the personal health services within its borders. It would also channelize all funds derived from social sources. A good deal of this responsibility, in turn, would be exercised through surveillance over the operation of HMOs.

The RHA should basically be responsible for assuring that all needed primary, secondary, and tertiary care services are available to all persons within its jurisdiction. So large a goal would not be achievable overnight, but the attainment of it would require, first of all, planning to acquire the needed health resources: facilities, manpower, and all the rest. This would entail not only the negative cast of planning, familiar under current CHP agencies (disapproving unnecessary hospital construction), but also affirmative actions to establish resources where they are deficient. The RHA, for example, would indicate to the National Department of Health its needs for primary care doctors, secondary care general hospitals in certain localities, or tertiary care cardiac surgeons. At the same time, it would have the power to prohibit construction of unnecessary health care facilities in the region (as under current "certificate of need" state hospital control laws), which might encourage unreasonably high utilization. By handling funds allocated under an NHI program, the RHA should have the economic wherewithal to support the functioning of properly needed resources. Moreover, the channelizing of all public funds for health care would give the RHA sanctions to enforce technical standards—for example, paying for certain surgical services only when done by properly qualified surgeons in appropriate types of hospital.

Much of the responsibility of RHAs, as mentioned, would depend upon the operation of HMOs, so that the promotion of new HMOs, especially in the early years, would figure prominently among their duties. Subsidy funds and technical advice would be given for this purpose from higher levels. Encouragement of the "group provider" model of HMO will often require construction funds for ambulatory care centers, which should also be forthcoming from state and national levels. Many such centers, on the other hand, could doubtless be built on the basis of local initiative and loans, in the same way that private group practice clinics or indeed voluntary hospitals have multiplied throughout the nation without public subsidy.

HMO Surveillance

With respect to HMOs there are two principal hazards that require surveillance: membership composition and quality of care provided. Regarding membership composition, so long as HMO financing is based on per capita payments calculated from the average experience in a region, it is important that the members represent an approximate cross-section of the local population. If a particular HMO enrolls selectively persons of low illness risk —favoring, for example, the young, the affluent, those without chronic illness—it could "offer" very generous benefits and yet earn excessive profits. To guard against this form of abuse—well recognized in the commercial health insurance field—there would have to be criteria for monitoring membership composition. Also a mandatory "open enrollment period" each year is a device, required in the new federal legislation, for enabling persons of any degree of illness risk to enroll in any HMO.

The second hazard of poor quality care is more difficult to control, but various approaches are possible. Evaluation can be conducted on the levels of what Avedis Donabedian has epitomized as structure, process, and outcome.[33] Just as the open-market fee-for-service health care system, linked with insurance, yields the hazard of over-servicing, the HMO pattern can result in poor quality care through under-servicing.*

Monitoring the "structure" of health service in HMOs will require the application by the RHA of criteria (presumably issued by the National Department of Health) on the input of resources: the manpower, facilities, equipment, etc. Appropriate ratios of these resources must be expected, including proper qualifications of medical specialists, nurses, technicians, and all the rest. Adequate hospital or health center equipment, drugs, and supplies must be expected. The location of resources, in relation to the residences of HMO members, so that care is physically accessible, is also part of the surveillance of "structure."

"Process" surveillance or evaluation entails information on rates of utilization of all types of health service—such as physician encounters, prescribed drugs, hospital admissions and days, technical tests—in relation to reasonable norms. It also requires "medical audit" techniques, through record analysis or actual observation, to determine whether preventive, diagnostic, and treatment procedures are being carried out in a manner consistent with prevailing scientific opinion. Such review, of course, can be very

---

*Quality assurance mechanisms are also required in the 1973 HMO Act.

laborious and expensive, so that it must be carried out on a sampling basis. Moreover, regular self-auditing should be expected within each HMO.

Monitoring of health service "outcomes" or end-results in HMOs is the most difficult task, but methods must be developed to do this. The problem, of course, is that rates of mortality, morbidity, or disability depend on many factors outside of the health services provided. Statistical adjustments can be made for these influences—demographic, environmental, etc.—in determining outcome measures of an HMO. As a sort of proxy for health status outcome, measurements of the satisfaction or grievances of HMO members can also be made.[34]

Other Surveillance Responsibilities

In practice, all three of these approaches to evaluation of the quality of care provided by HMOs should be carried out simultaneously and continuously. But what about the population in a health region not enrolled in HMOs? The Regional Health Authority, of course, must carry equivalent responsibility for monitoring the quantity and quality of services received by these people. Conceptually, as suggested earlier, the non-HMO population must be considered as the "social remainder" of people in the region for whom direct surveillance of care is done by the RHA. To calculate ratios of resources and rates of services, so essential to evaluation, population denominators derived from census counts (minus the HMO members) will have to be used. To carry out medical audits or their equivalent on services rendered to non-HMO persons, we must rely on reviews of performance on a sample basis, both in hospitals and in private practitioner offices. Expectation of such surveillance can no longer be considered utopian, since the enactment in late 1972 of P.L. 92-603, with its provision for Professional Standards Review Organizations (PSROSs) in each local area under the Medicare law.[35] We would envisage the PSRO function extended to the full population outside of HMOs and absorbed within the official role of the Regional Health Authority.

To permit social controls both within HMOs and outside them, a much more comprehensive and uniform system of health records than we now have will be necessary. The operation of a national health insurance program would probably require more systematized records in any case, but the information demanded on records should go beyond the requirements of fee payments. Several systems of medical records have been developed recently, through which basic and uniform information on diagnosis, diagnostic procedures, and treatment can be indicated in a relatively simple and codifiable manner.[36]

The findings of quality review procedures within each health region should provide a basis for both regulation and public education. The

Regional Health Authority should be free to make on-the-spot inspections of all health facilities as well as individual practitioner premises, both routinely and on the basis of statistically suspicious clues or patient grievances. Beyond such policing, the population as a whole should be informed regularly of information accumulated on the quality of services throughout the system. Only in this way can accountability of health service providers be achieved. Only by such policies can one expect the mechanism of competition, implied in the whole HMO strategy, to operate effectively toward protection of consumer interests.

Special importance attaches to the monitoring of resources for tertiary-level care in each Health Region. As suggested earlier, these super-specialty or long-term care activities would ordinarily serve the members of several HMOs as well as the non-HMO population. If, as we advocate, these services are financed from general revenues, their surveillance may be easier, but whether so financed or not, tertiary care performance must be subject to RHA controls. The necessary skills for monitoring these services may require consultative assistance from above the level of the health region, at the state or even the national Department of Health.

The controls over quality exercised by the Regional Health Authority must not, however, be limited to policing and public education. The RHA role in resource planning has been mentioned. It should also have functions in the sphere of professional education and administrative consultation. The RHA should promote programs of continuing education for all types of health personnel, to be offered by universities, hospitals, professional societies, or even by the RHA itself. In a future realistic system, such lifelong learning of health care providers ought to be a condition of continuing licensure, and local organizational steps should make this feasible.

Consultation to HMOs, hospitals, health centers, to health units in industries or schools, or to any other categorical health agencies focusing on special local problems should also be a function of RHAs, aided by State Departments of Health. In the early years especially, one may expect a great need for consultation on the problems of organizing new HMOs. The tasks of mobilizing providers, enrolling members, establishing administrative procedures, and all the other HMO requirements will need consultation. If federal subsidies for start-up costs of establishing new HMOs are provided, they should be funneled through RHAs.

Along with quality controls in a health care system must also go cost controls. For the most part, one may expect these to be built into the mechanisms of a national health insurance program. For the HMO population, of course, cost controls are largely achieved by the inherent capitation payment pattern. For services to the rest of the population, other administrative procedures would be necessary. Hospital costs should be subject to maximum limits that are achievable in various ways: by prospective budgeting (with prior budget review) under an insurance reimbursement system, by statutory "Hospital Rate Boards" in each state, by scheduled maximum charges for each item of service applied by the paying agency, or by combinations of methods.[37] Medical or allied practitioners paid on a fee-for-service basis should be subject to the constraints of maximum fee schedules; the "usual and customary fee" rule under Medicare invites cost escalation and should be eliminated under any program covering the general population and assuring doctors and others fair remuneration. Within each health region, moreover, the payment for services to non-HMO members should be subject to the constraint of the overall fiscal allotment to the region; thus, providers choosing fee remuneration may have to accept the possibility of proration of fees below 100 percent, in proportion to the total funds available each year or each quarter-year.

A final task of the Regional Health Authority would be to promote shared services among HMOs and among health facilities within its borders. Economies of scale as well as protection of quality standards can often be achieved by joint purchase of supplies, coordinated training and recruitment of personnel, and by operation of certain services on a centralized basis.[38] The latter could range from highly sophisticated laboratory procedures or computerized data analyses to housekeeping tasks, such as certain aspects of kitchen or laundry operations in hospitals.

While these are the principal forms of social control to be exercised at the state and regional health levels, special problems will doubtless arise. The RHA would be expected to cope with these, seeking advice and assistance from the state and national Health Departments when necessary. Likewise, the RHA would be the channel of feedback to the state and national levels on problems requiring new actions in the production or allocation of resources or in the stipulation of standards. Acting within policies and standards from the national and state Health Departments, the RHA would oversee the day-to-day operations of the whole health care system within its area—both within the HMOs and outside them.

ADJUSTMENTS TO THE PAST AND FUTURE

The above account of planning, delivery patterns, financing, and controls is believed to offer a realistic proposal for improving our national system of personal health services. It aims to strike a reasonable balance between the needs for systematic rationalization and the demands of the largely free market political economy in America.

What then would happen to all the organized programs for planning, financing, delivering, and controlling health services that now exist? There can be no dogmatic answer, but we believe that in general their functions would gradually become absorbed into the new system. The planning, now identified in part with "comprehensive health planning" (CHP) bodies, would become a function of National and State Health Departments and the Regional Health Authorities—but on a broader scale than seen today. As we have emphasized, planning must come to involve affirmative actions to fill needs as well as negative actions to prohibit the establishment of unnecessary or redundant resources in an area.

The countless categorical programs for health care financing or delivery or both, focused on special population groups or special disorders, would be largely replaced by activities of more comprehensive scope. Financing would, in large part, be covered through national health insurance. Delivery of care would, for most primary and secondary level services, come increasingly under the umbrella of health maintenance organizations (HMOs). In the transition process, the various categorical service programs would gradually diminish until their "market" of clients became too small to permit survival.

The well-baby examinations of a Health Department clinic or the venereal disease treatments of a youth-sponsored "free clinic" would be done in the HMO that served the total needs of these people, or by private practitioners in the non-HMO sector of each Health Region. To retain the benefits of public health nursing, health education, or epidemiological follow-up, personnel with these skills would be engaged by HMOs. Indeed these ancillary services of HMOs, not so feasible under the solo practice medical care model, would add strength to the movement for HMO expansion through the group provider model. The same sort of absorption of specialized services into a mainstream HMO movement would apply to mental health services, emergency care, family planning, and other categorical programs now permeating our pluralistic system. Emergency care would illustrate a class of service in which the Regional Health Authority could well promote coordinated actions among several HMOs.[39]

Regarding the existing voluntary health insurance plans, now engaged only in fiscal support and not in service delivery—the Blue plans and commercial carriers—the future role is not so clear. It would depend largely on the form of national health insurance that is enacted. As discussed earlier, these agencies under one approach would continue to operate and carry the risks (with mandatory enrollment of the population); under another approach they would serve simply as fiscal intermediaries (as under Medicare), without carrying insurance risks; under still another approach they would offer, as in Canada today, supplemental insurance benefits not offered by the statutory program.

Agencies of government engaged solely in fiscal support, such as state or local welfare departments (Medicaid), would presumably be relieved of all health-related responsibilities, once funds for their beneficiaries became available through a national mechanism. Other government agencies, like the Veterans Administration, would have little justification for health care financing or delivery, once their services were available equitably to all persons on a "hometown" basis. Workmen's compensation for industrial injuries, now entirely financed by employers, would make sense for cash benefits, but medical care for such cases should, as in Britain, be absorbed into the main health care system.

Absorption of current social control functions of governmental and voluntary bodies into the future realistic system may entail more complex dynamics. As noted earlier, we propose greater flexibility of state government professional licensure, as well as incorporation of these functions into State Health Departments. The standard setting and implementation of voluntary bodies, such as the Specialty Boards of the American Medical Association or the Joint Commission on Accreditation of Hospitals, on the other hand, belong properly within the purview of a National Department of Health. Indeed, this would be necessary if the national planning objectives, discussed earlier, are to achieve a rational distribution of all specialties, hospital facilities, etc., in relation to local population needs. Programs for quality promotion, such as the Regional Medical Program (RMP) — presumably to be eliminated in any case under the Presidential budget for 1973-1974 — would become absorbed into the regular functions of the Regional Health Authorities. Likewise for PSRO responsibilities.

Numerous voluntary health agencies would doubtless continue to operate either to provide supplemental services — for example, for mental health care — not adequately provided by the main system, or to serve as watchdogs in the sociopolitical arena. Likewise, there is no doubt that some few affluent persons would remain entirely outside an organized health care system — whether through HMOs or not — and seek care entirely in the private sector. With personal wealth, they would not hesitate to "pay twice" (once through national insurance or taxes and secondly through their own pockets), just as affluent families now send their children to private elementary schools, while public ones are freely available. If the public system has adequate resources and standards, the size of this private sector should gradually diminish and not entail serious inequities.

Everything depends, of course, on the general political climate of the coming decade. The assumption we make is that national health insurance of some type will largely, if not entirely, eliminate financial barriers to health care for virtually everyone. It will also provide the indispensable leverage for changing the delivery system to a more efficient and effective model.[40] By designing that system around HMOs, covering an increasing proportion of the U.S. population and operating within a framework of Regional Health Authorities, we believe that such a system would constitute a politically realistic blend of rational planning and local enterprise appropriate to American culture in the 1970s.

While prophecy is always hazardous, of one thing we can be quite certain. Whatever laws are passed will, with time, be amended as experience is gained. The American strategy in health services is to make a start, to render issues visible, and to count on the fact that problems tend to generate their own reforms. This has been the health service story of the past, and it will probably so continue in the future.

NOTES

1. Anderson, Odin, "Planning Health Services, American Style," *Med. Care*, Vol. 7, pp. 345-347, Sept.-Oct. 1969.

2. McNerney, Walter J., "Health Care Reforms—The Myths and Realities," *Am. J. Public Health*, Vol. 61, pp. 222-232, Feb. 1971.

3. Roemer, Milton I., " 'Socialized' Health Services in Saskatchewan," *Social Research*, Vol. 25, pp. 87-101, Spring 1958.

4. Lerner, Monroe, and Odin Anderson, *Health Progress in the United States 1900-1966*, Chicago: University of Chicago Press, 1961.

5. Ellwood, Paul M., Jr., "Health Maintenance Organizations: Concept and Strategy," *Hospitals*, Vol. 45, pp. 53-56, March 16, 1971.

6. Myers, Robert J., *Medicare*, Homewood, Illinois: Richard D. Irwin, 1970.

7. McNerney, Walter J. and Donald C. Riedel, *Regionalization and Rural Health Care*, Ann Arbor: University of Michigan, 1962.

8. Roseman, Cyril, "Problems and Prospects for Comprehensive Health Planning," *Am. J. Public Health*, Vol. 62, pp. 16-19, Jan. 1972.

9. U.S. National Advisory Commission on Health Manpower, *Report*, Washington, D.C.: Government Printing Office, 1967.

10. U.S. Dept. of H.E.W., Public Health Service, *Health Resources Statistics: Health Manpower and Health Facilities, 1971*, Washington, Feb. 1972.

11. Hershey, Nathan, "An Alternative to Mandatory Licensure of Health Professionals," *Hospital Progress*, Vol. 50, p. 73, March 1969.

12. "Health Personnel Will Be Assigned to Critical Manpower-Lacking Areas," *Medical Tribune*, June 28, 1972.

13. Coggeshall, Lowell T., *Planning for Medical Progress through Education*, Evanston, Illinois: Association of American Medical Colleges, 1965. Also: Citizens Commission on Graduate Medical Education (John S. Millis, Chairman), *The Graduate Education of Physicians*, Chicago: American Medical Association, 1966.

14. Roemer, Milton I., "Health Needs and Services of the Rural Poor" in *Rural Poverty in the United States*, Washington: National Commission on Rural Poverty, 1968, pp. 311-332.

15. Center for Health Administration Studies, *Public Control and Hospital Operations*, Chicago: University of Chicago (Fourteenth Annual Symposium on Hospital Affairs), 1972.

16. U.S. Senate, Subcommittee on Monopoly, *Task Force on Prescription Drugs: Report and Recommendations*, Washington, 1968.

17. U.S. Dept. of H.E.W., *A Report to the President on the Research Programs of the National Institutes of Health*, Washington, 1967.

18. Ellwood, Paul M., Jr., "Implications of Recent Health Legislation," *Am. J. Public Health*, Vol. 62, pp. 20-23, Jan. 1972.

19. MacLeod, Gordon K. and Jeffrey A. Prussin, "The Continuing Evolution of Health Maintenance Organizations," *New Engl. J. Med.*, March 1, 1973.

20. Public Law 92-603, *Social Security Amendments of 1972*, 92nd Congress, H.R. 1, Oct. 30, 1972.

21. American Public Health Association, "Health Maintenance Organizations: A Policy Paper," *Am. J. Public Health*, Vol. 61, pp. 2528-2536, Dec. 1971.

22. Roemer, Milton I., Statement before U.S. House of Representatives, Subcommittee on Public Health and Environment, *Hearings on Health Maintenance Organizations,* Part 2, Washington, Apr. 1972, pp. 567-594.

23. Shain, Max and Milton I. Roemer, "Hospitals and the Public Interest," *Public Health Reports,* Vol. 76, pp. 401-410, May 1961.

24. Anderson, O. E., J. H. Young, and W. F. Janssen, "The Government and the Consumer: Evaluation of Food and Drug Laws," *Journal of Public Law,* Vol. 13, pp. 189-221, 1964.

25. U.S. Senate Special Committee on Aging, *Long-term Institutional Care for the Aged,* Washington: U.S. Government Printing Office, 88th Congress, First Session, 1964.

26. Ross, Leonard, "The Urgent Need to Control the Quality of Prepaid Plans for Medical Care," *Los Angeles Times,* 25 January 1973.

27. Somers, Anne R., *Health Care in Transition: Directions for the Future,* Chicago: Hospital Research and Educational Trust, 1971.

28. U.S. Dept. of H.E.W., Health Maintenance Organization Service, *HMOs Financial Planning Manual,* Washington (undated), c. 1972.

29. Klarman, Herbert E., "Analysis of the HMO Proposal — Its Assumptions, Implications, and Prospects" in *Health Maintenance Organizations: A Reconfiguration of the Health Services System,* Chicago: University of Chicago Center for Health Administration Studies, 1971, pp. 24-38. See also Roemer, Milton I. and William Shonick, "HMO Performance: The Recent Evidence," *Health and Society,* Vol. 51, pp. 271-317, Summer 1973.

30. See for example: U.S. Senate Committee on Finance, *National Health Insurance: Brief Outline of Pending Bills,* Washington, 1971.

31. Robins, Leonard, "The Impact of Decategorizing Federal Programs: Before and After 314 (d)," *Am. J. Public Health,* Vol. 62, pp. 24-29, Jan. 1972.

32. Mountin, Joseph W., *Selected Papers,* Washington: Joseph W. Mountin Memorial Committee, 1956.

33. Donabedian, Avedis, "Evaluating the Quality of Medical Care," *Milbank Mem. Fund. Q.,* Vol. 44, p. 166, Part 2, July 1966.

34. Roemer, Milton I., "Evaluation of Health Service Programs and Levels of Measurement," *HSMHA Health Reports,* Vol. 86, pp. 839-848, Sept. 1971.

35. Editorial, "PSROs — Implications for the Medical Profession," *The Hospital Medical Staff,* Vol. 1, No. 12, Dec. 1972 (reprint).

36. U.S. National Center for Health Services Research and Development, *Guidelines for Producing Uniform Data for Health Care Plans,* Washington: DHEW Pub. No. (HSM) 73-3005, July 1972.

37. National Advisory Commission on Health Facilities, *A Report to the President,* Washington, Dec. 1968.

38. Blumberg, Mark S., *Shared Services for Hospitals,* Chicago: American Hospital Association, 1966.

39. American Medical Association, *Categorization of Hospital Emergency Capabilities,* Chicago: the Association, 1972.

40. Roemer, Milton I., "Social Insurance as Leverage for Changing Health Care Systems: International Experience," *Bull. N.Y. Acad. Med.,* Vol. 48, pp. 93-107, Jan. 1973.

Appendixes

APPENDIX I

Table 1. Federal agencies supporting health training: expenditures and numbers of students and trainees aided, authorized fiscal year 1972

Agency	Expenditure ($ million)	Numbers						
		Total	Medicine	Dentistry and other Professions	Nursing	Para-medical	Research	Other Health Manpower
H.E.W.	768	176,153	19,238	20,632	34,370	1,193	15,225	85,495
Labor	125	62,585				62,585		
Veterans	116	53,115	21,799	5,510	17,406	8,400		
Defense	88	16,719	3,239	1,263	2,470	5,955		3,785
A.I.D.	6	18,182	3,263	2,567	861	6,291	48	5,152
Environmental Protection	8	8,151		1,566		50	2	6,533
Other Agencies	18	3,996	22	31	250	230	156	3,303

1. The category, "Other Agencies," includes the National Science Foundation, Atomic Energy Commission, Department of Housing and Urban Development, National Aeronautics and Space Agency, etc.

2. The category, "Other Health Manpower," includes environmental and public health manpower and a wide variety of specialized manpower.

Source: *Special Analyses—Budget of the U.S. Government*, f.y. 1972. Tables K-5, p. 154 and K-17, p. 173.

Table 2.   National health expenditures: selected fiscal years, 1929-1972 ($ Millions)

	1928-29	1949-50	1964-65	1971-72
Total	$3,589	$12,028	$38,892	$83,417
Percent of Gross National Product	3.6%	4.6%	5.9%	7.6%
Per capita	29.16	78.35	197.81	394.16
Public	477	3,065	9,535	32,857
Percent of Total	13.3%	25.5%	24.5%	39.4%
Federal	98	1,362	4,625	21,560
Percent of Public	21%	44%	49%	66%
State/Local	379	1,703	4,910	11,297
Percent of Public	79%	56%	51%	34%
Private	3,112	8,962	29,357	50,560
Percent of Total	86.7%	74.5%	75.5%	60.6%
Personal Health Care				
Expenditures—Total	3,165	10,400	33,498	71,862
Public	282	2,102	6,958	26,757
Federal	85	979	2,840	17,746
State/Local	197	1,123	4,118	9,011
Private	2,883	8,298	26,540	45,105
Consumer Direct Payments	2,800	7,107	17,577	25,070
Insurance Benefits	—	879	8,280	19,000
Other	83	312	683	1,035

Sources: Cooper and Worthington "National Health Expenditures," Social Security Bulletin, Jan. 1973, Tables 1, 6, and 7.

Table 3. Federal health expenditures, by function amounts and proportions: selected years ($ millions)

	1950	1960	1965	1969	1972	Projected 1974
Total	$1,362	$3,507	$5,160	$16,316	$24,531	$30,323
Health Resources	302	1,017	1,807	3,057	4,281	5,042
percent	22%	28.9%	35%	18.7%	17.4%	16.6%
Research	73	510	1,040	1,476	1,776	2,147
percent	5.3%	14.5%	20.1%	9.0%	7.2%	7.0%
Training	n.a.	217	317	841	1,110	1,293
percent		6.1%	6.1%	5.1%	4.5%	4.2%
Construction	229	290	450	595	867	943
percent	16.8%	8.2%	8.7%	3.6%	3.5%	3.1%
Organization and Delivery	n.a.	n.a.	n.a.	145	528	659
percent				0.8%	2.1%	2.1%
Provision of Services	970	2,165	4,232	12,517	19,439	24,234
percent	74.5%	61.7%	82%	76.7%	79.2%	79.9%
Direct Care	965	1,701	2,022	2,895	4,026	4,475
percent	74%	48.5%	39.1%	17.7%	16.4%	14.7%
Funding of Care — Indirect	5	464	2,210	9,622	15,413	19,759
percent	0.5%	13.2%	42.8%	58.9%	62.8%	61.8%
Prevention and Control	89	326	418	741	810	1,047
percent	6.5%	9.2%	8.1%	4.5%	3.3%	3.4%

Sources: *Special Analyses, Budget of the U.S. Government*, 1967 to 1974.

APPENDIX II

Programs for Provision of Services for Specific Diseases

Mental illness

Governmental Agencies and Programs

Federal	**State**	**Local***
Dept. of Defense		
—Care of Military		
—hospital and outpatient psychiatric treatment of military and dependents at Defense facilities		
—Naval Hospital and Dispensary, Fort McArthur Army Hospital		
—CHAMPUS		
—hospital and outpatient psychiatric services for dependents of military		
Dept. of Health, Education, and Welfare (HEW)	Health and Welfare Agency	
—Health Services and Mental Health Administration	—umbrella agency for State Dept. of Mental Hygiene and other health related departments	

*Local: refers to multicounty region, county, city, or special districts in Los Angeles County.

Mental illness

Federal	State	Local
— Regional Office of HEW — provides coordination for mental health programs — National Institute of Mental Health — in-house research; contracts and grants for research in mental health; grants for improvement of care in state supported mental hospitals; training grants, studies of manpower needs and direct training programs; construction, staffing grants for Community Mental Health Centers; staffing grants to expand and innovate child mental health services; administers parts of 314 (d) grants to states for mental health services; statistics on mental health patients and out-patient psychiatric services	State Dept. of Mental Hygiene[1] — Short-Doyle, Lanterman-Petris-Short Acts — administers state hospitals for the mentally ill; finances 2 neuropsychiatric institutes for research, training, and care; finances and reviews Short-Doyle funds for community mental health programs; sets standards; conducts research, educational and training programs; licenses psychiatric facilities for care of mentally ill, including some board and care homes — Citizens Advisory Council — advises on all aspects of mental health programs including rules and regulations; mediates disputes between state and counties	L.A. County Dept. of Mental Health[2] — prepares annual Short-Doyle plan for mental health services and funds; provides emergency outpatient and inpatient psychiatric services at regional and public hospitals, child guidance clinics; contracts for services with private and voluntary hospitals; screens admissions to state mental hospitals; contracts with community mental health centers to provide services — Mental Health Advisory Board — reviews annual County plans (submitted to County Board of Supervisors and State Department of Mental Hygiene) — Tri-City Mental Health Authority — provides services through agreement with Depts. of Mental Health, Hospitals, in Pomona, Claremont, and La Verne

[1] Incorporated into new Department of Health in Health Treatment Systems Program, as of July 1, 1973.
[2] Incorporated into new unified Los Angeles County Department of Health Services.

Mental illness

Federal

State

State Health Planning Council
— reviews State Plan for community mental health

California Conference of Local Mental Health Directors
— advisory to State Dept. of Mental Hygiene in setting standards for local mental health programs

UCLA Neuropsychiatric Institute
— center for research, training, and care of mental illness

Local

Interagency Committee on Mental Health
— informal advisory body of public and private agencies for mental health, on county plan for mental health

Community Mental Health Centers
— provide outpatient, emergency, inpatient services for mental health

Council of Mental Health Centers
— nonprofit association representing Community Mental Health Centers

L.A. County Health Dept.[2]
— operates joint mental health program to provide after care services to patients from mental hospitals; educational and preventive services

L.A. County Dept. of Hospitals[2]
— LAC-USC, Harbor General Hospitals; Olive View Hospital
— acute inpatient psychiatric care, psychiatric emergency services,

[2]Incorporated into new unified Los Angeles County Department of Health Services.

Mental illness

Federal	State	Local
		outpatient diagnostic care, treatment; centers for county mental health regions

—Antelope Valley Rehabilitation Center
  —long-term psycho-social rehabilitative care of male patients referred from county and state agencies

Psychiatric Court, Dept. 95 Superior Court
  —issues orders for evaluation of mentally disordered, chronic alcoholics, for contested 14-day intensive treatment of involuntary patients; hearings on post-certification treatment; appoints conservators

—Mental Health Counselor of Superior Court
  —visits patients held for 14 days; prepares and files petitions for evaluation and post certification treatment, screening; arranges

Mental illness

Federal

State

Local

conservatorships (by County Public Guardian)

County District Attorney
—Psychiatric Section represents people's interest in Dept. 95 of Superior Court in cases of civil insanity, mentally disordered sex offenders, alcoholic commitments and commitments to Cal. Narcotic Rehabilitation Center

L.A. County Public Administrator
—Public Guardian
—acts as guardian of persons under supervision of Psychiatric Court or in County institutions

County Probation Dept.
—operates 2 schools for emotionally disturbed girls; maintains psychiatric clinic at Juvenile Hall, places patients in and certifies homes

L.A. County Sheriff's Dept.
—authorizes emergency treatment and evaluation for involuntary patients;

Mental illness

State

Local

State Dept. of Public Health
—Bureau of Health Facilities Planning and Construction
  —approves funds and provides construction assistance to Community Mental Health Centers, state and county institutions

—Bureau of Health Facilities Licensing and Certification
  —licenses long-term psychiatric hospitals

responds to calls for assistance with disturbed persons

L.A. City Police Dept.
—responds to calls for assistance with disturbed persons, judges severity, transports to mental health facility for 72-hour evaluation by County Dept. of Mental Health or files petition with Superior Court

City Police Departments
—same functions performed by police departments in other cities in County

L.A. County Health Dept.
—Licensing Division
  —licenses mental health facilities in L.A. County by contract with State Dept. of Public Health

Mental illness

Federal

Community Health Service
— administers 314 (e) grants for comprehensive health centers and family health centers which provide preliminary mental health services

— Comprehensive Health Planning and Services
— reviews grants to states for 314 (a,b,c) funds, including mental health institutions and projects

— Migrant Health Service
— migrant health centers provide some mental health services

— Indian Health Service
— preventive and medical care for American Indians including mental illness provided at special facilities and through Indian community health programs

State

State Health Planning Council
— reviews State Plan for community mental health and applications for mental health facility construction

State Dept. of Public Health
— Office of Comprehensive Health Planning
— State Plan for Comprehensive Health Services; reviews, makes recommendations on, distributes 314 (a,b,c,e) health project grants for demonstration and training projects including mental health

State Health Planning Council
— reviews, makes recommendations on health project grant applications including mental health in California

Local

Regional Comprehensive Health Planning Agencies
— review, recommend on CHP grant applications

Comprehensive Health Planning Assn. of L.A. County
— reviews, acts on applications under CHP in L.A. County

13 projects throughout the State

Various Indian health aid projects in urban and rural areas, including 2 Indian Free Clinics

Mental illness

Federal	State	Local

— Federal Health Programs Service
  — administers PHS Hospitals—
    San Pedro in L.A. County; preventive
    services for large groups of
    federal employees including
    mental health diagnosis and
    some treatment
 	
— Maternal and Child Health
  Service
  — administers funds to states for
    MCH programs which include
    mentally ill; training grants for
    care
 	
— Health Care Facilities Service
  — Hill-Burton (Hill-Harris)
    — grants, loans, and loan
      guarantees for mental
      hospital construction and
      modernization; rehabilitation
      facilities, some to Community
      Mental Health Centers
	State Dept. of Public Health
	— Bureau of Maternal and Child
	  Health
	  — primary mental illness prevention
	    in maternal and child health
	    services and well child clinics
	  — Farm Workers Program
	    — direct health care services may
	      include mental health services
	— Bureau of Health Facilities Planning
	  and Construction
	  — sets priorities for psychiatric
	    hospitals, administers loans under
	    Hill-Burton
	
	California Rural Indian Board
	— Health services project
		L.A. County Health Dept.
		— Bureau of Maternal and Child
		  Health
		  — clinics, preschool screening to
		    prevent, detect mental illness

Mental illness

Federal

- Nat'l Institutes of Health
- Nat'l Inst. of Neurological Diseases and Stroke
  - specialized research on neurological disorders including those affecting mental health.
  e.g., epilepsy, muscular dystrophy, spinal cord injury, stroke

State

- Bureau of Health Facilities Licensing and Certification
  - Licenses long-term psychiatric hospitals, nursing homes and intermediate and other care facilities

- Office of Comprehensive Health Planning
  - advises SDPH on Hill-Burton

State Health Planning Council
  - reviews applications, advises SDPH on Hill-Burton, mental health facility construction

State Dept. of Mental Hygiene
  - receives research grants from NINDS

Local

Regional Comprehensive Health Planning Agencies
  - review, recommend on facility construction grants

Comprehensive Health Planning Assn. of L.A. County
  - reviews, acts on applications under CHP in L.A. County

L. A. Depts. of Hospitals and Mental Health and various community hospitals receive research grants from NINDS

Mental illness

Federal	State	Local

— Nat'l Inst. of Child Health and Human Development
  — research on behavioral problems; training
 	
— Office of Child Development
  — Bureau of Head Start and Early Childhood
  — financial assistance to local agencies to provide comprehensive preschool child development programs including medical and psychological screening and treatment
 	
— Office of Education
  — Bureau of Education for the Handicapped
  — special educational assistance for handicapped children including mentally disturbed
	Dept. of Education
	  — Instruction for the Educationally Disadvantaged Student
	  — Head Start preschool education program
	
	Dept. of Education
	  — Bureau of Special Education: Educationally Handicapped and Mentally Exceptional Children
	  — standards and funds for special classes and services to emotionally handicapped; Diagnostic Schools for the Neurologically Handicapped
		Community Action Agencies in Los Angeles, Compton, Long Beach, and Pasadena
		  — Head Start programs provide medical exams, follow-up care, and mental health services
		
		Diagnostic School for the Neurologically Handicapped, Southern California
		  — diagnosis of neurological disorders; education and treatment; training of professional personnel
		
		L.A. County Supt. of Schools
		  — supervises, coordinates special education programs in school districts within the county

Mental illness

Federal

—Social and Rehabilitation Service
—Assistance Payments Admin.
— public welfare assistance includes temporary care or hospitalization for needy mentally ill children and adults including continuing hospitalization for the aged

—Medical Services Admin.
—Medicaid
— medical care for the categorically and medically needy; payment for care for mentally ill over 65

State

State Dept. of Social Welfare
—administers state-federal welfare assistance programs, certifies facilities for recipients of federal disability payments; licenses certain residential care facilities

—Division of Community Service
— placement, follow-up, after care services to patients discharged from community mental health centers

State Dept. of Health Care Services
—Medi-Cal
— provides funds, supervises program of categorically and

Local

L.A. City Unified School Dist.
—Mental Health Services Section and PTA Guidance Clinics
— conducts clinics in 5 districts, upon referral from school nurses or administrators for diagnostic and outpatient services

Mental illness

Federal	State	Local

medically indigent including funds for AFDC children requiring care, including mentally disturbed

State Dept. of Health Care Services
— Regional Office
— supervises Medi-Cal program in County, particularly Prior Authorization

State Dept. of Social Welfare
—supervises Medi-Cal eligibility determination

State Dept. of Public Health
— Bureau of Health Facilities Licensing and Certification
— certifies facilities for Medi-Cal participation including mental facilities

L.A. County Dept. of Public Social Services
—eligibility determination for Medi-Cal; placement in board and care facility or rehabilitation after release from mental health institutions

Mentalillness

Federal

— Community Services Admin.
— grants to states to provide
services to totally and
permanently mentally and
emotionally disabled, including
care of AFDC children,
placements in community
institutions

State

State Dept. of Social Welfare
— administers state-federal welfare
assistance programs, which may
include mentally ill children

State Dept. of Mental Hygiene
— Alternative Care Services Unit
— placement, follow-up care services
to patients from mental health
centers

Local

L.A. County Dept. of Public Social
Services
— ATD program of cash assistance
available for mental illness;
placement in board and care
facilities or rehabilitation after
release from mental institutions

— Protective Services Division
— intervenes in child abuse,
deprivation; placement for
emotionally disturbed children, or
if parents are emotionally
disturbed

Mental illness

Federal	State	Local

— Rehabilitation Services Admin.
  —grants to states for rehabilitation of mentally retarded, mentally, emotionally, and physically disabled
	Dept. of Rehabilitation
	  —rehabilitation for mentally ill including diagnosis, training, counseling; cooperative program with Depts. of Youth Authority and Corrections
		Fiscal Intermediaries

— Social Security Admin.
  —OASDHI
    — cash benefits to aged and disabled covers long-term disability, including mentally ill
  — District Offices
    — provide preliminary certification under OASDHI
	Dept. of Rehabilitation
	  — determines eligibility of disability benefits under contract with SSA	

— Bureau of Health Insurance
  — Medicare
    — hospital insurance payments for institutional care for mental illness in eligible psychiatric hospitals or psychiatric wards of general hospital		

— Food and Drug Admin. — tests, regulates drugs and devices used in treatment of mentally ill		

Mental illness

Federal	State	Local
Dept. of Housing and Urban Development —assistance through mortgage insurance of nursing homes, Model Cities' health centers, public hospital facilities, aid to housing of elderly and handicapped which may include service to mental patients or their aftercare		South Central Multipurpose Health Services Center
Office of Economic Opportunity —Office of Health Affairs — Neighborhood Health Centers provide some mental health care		
Small Business Administration —loans to privately owned hospitals, convalescent homes, including mental institutions		
Veterans Administration —inpatient clinic, outpatient services, and domiciliary care of mentally ill veterans; placement in community facilities		

Mental illness

Federal	State	Local
	Dept. of Veterans Affairs — care of Sick and Disabled Veterans psychiatric care included in care provided at Veterans Home California Youth Authority — admits wards to state mental hospitals for diagnosis, returns youths for rehabilitation and psychiatric follow-up Dept. of Corrections — Medical Services Division — psychiatric diagnosis and care of prisoners in correctional institutions — Parole and Community Services Division — psychiatric follow-up service for parolees including their families	

Mental illness

Selected Voluntary Organizations and Programs

Federal	State	Local
Nat'l Assn. for Mental Health —research into causes, treatment, cure and prevention of mental disease; bring about humane and beneficial legislation; community services; public and professional education Nat'l Committee against Mental Illness	California Assn. for Mental Health —coordinates similar activities at state level	Mental Health Assn. of L.A. County —promotes citizen support for mental health programs Council of Community Mental Health Centers Mental Health Development Commission —provides planning, coordination, and study among voluntary and public mental health agencies; conducts special studies and demonstrations for improved community mental health services and facilities Los Angeles Welfare Planning Council Welfare Information Service —Mental Health Resources Consultation Unit —program of special consultation on mental health problems and

Mental illness

Federal	State	Local
American Mental Health Foundation —research on better, less expensive methods for prevention and treatment of mental illness; advocates public understanding of mental illness and reforms in the selection of practitioners, professional education, and other aspects of mental health Recovery, Inc. —association of former mental patients and those with nervous disorders who meet for training in self-help aftercare		resources; education for professionals, patients, and families; publishes bulletin on out-patient psychiatric services Recovery, Inc., Greater Los Angeles District —groups for training in self-help aftercare

Mental retardation

Governmental Agencies and Programs

Federal	State	Local*
Office of the President	Health and Welfare Agency	
—President's Committee on Mental Retardation	—Office of Mental Retardation[1]	
— coordinates mental retardation activities of agencies; advises President on mental retardation	— coordinates mental retardation programs of state agencies; adopts standards, rules and regulations; prescribes payments; maintains	
Dept. of HEW		
—Secretary's Office of Mental Retardation Coordination		
— coordinates and evaluates HEW mental retardation activities, programs, policies, procedures; liaison with President's Committee		
— Mental Retardation Inter-agency Committee		
— composed of representatives of operating programs on mental retardation to provide communication, information		

*Local: refers to multicounty reg on, county, city, or special districts in Los Angeles County

[1]In 1973, changed to Office of Special Services—Developmental Disabilities Program.

Mental retardation

Federal	State	Local
exchange, and program development for agencies concerned with mental retardation —Health Services and Mental Health Administration — Nat'l Inst of Mental Health —hospital and staffing improvement grants, support of community care of mentally retarded, innovations for services to children	list of approved facilities; adopts state plan for retarded care (State Developmental Disabilities Planning and Advisory Council: —advises Sec'y of Human Relations Agency and State Health Planning Council on Mental Retardation programs and plan) State Dept. of Mental Hygiene —administers state hospitals for the mentally retarded; sets standards, licenses homes and resident facilities, conducts research, educational and training programs State Health Planning Council —reviews Dept. of Mental Hygiene's plans for community mental health and mental retardation, applications for mental health and facilities for the Developmentally Disabled construction	Long Beach Child Development Clinic —interagency clinic of Health Dept. for diagnosis of mental retardation in children under 5 with referral Comprehensive Health Planning Assn. of L.A. County —Mental Health – Mental Retardation Committee —advisory and planning for health agencies on health needs and priorities and assists review of facilities construction

Mental retardation

Federal

Regional Office of HEW
—coordinates mental retardation programs of federal agencies; provides information to Secretary's Office of M.R. Coordination

State

State Dept. of Public Health
—Bureau of Mental Retardation Services
   —maintains 14 Regional Mental Retardation Centers for services to mentally retarded

State Dept. of Social Welfare
—provides protective services and out-of-home placements for mentally retarded; certifies family care homes

Dept. of Rehabilitation
—cooperative program with State Dept. of Mental Hygiene for vocational rehabilitation counselors in state hospitals for the mentally retarded

Local

Regional Mental Retardation Program Board (Regional Developmental Disabilities Board)

Regional Center for the Mentally Retarded—operated by Children's Hospital of Los Angeles

L.A. County Dept. of Public Social Services
—placement for retarded children in residential care facilities

Mental retardation

Federal	State	Local
— Maternal and Child Health Service	State Dept. of Public Health	L.A. County Health Dept.
— administers funds to states for MCH and Crippled Children's programs: grants for staffing of mental retardation facilities, funds for improved institutional care, support of community care of retarded, research and training grants	— Bureau of Maternal and Child Health	— Bureau of Maternal and Child Health
	— conducts PKU testing program for detection of mental retardation; rubella prevention vaccination program	— operates special mental retardation clinics in 6 health districts, covers entire county in cooperation with Regional Mental Retardation Center in providing diagnosis and evaluation for children under 5; consults with physicians and parents
	— Crippled Children's Services	
	— sets standards for providers, arranges for provision of services for medically indigent, diagnosis, treatment, therapy	L.A. County Dept. of Hospitals
		— principal agent for Crippled Children's Service programs in County
— Health Care Facilities Service	State Dept. of Public Health	
— Hill-Burton	— Bureau of Health Facilities Planning and Construction	
— grants, loans, and loan guarantees for mental retardation facilities' construction and modernization; also for rehabilitation facilities	— approves funds and provides technical assistance in state and county institutions	L.A. County Health Dept.
		— Licensing Division
	— Bureau of Health Facilities Licensing and Certification	— licenses establishments for the handicapped and retarded children
	— licenses facilities for day care of mentally retarded	

Mental retardation

Federal	State	Local

Federal

—Nat'l Institutes of Health
 —Nat'l Inst of Neurological Disease and Stroke
  —research in mental retardation in connection with diseases of the nervous system; research in prenatal and postnatal factors related to development of children; training

—Nat'l Institutes of Health
 —Nat'l Inst. of Child Health and Human Development
  —research on mental retardation; supports mental retardation research centers, researchers, and training

—Office of Education
 —Bureau of Education for the Handicapped
  —special educational assistance for handicapped children

State

State Dept. of Mental Hygiene
 —Mental Retardation Hospitals
  —conducts research through grants from NINDS

UCLA Neuropsychiatric Institute
 —University affiliated Research Center
  —conducts Mental Retardation Research Program under grants from NINDS and NICH&HD

Dept. of Education
 —Bureau of Special Education
  —Educationally Handicapped and Mentally Exceptional Children
   —standards and funds for special

Local

County Superintendent of Schools
 —Special Education Programs and Classes
  —intermediary between State Dept. of Education and school districts.

Mental retardation

Federal	State	Local
including mentally retarded, learning disabled, and multihandicapped	classes and services to handicapped	in developing curricula for special education programs for handicapped—educable or trainable mentally retarded; runs Development Center for Handicapped Minors
(Nat'l Advisory Comm. on Handicapped Children —training teachers for handicapped)	Dept. of Rehabilitation —cooperative program with Dept. of Education for special education programs in school districts	
—Division of Research —establishes libraries for the handicapped; research programs; demonstration projects		
—Vocational and Technical Education —provides vocational education material and assistance for handicapped		
—Social and Rehabilitation Service —Assistance Payments Admin. —welfare assistance grants to states for categorically needy: mental retardation an eligibility factor in Aid to the Totally Disabled	State Dept. of Social Welfare —administers state-federal welfare assistance programs including ATD covering mentally retarded	County Dept. of Public Social Services —provides, contracts for services for Aid for the Totally Disabled —AFDC eligibility, social services, day care, placement for retarded children in residential care facilities

Mental retardation

Federal	State	Local

— Community Services Admin.
  —Child Welfare Services
    —services to AFDC recipients including mentally retarded: day care services, foster care, prenatal services to mothers to reduce incidence of mental retardation
 	
— Medical Services Admin.
  —Medicaid
    —medical care for categorically and medically needy; intermediate care, board and care, and public facilities used for mentally retarded
	State Dept. of Social Welfare
	  —administers AFDC program including protective services, out-of-home placement, certification of family care homes for mentally retarded
	
	(State Dept. of Mental Hygiene
	  —Alternate Care Services Unit
	    —has taken over placement and certification functions)
	
	Dept. of Health Care Services
	  —Medi-Cal
	    —provides funds and supervises program for categorically and medically indigent including funds to ATD mentally retarded eligibles and AFDC children requiring care
	    —provides prior authorization for services locally through Regional Office	

Mental retardation

Federal

— Rehabilitation Services Admin.
— Division of Developmental Disabilities
— grants to states for rehabilitation of mentally retarded or disabled; funds for professional personnel, new facilities, hospital improvement, training

State

State Dept. of Public Health
— Bureau of Mental Retardation Services
— maintains 14 regional mental retardation centers for diagnostic, counseling, and social services; contracts with agencies for services; establishes payments, performs guardianship services, hospitalization referral, care of mentally retarded discharged from state hospital; reviews project applications for mental retardation services in private sector

— Crippled Children's Service
— diagnosis, treatment; sets standards for providers; arranges for provision of services for medically indigent

Local

L.A. County Dept. of Public Social Services
— Medi-Cal eligibility determination for dependent children; placement for retarded in residential care facilities

Regional Mental Retardation Program Board
— operates or contracts with agencies for operation of regional center, develops service plan, coordinates and develops public and private facilities

Regional Center for the Mentally Retarded — Children's Hospital of Los Angeles
— counseling, diagnosis, pre-admission screening to state mental retardation hospitals, develops plan, purchases residential care, day care, medical services

L.A. County Dept. of Hospitals
— provides diagnosis and arranges treatment under CCS program

Mental retardation

Federal	State	Local
—Vocational Rehabilitation Services 　• grants to states for vocational rehabilitation of mentally retarded; facility improvement and training —Office of Research and Planning 　—research, planning, and evaluation; training for rehabilitation programs for mentally retarded —Social Security Admin. 　—OASDHI 　　—cash benefits to disabled cover long-term disability including mental retardation	Dept. of Rehabilitation 　—vocational rehabilitation programs for mentally retarded who are "educable" including diagnosis, training and counseling; provides vocational rehabilitation counselors to Regional Mental Retardation Centers; certifies workshops for mentally retarded Dept. of Rehabilitation 　—rehabilitation services to disabled including mentally retarded under Vocational Rehabilitation Program 　—determines state of disability under	

Mental retardation

Federal	State	Local
	OASDHI under contract with Social Security Administration	

Social Security Admin. District Offices
— preliminary certification of disability under OASDHI

Food and Drug Administration
— investigates drugs to prevent and treat conditions causing mental retardation

Dept. of Defense
— care of military
— hospital and outpatient psychiatric treatment of military and dependents at federal facilities, including mentally retarded

Veterans Administration
— care of mentally retarded veterans

Mental retardation

Selected Voluntary Organizations and Programs

Federal	State	Local
National Association for Retarded Children —program to improve the welfare of retarded persons and to promote a united attack on problems; research and education program for the public and for professionals	California Association for the Retarded —member of coordinating committee of State departments concerned with mental retardation	Exceptional Children's Foundation —provides training for mentally retarded children not accepted for special education by public schools; promotes coordinated system of workshops for training the retarded in L.A. County
	California Association for Neurologically Handicapped Children —assistance to children of substantially normal intelligence who have learning, perceptual, and behavioral disorders due to neurological impairment or brain dysfunction	California Association for Neurologically Handicapped Children—L.A. Chapter —distributes information on the neurologically handicapped child to public and professionals; promotes establishment of parent groups for helping children and for self-help; maintains speakers' bureau; provides scholarships to accredited teachers interested in the neurologically handicapped child
	California Council for Retarded Children —promotes welfare and education of mentally retarded children and adults	L.A. County Council for Retarded Children and Adults —Mental Retardation Information and Referral Service —information and referral service

Mental retardation

Federal	State	Local
American Association on Mental Deficiency —promotes welfare of mentally retarded persons; research on causes, treatment and prevention of mental retardation; publishes directory of residential facilities		for specific needs of mentally retarded; general information on mental retardation and on recreational programs for those over 16 Kennedy Child Study Center
National Rehabilitation Assn. —research, promotion, programs in rehabilitation of all disabled, including mentally retarded		
National Assn. of Sheltered Workshops and Homebound Programs —promotes sheltered workshops, rehabilitation programs	California Conference of Workshops for the handicapped	Sheltered Workshops —provide training and education for mentally retarded in sheltered workshops and training and development centers

Alcoholism

Governmental Agencies and Programs

Federal	State	Local*

Dept. of Health, Education, and Welfare — Health Services and Mental Health Administration
— Nat'l Inst. of Mental Health
— Nat'l Institute on Alcohol Abuse and Alcoholism
  — develops and conducts comprehensive health, education, training, research, and planning activities for prevention, treatment, and rehabilitation of alcoholics; formula grants to states, project grants to public and private agencies, community mental health centers
	Health and Welfare Agency
	— Office of Alcoholism[1]
	  —oversees and coordinates state alcoholism programs; develops state plan, budget
		L.A. County Health Dept.
		— Coordinator of Alcohol Programs
		  — coordinates county alcohol programs and voluntary and public agencies

	Dept. of Mental Hygiene
	— Division of Local Programs
	  — consultant to county and voluntary agencies on alcoholism; treats chronic alcoholics in state mental hospitals; supervises Short-Doyle outpatient clinics which may treat alcoholics; research
		County Dept. of Mental Health
		  — emergency treatment, screening and referrals to Diagnostic, Evaluation and Referral Centers for voluntary patients, sponsors voluntary rehabilitation for chronic alcoholics; contracts for services with Community Mental Health Centers

— Nat'l Advisory Council on Alcohol Abuse and Alcoholism
  — advises, consults; reviews and
		Community Mental Health Centers
		  — psychiatric treatment which may include alcoholism as a factor in mental illness

		Los Angeles County Committee on Alcoholism — advisory to Board of Supervisors and

*Local: refers to multicounty region, county, city or special districts in Los Angeles County.
[1]1973. Office of Special Services — Alcoholism Program.

Alcoholism

Federal	State	Local
recommends on project grants; research, information to agencies and public		County Health Department on alcoholism
		L.A. County Depts. of Health and Mental Health — joint program for mental treatment and diagnosis including alcoholism
	State Dept. of Public Health — Bureau of Health Facilities Licensing and Certification — licenses alcoholic hospitals and rehabilitation facilities	
	Dept. of Rehabilitation — McAteer Alcoholism Program — alcoholic rehabilitation plans, research; assists other departments; plans community rehabilitation programs, reviews and helps finance local programs, provides vocational rehabilitation restorative services, training, maintenance and job placement	L.A. County Health Dept. — Alcoholic Rehabilitation Clinic, joint program of State Dept. of Public Health and State Dept. of Rehabilitation, providing medical care for alcoholism including antabuse, social work, education, rehabilitation counseling, referrals to halfway houses, furnishes services to rehabilitation centers

Alcoholism

Federal	State	Local
		— Diagnostic, Evaluation and Referral center (DER) — joint program with State Dept. of Rehabilitation provides diagnosis evaluation, and referral to proper agency; some counseling — Harbor Light Clinic Alcoholism Program — joint program with Salvation Army provides medical service, counseling, residence, and meals for indigents Dept. of Hospitals — detoxification at LAC-USC Medical Center; inpatient treatment at Long Beach General, Harbor General and El Cerritos Hospitals; joint program with State Dept. of Rehabilitation on rehabilitation: rehabilitation at Antelope Valley Rehabilitation Centers L.A. City Receiving Hospital — sedation; sends alcoholics to County Hospital, mental wards, or jail

Alcoholism

Federal	State	Local
— Indian Health Service — collaborative program with NIAAA, Bureau of Indian Affairs (Dept. of Interior), OEO, Social and Rehabilitation Service, funding Indian community alcoholism programs including research and treatment — Social and Rehabilitation Service — Rehabilitation Services Admin. — grants to states for rehabilitation programs, including alcoholism		Long Beach Health Dept. — special medical care and counseling program for alcoholics Pasadena Health Dept. — maintains alcoholism center for medication, counseling therapy for alcoholics; emergency center for detoxification and acute treatment of alcholics Indian Lodge, L.A. County — provides alcoholism program for Indians in County (services also at Indian Free Clinics)

Alcoholism

Federal	State	Local

— Community Services Admin.
  — grants to states to provide services to disabled under ATD and dependent children (AFDC)
 	
— Medical Services Admin.
  — Medicaid
  — payment for medical care for the categorically and medically needy
	State Dept. of Rehabilitation
	  — rehabilitation services provided under Vocational Rehabilitation including alcoholics
	
	State Dept. of Social Welfare
	  — welfare assistance to alcoholics who have dependent children or other disabling conditions due to alcoholism; provides referral service and case finding; licenses board and care facilities
	
	Dept. of Health Care Services
	  — Medi-Cal
	  — payments to private providers for medically needy alcoholics eligible for medical assistance
	
	Dept. of Social Welfare
	  — Medi-Cal eligibility determination
		L.A. County Dept. of Public Social Services
		  — counseling and general relief, through unattached men's center for male alcoholics, referral to DER; supports halfway houses; refers to ATD if unemployable, determines ATD, AFDC eligibility; licenses board and care facilities
		
		Half-way Houses
		  — board and room facilities, some supervised medication; AA meetings

Alcoholism

Federal	State	Local
		L.A. County Health Dept. — Licensing Division — performs licensing functions for State Dept. of Public Health
		Community Action Agencies —serve alcoholics
	State Dept. of Public Health — Bureau of Health Facilities Licensing and Certification — certifies facilities for Medi-Cal participation; licenses alcoholic rehabilitation and hospital facilities and laboratories for testing for alcoholism	
	Business and Transportation Agency — Office of Transportation Safety Coordinator — coordinates activities of state and local agencies in highway safety in which alcoholism is a factor; reviews grants for projects; develops legislation and methods to reduce alcohol-caused accidents	
Office of Economic Opportunity — Division of Alcoholism, Addiction and Mental Health Services — project grants to community agencies to discover and treat alcoholism and promote rehabilitation		
Dept. of Transportation — Federal Highway Admin. — Nat'l Highway Safety Bureau — research grants to states to develop comprehensive highway safety programs including alcoholism; alcoholism related projects in education, identification of drinkers, referral for treatment		

Alcoholism

	Federal	State	Local
		Dept. of Motor Vehicles — identifies alcoholic drivers; monitors violations, revokes or suspends licenses of alcoholics	L.A. County Sheriff's Dept. — alcoholic inmates detoxified and given treatment; AA and YMCA group discussions at Central County Jail
		California Highway Patrol — involved in Dept. of Transportation highway safety study of alcoholism and safety; apprehends and refers drunk drivers	So. Cal. Permanente Medical Group — program for federal employees for treatment, antabuse, nutrition, and counseling of alcoholics under contract for U.S. Civil Service Commission
	U.S. Civil Service Commission — develops prevention, treatment, and rehabilitation program among federal civilian employees		
	Veterans Administration — comprehensive health services to veterans including alcoholism at Veterans' facilities	Dept. of Education — Div. of Health Education — consultation and educational materials to school districts on alcoholism, drug abuse	

Alcoholism

State	Federal	Local
	Dept. of Corrections — conducts some rehabilitation for alcoholics, including voluntary AA meetings, group and individual therapy; 20 bed pilot program **Dept. of Youth Authority** — counseling and voluntary AA available at some institutions **Dept. of Employment** — State Disability — medical benefits payments for disability insurance claims resulting from alcoholism **Dept. of Justice** — California Council on Criminal Justice — Narcotics, Drug and Alcohol Abuse Task Force — evaluates state and local programs for control and prevention of alcohol abuse; funds local programs dealing with alcoholism	**L.A. County Superior Court** — recommends persons for treatment **County Probation Dept.** — arranges treatment and counseling for parolees **County Adult Authority** — arranges counseling and education for alcoholics **County Dept. of Personnel** — emergency and crisis medication for alcoholic county employees; counseling and follow-up

Alcoholism

Selected Voluntary Organizations and Programs

Federal	State	Local
National Council on Alcoholism — program for control and prevention of alcoholism through education; community services; promotion of research; provides services for a broad public health program on a national level Alcoholics Anonymous (A.A.) — provides services to help treat alcoholics and for community services — Al-Anon — provides services for family groups, relatives, and friends of alcoholics		Local Councils on Alcoholism — Alcohol Council of Greater Los Angeles — education, information, and referral, direct service to industry in establishing programs; coordination of community resources for alcoholics; publishes directory of community resources — Pasadena Council on Alcoholism — public education; training of personnel; casefinding, information and referral; encouragement of industry programs; coordination services A.A. Central Office publishes directory of meetings and provides information on groups located in L.A. County — A.A. groups for alcoholics — Al-Anon family groups — Alateen groups for children of alcoholics

Alcoholism

Federal	State	Local
American Council on Alcoholic Problems — education for prevention of alcoholism	California Council on Alcoholic Problems — education for prevention of alcoholism	Salvation Army, Divisional Headquarters for Southern California — supervises all program services and institutions in Southern California, including those for alcoholics — Harbor Light Center for Alcoholics provides treatment and rehabilitation of alcoholics, including alcoholic clinics and follow-up services; employment counseling and placement and contacts with families CARD (Counselors on Alcoholism and Related Disorders) — organization of recovered alcoholics and others working with alcoholics Private Hospitals — provide various kinds of treatment for alcoholism including detoxification, counseling, psychiatric treatment

Drug abuse

Governmental Agencies and Programs

Federal	State	Local*

Office of the President
—Special Action Office for Drug Abuse Prevention
  — coordinates programs on drug abuse in federal agencies
 	
Nat'l Advisory Council on Drug Abuse and Dangerous Drugs
—advises Special Action Office for Drug Abuse Prevention, approves, evaluates drug abuse grant programs
 	
(**Commission on Marijuana and Drug Abuse:**
—joint congressional and presidential appointed commission published findings of study and recommendations in 1972)
 	
Dept. of Health, Education, and Welfare (HEW)
—Office of the Secretary provides coordination program
	California Interagency Council on Drug Abuse
	—advisory to the Governor on narcotics and dangerous drug abuse; proposes programs
	
	Health and Welfare Agency
	—Office of Narcotics and Drug Abuse[1]
	  — coordinates interdepartmental activities in drug abuse, develops	

*Local: refers to multicounty region, county, city, or special districts in Los Angeles County.

[1]In 1973, changed to Office of Special Services—Narcotics and Drug Abuse Program.

Drug abuse

Federal	State	Local
evaluation, and recommends on control of drugs	state plan, promotes research and legislation; assists state and local agencies in developing programs	County Interdepartmental Committee on Drug Abuse —coordinating committee plans, evaluates county drug abuse programs
— Health Services and Mental Health Administration — Division of Narcotics Addiction and Drug Abuse — maintains 2 hospitals and clinical research centers for diagnosis, treatment, and rehabilitation of narcotics addicts under civil commitment	Dept. of Mental Hygiene —operates specialized programs at 2 state hospitals, treatment at 7 hospitals, funds methadone clinics, local programs providing services to drug patients; research; evaluates treatment programs; inservice training programs, funds several drug abuse education and prevention programs throughout the state	County Dept. of Mental Health —consultation and technical assistance to public and voluntary agencies involved in drug abuse control; contracts with Community Mental Health Centers for service to drug abusers
— Narcotics Rehabilitation Branch —grants to community agencies for staffing of treatment and rehabilitation programs; contracts with local agencies for after care services to patients, vocational	Dept. of Public Health —maintains resource file of information on drug abuse, provides technical consultation to, supports drug abuse projects, conducts health education on drug abuse, licenses drug manufacturers	County Dept. of Hospitals —LAC-USC, Harbor General Hospitals provide emergency detoxification and medical care County Health Dept. —maintains clinics for out-patient detoxification, group therapy, medical assistance; inservice training, education

Drug abuse

Federal

rehabilitation; staffing grants to 23 special narcotic addict treatment centers to provide detoxification, institutional and after-care services

State

Dept. of Rehabilitation
—vocational rehabilitation of drug addicts, by contract in halfway houses, in conjunction with other agencies, e.g., with Model Cities Program in Watts

Dept. of Corrections
—maintains California Rehabilitation Center and outpatient clinics for addicts; also half-way houses for addicts committed to the Department; conducts research; checks parolees

California Youth Authority
—establishes narcotic treatment control units in correctional

Local

County Dept. of Community Services
—community education, referral to assist addicts and families in obtaining detoxification, rehabilitation, counseling, jobs; consultations to establish drug abuse programs

County Dept. of Community Services
—Commission on Youth
—advisory to Board of Supervisors

Local

Dept. of HEW Regional Office
—coordinates HEW drug abuse programs

Drug abuse

Federal	State	Local
	institutions; experimental community control programs, research, information	on problems of youth including narcotic addiction sponsors education and planning
	Narcotic Addict Evaluation Authority —independent body within Dept. of Corrections and Youth Authority, responsible for releasing patients to out-patient status —Narcotics Rehabilitation Advisory Council 　—advises governor and officials concerning treatment of addicts; reports annually on studies at California Rehabilitation Center	L.A. City Unified School Dist. and other school districts —drug education programs in health education
—Office of Education 　—Office of Communications 　　—drug abuse education program in schools and communities through project grants, training teams	Dept. of Education —compiles and evaluates drug abuse education projects in the state, with State Dept. of Public Health; consultations with school districts on drug programs; training of educational personnel and community representatives	

Drug abuse

Federal	State	Local
Office of Education	California State University and Colleges	
— Division of Manpower and Training	—teach courses, conduct seminars on drug abuse	
— administers grants to educational institutions for courses in prevention, treatment and rehabilitation	University of California	
Nat'l Action Committee	— Drug Abuse Information Project; Neuropsychiatric Institutes conduct research on use and prevention of drug abuse	
— advisory committee providing technical assistance to drug abuse programs; evaluation		
Social and Rehabilitation Service		
— Rehabilitation Services Admin.		
— grants to states for special rehabilitation projects for drug addicts; vocational rehabilitation program includes drug addicts		
— Medical Services Admin.	Dept. of Health Care Services	
— Medicaid provides payment for medical care for the categorically and medically indigent	— Medi-Cal	
	— drug addicts who are eligible receive medical care assistance under Medi-Cal	

Drug abuse

Federal	State	Local
		L.A. County Dept. of Public Social Services—determines eligibility for Medi-Cal
	State Dept. of Social Welfare —Medi-Cal eligibility determination	
	California State Board of Pharmacy —establishes standards for filling narcotics prescriptions; inspects records; examines, licenses and regulates the transportation, distribution, and prescription of controlled drugs and narcotics; provides drug information to colleges	
Dept. of Justice —Bureau of Narcotics and Dangerous Drugs —control of illegal narcotics supplies and regulation of legal trade in drugs; training program for law enforcement officers	Dept. of Justice —Bureau of Narcotic Enforcement —enforces laws regulating use and manufacture and sale of drugs; inspects agencies permitted to prescribe drugs; program to combat illegal traffic —Research Advistory Panel —approves research projects on drug abuse, releasing drugs for use in projects	
—Bureau of Prisons —treatment in prisons for narcotics offenders, including psychiatric contracts for outpatient treatment		

Drug abuse

Federal	State	Local
— Law Enforcement Assistance Agency —education and narcotics prevention; training program for state and local law officers; supports programs of narcotics prevention, crime detection, and research	—California Council on Criminal Justice —Narcotics, Drug and Alcohol Abuse Task Force —evaluates state and local programs for control and prevention of narcotics and alcohol abuse; funds local control and preventive programs	County Dept. of Community Services —Narcotics and Dangerous Drugs Commission —reviews existing legislation, recommends enforcement and programs to Board of Supervisors, assists education
	—Bureau of Criminal Identification and Investigation —registers persons convicted of violating state narcotics law; informs local law agencies	County Sheriff —enforces narcotics and drug abuse laws
	California Highway Patrol —trains officers in narcotics and drug abuse; enforces Vehicle Code on driving under the influence of drugs	Los Angeles City and Other City Police Depts. —Juvenile Narcotics Unit —enforces narcotics and drug abuse laws

Drug abuse

Federal	State	Local

Dept. of Housing and Urban
Development
—Model Cities Administration
— special programs on drug abuse in
model cities, including Watts in
East Los Angeles

Office of Economic Opportunity
—Division of Alcoholism, Addiction,
and Mental Health Services
— treatment, education, research on
drug abuse in poverty areas

Economic and Youth Opportunities
Agency (EYOA)
—Narcotics Prevention Project
— information, counseling,
organization by ex-addicts for
community; contracts for
detoxification beds, rehabilitation
in 3 Chicano neighborhoods

Dept. of Defense
—inpatient and outpatient treatment,
rehabilitation for drug abusers in
military; referral of discharged
addicts for care—primarily to the
VA through a cooperative program;
research, training

Drug abuse

Federal	State	Local

Veterans Administration
—inpatient, outpatient care of veterans with drug problems; research

Dept. of Motor Vehicles
—may refuse to issue license, suspend license, or place on probation anyone driving when on drugs

Selected Voluntary Organizations and Programs

American Social Health Assn.
—program on drug abuse and dependence includes public education; consultation services to narcotics treatment and rehabilitation projects; assistance to legislative groups planning new drug abuse laws

Narcotic Symposium of California

Los Angeles Chapter, Narcotic Symposium of California
—Boyle Heights Center Narcotic Prevention Project

Drug abuse

Federal	State	Local
		— provides information services; rehabilitation, job training, and employment support to Boyle Heights residents with narcotics problems; counseling services to families; educational program
		Narcotics Anonymous —assistance to persons with narcotics problems; provides literature and list of meeting places
		NAR-NON —assistance to families of narcotics addicts
		Narcotics Information Service
		Free Clinics —offers drug abuse programs and guidance
		Federation of Community Coordinating Councils of L.A. —95 community coordinating councils and area associations join to sponsor local and countywide efforts to deal with narcotics and drug abuse as part of major juvenile delinquency program

Drug abuse

Federal	State	Local
		L.A. City Citizens Narcotic and Dangerous Drug Committee —study committee on drug abuse Synanon —self-help group treatment and rehabilitation centers for narcotics users Half-way Houses —for discharged narcotics users

INDEX